# MARITAL THERAPY

## A COMBINED
## PSYCHODYNAMIC – BEHAVIORAL APPROACH

CRITICAL ISSUES IN PSYCHIATRY
An Educational Series for Residents and Clinicians

*Series Editor:* Sherwyn M. Woods, M.D., Ph.D.
*University of Southern California School of Medicine*
*Los Angeles, California*

A RESIDENT'S GUIDE TO PSYCHIATRIC EDUCATION
Edited by Michael G. G. Thompson, M.D.

STATES OF MIND: Analysis of Change in Psychotherapy
Mardi J. Horowitz, M.D.

DRUG AND ALCOHOL ABUSE: A Clinical Guide to
Diagnosis and Treatment
Marc A. Schuckit, M.D.

THE INTERFACE BETWEEN THE PSYCHODYNAMIC AND
BEHAVIORAL THERAPIES
Edited by Judd Marmor, M.D., and Sherwyn M. Woods, M.D., Ph.D.

LAW IN THE PRACTICE OF PSYCHIATRY
Seymour L. Halleck, M.D.

NEUROPSYCHIATRIC FEATURES OF MEDICAL DISORDERS
James W. Jefferson, M.D., and John R. Marshall, M.D.

ADULT DEVELOPMENT: A New Dimension in Psychodynamic Theory
and Practice
Calvin A. Colarusso, M.D., and Robert A. Nemiroff, M.D.

SCHIZOPHRENIA
John S. Strauss, M.D., and William T. Carpenter, Jr., M.D.

EXTRAORDINARY DISORDERS OF HUMAN BEHAVIOR
Edited by Claude T. H. Friedmann, M.D., and Robert A. Faguet, M.D.

MARITAL THERAPY: A Combined Psychodynamic–Behavioral Approach
R. Taylor Segraves, M.D., Ph.D.

TREATMENT INTERVENTIONS IN HUMAN SEXUALITY
Edited by Carol C. Nadelson, M.D., and David B. Marcotte, M.D.

A Continuation Order Plan is available for this series. A continuation order will bring delivery of each new volume immediately upon publication. Volumes are billed only upon actual shipment. For further information please contact the publisher.

# MARITAL THERAPY

## A COMBINED
## PSYCHODYNAMIC – BEHAVIORAL APPROACH

R. Taylor Segraves, M.D., Ph.D.

*University of Chicago*
*Chicago, Illinois*

Plenum Medical Book Company
New York and London

Library of Congress Cataloging in Publication Data

Segraves, R. Taylor, 1941 –
  Marital therapy, a combined psychodynamic–behavioral approach.

  (Critical issues in psychiatry)
  Bibliography: p.
  Includes index.
  1. Marital psychotherapy. I. Title. II. Series. [DNLM: 1. Marital therapy. WM 55
S455m]
  RC488.5.S43  1982                      616.89'156                      82-16653
  ISBN 0-306-40936-4

© 1982 Plenum Publishing Corporation
233 Spring Street, New York, N.Y. 10013

Plenum Medical Book Company is an imprint of Plenum Publishing Corporation

All rights reserved

No part of this book may be reproduced, stored in a retrieval system, or transmitted
in any form or by any means, electronic, mechanical, photocopying, microfilming,
recording, or otherwise, without written permission from the Publisher

Printed in the United States of America

# Foreword

This book is welcomed to the series as a truly unique contribution to the literature on marital therapy. It is written for the empirically oriented psychotherapist, regardless of his or her discipline, who encounters patients with marital discord and has been distressed by the absence of an acceptable conceptual model for treatment. Psychoanalysis, behavior therapy, general system theory, and social learning theory have all made important contributions to treatment. But all too often these approaches have focused either on individual psychopathology or on the formal elements of marital interaction. This volume is the first to propose an approach to marital therapy which is clinically sophisticated, empirically based and which integrates important elements of seemingly disparate theoretical systems. The result is a cognitive-behavioral model for the treatment of marital discord which borrows from both psychoanalytic and behavioral contributions by translating them into the language of cognitive social psychology.

The author documents the toll in human suffering as well as the ubiquitous nature of marriage-related problems. Despite the frequency with which marital dissatisfaction and discord are encountered in clinical practice, an amazingly high percentage of mental health professionals have received inadequate training in either the theory or technique of effective clinical intervention. The absence of a conceptual framework linking individual psychopathology to interactional difficulties has worsened the problem for clinicians interested in conjoint treatment.

The author devotes several chapters to a thorough review of the contributions of psychoanalytic theory, general system theory, and behavioral marital therapy. There is an evenhanded and thoughtful review of these various contributions, the manner in which each has influenced the other, and the similarity of many hypotheses which differing schools agree upon but express in different language. The seeming dichotomy between behavioral and psychodynamic therapy may be partially an artifact and there is a review of the contributions which suggest that a clinical integration is not only possible but useful.

From this base, the author's psychodynamic-behavioral model for the treatment of chronic marital discord is developed. A linkage is made between psychopathology and interactional data, and this aids in understanding the enduring nature of maladaptive interactional patterns. His clinical presentations demonstrate that marital partners form cognitive templates or schemas, roughly equivalent to the psychoanalytic conceptualization of transference, for the perception of each other. These schemas are often negative, distorted, and at variance wth the spouse's personality. The problem for the clinician is that he or she is often faced with a bewildering complexity of observable behavioral abnormalities and distorted schemas. An important technical maneuver involves the disruption of chronic maladaptive interactional patterns which confirm the distorted inner representational models, after which interpretation is used in the service of discrimination learning.

Moving from theory to clinical practice, the author provides a scholarly and intellectually sound road map for effective therapeutic intervention in the conjoint treatment of couples. Synthesis and integration are apparent at both the theoretical and technical levels, a welcomed departure from the parochial and/or theoretically radical presentations which have too often been characteristic in this field.

Sherwyn M. Woods, M.D., Ph.D.
*Series Editor*

# Preface

This book is the result of years of struggle by the author to evolve clinically responsible and empirically based approaches to the treatment of interpersonal difficulties. During my development as a psychotherapist, I often became discouraged when my observations did not fit those of my teachers or of then-existing theories. This happened first when I, as a behaviorally oriented psychologist, noted with irritation that many of my patients spontaneously discussed matters better suited for analytic models of therapy. Later, as a dynamically trained psychiatrist, I noted that behavior therapy often provoked internal psychological change in patients. It began to appear that the therapies were not as dissimilar in their effects as current theory suggested. More recently, as a marital therapist, I often observed that behavioral change in one spouse produced profound internal psychological change in the other spouse. This book is the result of my observations of these clinical phenomena, which do not fit any of the current theories of psychotherapy.

Throughout this struggle, Dr. Jarl Dyrud, professor in the Department of Psychiatry at the University of Chicago, has had a marked influence on my thinking and development. Initially as a teacher and clinical supervisor and subsequently as a colleague, he provided the constant reminder that clinical theory should be regarded merely as a temporary approximation to explanation. As a role model, he communicated the message that clinicians and scholars have to bear the discomfort of attending to the full complexity of the phenomena being observed, especially when the data observed do not fit one's favorite theory. He also provided an often necessary reminder that one must avoid premature theoretical closure and a retreat to theoretical orthodoxy. Such a retreat is a disservice to our patients and students as well as an act of personal dishonesty.

I would also like to acknowledge the influence of Professor H. J. Eysenck, my Ph.D. supervisor some 10 years ago. Although Professor Eysenck will probably disagree with many of the conclusions reached in this text, his influence is clearly present. This text is a result of Professor Eysenck's impressing upon his students at the Institute of Psychiatry of the University of London the tenet that clinical and research activities should not be viewed as separate undertakings. Empirical foundations for clinical activities are both necessary and possible. However, this foundation need not take the form of radical behaviorism. Hypothetical constructs are perfectly acceptable in scientific theory as long as they follow the basic principles of good theory constructions. He would even agree with the author that the problem with psychoanalytic theory has more to do with the structure of that theory than with its content.

# Acknowledgments

I would especially like to thank Dr. Daniel X. Freedman, Chairman of the Department of Psychiatry at the University of Chicago, for his help and encouragement during the preparation of this manuscript. His contribution was twofold: First, he created an academic climate in which eclectic approaches to psychiatric problems were encouraged and fostered. Throughout my academic career, he emphasized that psychopathology is multidetermined, involving the interplay of biologic, psychologic, and social factors. More important, I am indebted to Dr. Freedman for his example of personal integrity in the pursuit of knowledge. While writing this text on marital therapy (a topic of lesser importance in many academic circles) I was repeatedly reminded that he pursued biological research at a time when psychoanalysis dominated academic psychiatry.

Two colleagues were especially helpful in critically reviewing this text. I would like to express my thanks to close friends and colleagues, Dr. Lolita Ang at the Illinois State Psychiatric Institute, and Dr. Thomas Garrick at the Department of Psychiatry, University of California, Los Angeles.

Last but not least, I wish to express my appreciation for laborious and patient persistence during the preparation of this manuscript to Ms. Runae Hartfield and Ms. Amelia Spenser.

# Contents

CHAPTER 1
**Current Status of Marital Therapy**    **1**

Psychoanalytic Treatment of Marital Discord ........................... 4
Behavioral Treatment of Marital Discord ............................... 5
Beginning Rapprochement ............................................. 7
An Integrated Approach................................................ 9
Clinical Ramifications ................................................ 14
Overview............................................................. 17
References ........................................................... 18

CHAPTER 2
**The Relationship of Marriage to Psychological Well-being**    **21**

Marital Status and Mental Health Service Usage ....................... 22
Marital Status and Psychiatric Hospitalization......................... 24
Marital Status and Outpatient Clinic Usage .......................... 26
Psychological Well-being and Marital Status........................... 28
Marital Status and Alcoholism ........................................ 31
Suicide and Marital Status............................................ 32
Marital Status and Mortality ......................................... 34
Marital Discord, Psychiatric Impairment, and
       Mental Health Service Usage.................................. 36
Divorce, Marital Discord, and Children............................... 40
Sex and Marital Status Differences in Psychopathology .............. 45
Explanatory Hypotheses............................................... 46
Trends in Divorce Rates .............................................. 49
Response of Mental Health Professionals ............................. 50
References ........................................................... 51

CHAPTER 3
**Psychoanalytic Theory and Marriage**                                    58

Classical Psychoanalytic Theory and Practice..........................61
Retranslation....................................................................63
Minor Modifications of Orthodox Analytic Treatment.................64
Psychoanalytically Oriented Conjoint Marital Therapy ...............65
Object-Relations Theory .....................................................67
Object-Relations Marital Therapy........................................69
Comment and Critique ......................................................70
References ......................................................................73


CHAPTER 4
**General System Theory and Marriage**                                    76

General System Theory.......................................................78
Cybernetics .....................................................................82
Don Jackson ....................................................................83
Jay Haley.........................................................................87
Virginia Satir and Marital Therapy ......................................90
Comment and Critique ......................................................91
References ......................................................................93


CHAPTER 5
**Behavioral Marital Therapy**                                            96

Behaviorism and Behavior Therapy ......................................99
Behavior Therapy .............................................................103
Basic Concepts in Behaviorial Marital Therapy......................107
Treatment.......................................................................110
    Positive Reinforcement Exchange Procedures ...................111
    Communication .........................................................113
Comment and Critique ......................................................116
References ......................................................................120


CHAPTER 6
**Inner Worlds, External Reality, and Interactional Systems**            126

Current Status .................................................................127
Requirement of a Theory....................................................129
Behavioral Change and Inner Representational Events..............130

Inner Representational Events and Social Behavior ................. 135
Description of Inner Representational Events ......................... 137
Psychoanalytic Concepts and Cognitive Theory ..................... 141
How Schemas are Self-sustaining ..................................... 142
Summary .................................................................... 144
References ................................................................. 145

CHAPTER 7
**An Integrative Model**                                    **148**

Basic Assumptions ........................................................ 150
  Interpersonal Consistency ............................................ 150
  Person–Environment Interaction ..................................... 153
  Behavior as a Function of Perceived Environment ............... 154
  Nature of Cognitive Events ........................................... 155
  Psychotherapy as a Social Influence ............................... 157
  Choice of Therapeutic Intervention ................................ 160
An Integrative Model ..................................................... 161
  Definition ................................................................ 162
  Cognitive Factors in Marital Discord ............................. 165
  The Clinical Context .................................................. 169
  Hypothesis One ......................................................... 171
  Hypothesis Two ......................................................... 173
  Hypothesis Three ....................................................... 175
  Hypothesis Four ........................................................ 177
  Relationship of Cognitions to Interpersonal Behavior .......... 178
  Hypothesis Five ........................................................ 178
  Hypothesis Six .......................................................... 180
  Properties of Interactional Systems ............................... 182
  Hypothesis Seven ....................................................... 182
  Hypothesis Eight ....................................................... 183
  Mechanism of Change .................................................. 185
  Hypothesis Nine ........................................................ 186
  Hypothesis Ten .......................................................... 187
Conclusions ................................................................. 188
References ................................................................. 189

CHAPTER 8
**Clinical Application**                                    **197**

Conceptual Overview ..................................................... 197
Indications ................................................................. 209

Length of Therapy ..................................................210
Technical Considerations ...........................................211
Goal of Therapy ....................................................213
Stages of Therapy ..................................................214
    Early Phase (Entrance into Therapy) ...........................214
    Middle Stages..................................................223
Comment ............................................................235
    End Stage .....................................................238
Comment ............................................................242
Clinical Wisdom.....................................................242
Comments ...........................................................250
Differing Needs of Researchers and Clinicians ......................251
References .........................................................253


CHAPTER 9
**Case Illustration**                                                **255**

Brief History of the Relationship...................................255
Brief Personality Sketch of Mrs. P .................................257
Mr. P ..............................................................258
Entrance into Therapy ..............................................259
Course of Therapy ..................................................260
    First Session .................................................260
    Negotiation Training...........................................264
    Modifying Specific Interactional Problems .....................271
    Specific Communication Problems................................272
    Further Modification of Interaction ...........................274
    Cognitive Restructuring .......................................282
    A Return to the Past ..........................................286
    Discrimination Training........................................289


**Index** ..........................................................297

# Current Status of Marital Therapy

A major obstacle to clinicians interested in marital therapy is the absence of an acceptable conceptual framework to guide their interventions and organize their perceptions (Manus, 1966; Olson, 1975). The clinician treating relationship disturbances is quickly faced with a baffling complexity of data: each spouse's personal history and signs of psychopathology, the history of the shared relationship and the individual meanings of shared events, current observable patterns of interactions between spouses. In order to make effective interventions, the clinician needs a conceptual framework to organize his perceptions and therapeutic interventions. The need for a theory of marital therapy is acutely felt because, in the midst of rapid bombardment with overwhelming data in the usual marital therapy session, the therapist must consider both past and current determinants of the discord, the individual and interactional data, and the interplay of internal psychological representational systems with recurring maladaptive behavior patterns. The absence of an adequate theory of marital therapy may partially explain the relative lack of activity in this clinical area by many therapists (Segraves, 1978). Similarly, the absence of a theoretical system that relates therapeutic interventions into marital interaction systems with individual psychopathology may account for the tendency of many psychotherapists to regard marital therapy as a more superficial, less meaningful intervention.

Three main theoretical systems—general system theory, psychoanalytic theory, and behavioral marital therapy—have influenced the practice of marital therapy (Prochaska and Prochaska, 1978). Each of these theoretical systems offers the clinician a unique vantage point of observation, a differing set of explanatory concepts, and a suggested format for therapeutic interventions. These partial theories of marital therapies tend to focus on one class of events, to the relative exclusion of other classes of events (Segraves, 1978). The concepts and techniques of the partial theories frequently appear incompatible with one another, and the degree of possible overlap that may exist in psychodynamic, behavioral, and general system approaches to marital therapy is obscured by the absence of common terminology and by unnecessary polemical disputes among representatives of the various therapeutic schools (e.g., Gurman and Knudson, 1978; Jacobson and Weiss, 1978).

The principal theoretical gap appears to lie between the theoretical schools emphasizing individual psychopathology and interpretive approaches and those, such as general system theory and behavioral marital therapy, that advocate direct modification of problematic interpersonal behavior. Marital therapy models derived from psychoanalytic theory provide the clinician with a framework to understand the contribution of individual past experiences to the genesis of marital discord (Martin, 1976). Unfortunately, these models are deficient in explaining the role of current interpersonal forces in maintaining individual psychopathology. An even more glaring deficiency of these models is that they do not provide the clinician with a conceptual orientation to understand the impact of behavioral change in the marital interaction system on the individual psychology of each of the spouses. These models tend to limit the therapist to activities designed to engender insight in the marital partners as to the unconscious origins of their conflict (e.g., Dicks, 1967). Other major approaches to marital therapy, such as behavioral marital therapy or approaches derived from general system theory, stress the importance of modifying current observable maladaptive behavior patterns. Therapists influenced by general system theory, such as Don Jackson (1965), have described the repetitive sequences of behavior patterns in disturbed couples and have devised clinically sophisticated techniques to interrupt these sequences of maladaptive behavior. Behavioral marital therapists stress the importance of modifying a different class of maladaptive interpersonal behavior (O'Leary and Turkewitz, 1978). Therapists firmly bound to either behavioral marital therapy or general system theory do not have a conceptual framework to appreciate the role of individual personality disturbances in the genesis of marital discord and thus are limited in their understanding of marital discord and the range of therapeutic interventions. At one extreme, individual psychopathology models have tended to view the married individual almost as a social isolate with his or her own encapsulated psychopathology independent of the spouse. At the other extreme, behavioral marital therapy and general system theory tend to view marital individuals as totally socially reactive beings, almost devoid of individual pasts and personalities separate from the spouse and marriage. Clearly, both approaches exclude significant contributions to the understanding and treatment of marital discord from their theoretical perspective. Clinical reality resides somewhere between these two theoretical extremes.

A therapist of any of the three main theoretical orientations toward marital therapy is limited either to interventions focused on modifying individual psychopathology or to interventions focused on modifying interactional behavior. In the actual clinical situation, the therapist needs to be able to shift between individual and interactional levels of interventions and to conceptualize how interventions at one level will influence events at a different level. The therapist needs to be able to predict the probable intrapsychic impact of a given intervention in the interactional pattern. None of the current partial theories of therapy gives the clinician this flexibility. The current partial theories thus can be characterized as compartmentalizing reality in quite artificial ways.

Another difficulty with current models of marital therapy is the absence of an empirical data base to support the assumptions of many marital therapists (Olson, 1975). General system theory and psychodynamic models of marital therapy are formulated in such a manner that empirical validation or invalidation is virtually impossible. Behavioral marital therapy is unique, with its emphasis on explicitly stating basic assumptions and empirically evaluating treatment efficacy. However, many of the basic assumptions of the behavioral model have not been validated (Jacobson and Martin, 1976). One glaring deficiency of the behavioral model is its neglect of the contribution of individual psychopathology to marital discord. Numerous well-conducted prospective studies have found that personality predispositions existing prior to marriage do contribute significantly to marital adjustments (e.g., Kelly, 1939; Adams, 1946; Burgess and Wallin, 1953; Bentler and Newcomb, 1978). Thus, a model of marital therapy, supposedly concerned with empirical support of its basic tenets, excludes an established etiologic factor from its consideration.

As a result of the current theoretical situation, many experienced clinicians have evolved treatment models from personal trial and error. In many cases, these clinicians freely borrow assumptions and techniques from various theoretical camps without being disturbed by this (e.g., Fitzgerald, 1973; Sager, 1976). Although many of these clinicians may be gifted and effective therapists, they frequently don't record their observations or even explicitly acknowledge the basic assumptions underlying their interventions. The resulting approach usually consists of expert clinical wisdom gained after years of individual clinical trial and error mixed with faulty, poorly conceptualized procedures and assumptions. Their wisdom is primarily transmittable by personel contact and apprenticeship and thus has minimal impact. The evolution of an explicit theoretical system for the conduct of marital therapy is important in that it can be readily disseminated, examined, and modified.

## PSYCHOANALYTIC TREATMENT OF MARITAL DISCORD

Psychoanalysis evolved as a methodology and a conceptual system to be employed in both the study and the treatment of individual psychological abnormalities. Marriage and marital discord *per se* have never been a primary interest of the psychoanalytic community. The psychoanalytic model stresses the role of psychopathology in the individual marital partners as primarily responsible for marital conflict. This model hypothesizes that unresolved early conflicts occurring in the family of origin of the individual spouses are unconsciously replayed in current interpersonal relationships, including marriage. This model strongly emphasizes the role of the past experiences, subjective experiences, and unconscious motivations in individuals (e.g., Brody, 1961). From this theoretical perspective, the treatment of choice for marital disturbances is separate individual psychoanalysis for one or both spouses. The assumption is that marital disturbances will abate when the disturbed spouses resolve their individual difficulties. Individual psychotherapy is preferred to conjoint psychotherapy, as the theoretical model emphasizes resolution of the transference neurosis as one of the major curative mechanisms in psychoanalysis (Kaplan, 1976). In other words, the unconscious perceptual distortions and motivations underlying disturbed intimate relationships in current life will also occur in the therapist's office. As the therapist is a more neutral participant than the spouse or other family members, the transference neurosis, once evolved, can be examined and resolved in the safety and objectivity of this therapeutic relationship. Once the patient is fully conscious of the complex chain of internal eliciting stimuli for his or her disturbed behavior pattern, and this behavioral sequence has less emotional autonomy and intensity, the patient should be able to self-regulate his or her own behavior in future intimate relationships (Offenkrantz and Tobin, 1975).

This model has an appealing logic, and most eclectic therapists are probably aware of individual cases where successful psychotherapy of one or both spouses has contributed significantly to the success of a previously disturbed relationship (Sager et al., 1968). However, in many cases, this treatment approach is unsatisfactory. Most psychoanalytic therapists with a serious interest in the treatment of marital disturbances have modified the traditional psychoanalytic model (e.g., Sager, 1976). In couples with a fairly lengthy history of chronic difficulties in marriage, it is frequently impossible to disentangle reality problems from transference distortions. Similarly, many couples tend to view individual psychotherapy of each spouse as an expensive, lengthy, and roundabout way to resolve the presenting difficulty. Thus, most psychoanalytically oriented marital therapists have made significant modifications of the basic analytic paradigm in order to treat relationship disturbances. These modifications have included adjustment of the basic treatment paradigm from traditional individual therapy to a conjoint treatment format. Most current psychoanalytically oriented marital therapists would probably best be described as eclectic therapists with a psychodynamic bias (e.g., Nadelson, 1978; Martin, 1976).

Psychoanalytically oriented therapists have tended to stress the importance of higher level abstractions as explanatory concepts, such as psychic structure, unconscious motivation, internalized objects. Most psychoanalytic hypotheses are stated in essentially untestable forms. Also, many psychoanalytic hypotheses and formulations are stated in a language form that is most often alien to social scientists. For these reasons, many empirically oriented therapists have tended to dismiss the writings of analytic therapists as useless or, at best, of minor historical interest. This is unfortunate, as many analytically oriented therapists are highly skilled clinicians and represent the only school of thought to have articulated how the individual personalities of the spouses can interact and cause marital discord. The absence of exchange of ideas and information between the opposing theoretical orientations is unfortunate, as each offers a valuable vantage point of observation.

## BEHAVIORAL TREATMENT OF MARITAL DISCORD

In many ways, behavioral approaches to the treatment of marital discord appear to be the polar opposite of psychodynamic approaches. Whereas analytic therapists tend to view determinants of present behavior as residing in the unconscious past of individuals, behavioral marital therapists tend to emphasize that the important determinants of behavior are current and reside outside of the individual in the interpersonal environment (Goldiamond, 1965). With a strong emphasis on operationally defining concepts and empirically testing procedures and hypotheses, these therapists have tended to focus their attention on modifying current, observable behavior patterns. The inner meanings and past origins of these behavior patterns receive scant, if any, attention. They also employ a language system alien to the dynamic therapist, speaking of reinforcement and stimulus control rather than of unconscious incestuous wishes.

Most behavioral marital therapists have been influenced by social exchange theory, which posits that in social interactions the individuals involved, regardless of their past histories, will tend to try to maximize individual rewards and to minimize personal costs (O'Leary and Turkewitz, 1978). Thus, most behavior therapists have hypothesized that certain characteristics of social exchange systems are more conducive to marital happiness than others. They postulate that happy marriages are characterized by a greater frequency of positive exchanges, a relative equity between partners in this process, and the absence of coercion (Greer and D'Zurilla, 1976). Indeed, some evidence exists to support these hypotheses. Working from these basic assumptions, the behavior therapist's goals are naturally to teach the couple ways to alter their behavior and thus to negotiate a relationship in which both spouses' reinforcements are maximized. It is assumed that each spouse has within his or her repertoire most of the reinforcing behaviors that the other spouse desires and that both spouses would find a higher rate of reinforcement exchange more satisfying. Thus, most behavioral marital therapists would attempt to get each spouse to state explicitly his or her preferred behaviors from the opposing spouse and then would negotiate an equitable exchange of positive reinforcement from marital relationships and teach more satisfactory communication skills. It is important to realize that most statements by spouses are accepted at face value, and questions about ambivalence, fears of intimacy, fears of loss of control, and perceptual distortions of the mate's personality are not considered by most behavioral marital therapists (e.g., Jacobson, 1972).

The simplicity of this approach and the seeming clinical naïveté of behavioral marital therapists has led many dynamic therapists to dismiss their therapeutic efforts outright, if not to regard them with abhorence. This neglect of the contribution of behaviorally oriented therapists by psychodynamically oriented clinicians is unfortunate, as behavioral marital therapy represents the only serious attempt within the field to operationalize critical concepts and to empirically test procedures and hypotheses. Part of the seeming irreconciliation between the two models is the assumption of the lack of an interrelationship between behavior and inner psychological events, or the assumption that change in one sphere somehow takes precedence over change in the others.

It is a common clinical occurrence when one observes a couple interlocked in a recurring behavioral sequence, the reality of which reinforces each spouse's inner view of the other. On occasion, reciprocity training can be a highly effective way to begin disrupting these sequences of behavior and to force the spouses into new experiences of each other and themselves. In these cases, changes in superficial behavior can have far-reaching repercussions in the emotional lives of both spouses. The unfortunate polarization of therapists into artifically created theoretical camps has resulted in a situation where few therapists are able to appreciate the interplay between behavioral change and inner psychological reality.

## BEGINNING RAPPROCHEMENT

One of the primary theoretical gaps in the treatment of marital discord is the dichotomy between behavioral and psychodynamic approaches (Segraves, 1978). A similar situation existed in the field of individual psychotherapy until the recent past (Segraves and Smith, 1976). A brief diversion to consider the resolution of a similar theoretical polarity in the field of individual psychotherapy may be warranted. Rather than viewing marital difficulties as distinct in nature from the types of difficulties for which individuals seek psychotherapy, one can view marriage as an opportunity to observe individual interactional difficulties in a meaningful relationship freely chosen and evolved of its own accord in the natural environment. Marriage can also be viewed as an ideal context in which to study the interface between the inner representational realities of the individual spouses and the external reality of a behavioral interaction with an intimate other.

In the recent past, there was a heated polarization of viewpoints between individual psychotherapists of psychodynamic and behavioral schools of thought. A considerable literature evolved that centered around attacks by representatives of one school of thought on the results and putative flaws of the opposing theoretical system (Breger and McGaugh, 1965; Eysenck and Rachman, 1965). Although vestiges of the old polemics remain, numerous clinicians have noted that the debates often seemed to serve political as well as scientific motivations (London, 1972). Other clinicians have noted that the polarization of viewpoints was partially an artifact of the theoretically orthodox, who minimally comprehended the theoretical concepts of the opposing schools of thought (Hunt and Dyrud, 1968; Birk and Brinkley-Birk, 1974; Segraves and Smith, 1976).

Historically, it is important to note that the original impetus for the developmental of a behavioral school of psychotherapy was the growing dissatisfaction among academic psychologists with the field of clinical psychology (Eysenck and Rachman, 1965). Prior to the advent of behavior therapy, psychodynamic theory was the main theoretical force in clinical psychology. Psychodynamic theory, with its emphasis on exploring the relationships involving poorly defined higher level abstractions about mental functioning and structure, appeared forever irreconcilable with the discipline of experimental psychology. Thus, the evolution of behavior therapy treatment approaches that were at least loosely linked to empirical principles and the language of experimental psychology and learning theory were greeted with an enthusiastic reception by this group of academic psychologists. It was hoped that a true science of psychotherapeutic interventions could be evolved. In reaction against the dangers of mentalism, as represented by psychoanalytic theory, this movement originally took the form of strict behaviorism. It was concerned solely with the study of observable behavior, and data suggesting information about the organization of mental events were excluded from consideration, if not from awareness (Eysenck and Beech, 1971). As this movement acquired popularity among practicing clinicians, a counterswing began. Clinical psychologists were impressed with the absolute clinical necessity of utilizing data that they could infer about internal psychological functioning in their patients (e.g., Lazarus, 1971). The dilemma was how these data could be utilized without appealing to psychoanalytic theory and thus returning to the previous pitfalls of mentalism. The current popularity of social learning theory (Bandura, 1977) and cognitive behaviorism (Meichenbaum, 1977; Mahoney, 1974) are an outgrowth of this conflict.

Clinical theorists are again tackling the problem of identifying inferred organismic variables that affect behavior and attempting to study these variables empirically. This new approach appears to be walking a tightrope between the extremes of mentalism and behaviorism. Internal cognitive emotional events are again an object of study. However, explanatory concepts are generated at a much lower level of abstraction and there is a notable attempt to link these inferred variables with observable events.

At the same time that these events are occurring in academic psychology, analogous events are occurring within the field of psychiatry. Psychiatric clinicians, whose backgrounds usually include a greater emphasis on psychoanalytic theory and practice, have been attracted to the application of behavior therapy approaches to the treatment of specific syndromes (e.g., Brady, 1969; Marks and Gelder, 1967). At first, it appears, there were two separate treatment strategies, one applicable to the correction of specific behavioral abnormalities and the other applicable to the correction of internal psychological misfunctioning. However, with greater exposure to the application of behavioral treatment approaches, more and more of these clinicians began observing that behavioral change was frequently associated with the evocation of mental imagery and early childhood memories, which psychoanalytic theory posits as etiologically related to the behavioral abnormalities (Feather and Rhoads, 1972). In certain cases, successful behavioral treatment of an isolated symptom appeared to open the way for the patient's subjective reorganization of his or her views of the world. These observations led many psychiatric clinicians to conclude that behavior has its internal cognitive referents and that change in behavior may lead to internal symbolic change (Birk and Brinkley-Birk, 1974; Segraves and Smith, 1976). In particular, it appears that symptomatic behavior occurs in clusters, which consist of interrelationships between external behavior and internal cognitive-emotional events, and that significant psychotherapeutic change could be induced in either sphere.

It would appear that developments in both clinical psychology and psychiatry have opened the way for a new approach to the study of human difficulties in living. In particular, there appears to be a readiness for a careful denotation and study of the links between observable behavioral abnormalities and inferred internal psychological variables (intervening organismic variables). This approach is different from previous psychoanalytic approaches in that lower level explanatory concepts are employed and the observable behavioral referents for these concepts are explicitly stated. This change allows the empirically oriented clinician to again consider the interrelationship between a patient's subjective reality and his objective behavior in life.

## AN INTEGRATED APPROACH

The previously discussed integrative developments in the field of individual psychotherapy help to lay the groundwork for a similar beginning theoretical integration of the differing approaches to the treatment of marital discord. It seems obvious that the pleasure of an individual in marriage is partially the function of the external reality of the behavior of one's spouse. It also seems obvious that one's pleasure in marriage is partially a function of one's perception of one's spouse and that past experiences influence the nature of that perception. A third dimension known intimately by marital therapists is that the behavior of one's spouse toward oneself is partially determined by one's behavior toward that spouse. In many instances, the complaining spouse may repetitively provoke the offensive behavior that is then complained about. This mechanism is aptly captured in a discussion by an analytically oriented therapist, Selwyn Brody, who treated marital discord by simultaneous individual psychotherapy of each of the spouses: "While the wife feels unloved and has never felt consistently loved, she compensates by romantic daydreaming of an ideal lover. The more the husband feels rejected, the more recalcitrant he is about modifying careless—even repulsive personal habits which readily justify some of his wife's behavior. In effect, while contemptuously blaming him, she successfully provokes him to remain as he is, so she can continue to be as bitterly hopeless and suicidal as she is" (Brody, 1961, pp. 100–101).

Clearly, a useful theory of interpersonal therapy has to encompass complex observations. It needs to address the inner psychological worlds of both spouses, the relationship of inner psychological events in each spouse to that spouse's behavior toward his or her mate, and the role that each spouse's behavior plays in eliciting the mate's behavior. It also needs to address the role the mate's behavior plays in maintaining the other spouse's inner psychological state. By necessity, such a theory has to bridge data currently subsumed separately by behavioral and psychodynamic models of therapy. It needs to specifically relate inner psychological events to observable interpersonal behavior. Ideally, this theory should also be in a language form allowing for public verification or rejection. I believe that such a beginning synthesis is possible and that it is possible to evolve a therapeutic model that acknowledges the complexity of the phenomena involved, yet is still publicly verifiable. A major part of achieving theoretical synthesis is in choosing a language system that relates inner psychological events to observable behavior in a systematic manner.

Although no current theories of psychotherapy meet these criteria, work in the field of cognitive social psychology has laid the groundwork for such a synthesis. In the 1950s, George Kelly (1955) evolved a theoretical system linking inner psychological events to interpersonal behavior. Kelly suggested that much of psychopathology could be understood by examining a patient's personal construct system, his idiosyncratic way of viewing the world. In particular, he stressed the importance of constructs (expectations or cognitions) about significant others in the patient's personal world. He suggested that a neurotic's suffering was often less the result of external events in the real environment than the result of the patient's experience (way of construing) those events. Kelly recommended that the goal of therapy was to change the patient's way of construing the universe, i.e., his inner representational system. It is of note that Kelly should be considered the father of cognitive behavior therapy. He suggested that a therapist should help the patient to have life experiences discrepant with the patient's inner representational world. If such life experiences could be maintained, the patient would undergo permanent inner psychological change. Kelly outlined a form of therapy, fixed role therapy, which was based on the assumption that behavior change could be used as a therapeutic tool to elicit inner psychological change. Even more important, Kelly evolved a methodology, the construct repertory test, to operationalize these interpersonal construct systems. In effect, he described a methodology for systematically measuring a patient's inner representational world.

Kelly's contribution has been complemented (1) by interpersonal theorists (e.g., Leary, 1957) who have demonstrated how a patient's interpersonal behavior may reliably serve to elicit from others responses that are confirmatory to the patient's distorted world view and (2) by contemporary social psychologists (e.g., Stotland and Canon, 1972; Carson, 1969) who have more systematically related inner psychological events to interpersonal behavior. These theorists have conceptualized the reciprocal interrelationship between inner representational reality and the interpersonal environment. The relationship of work in cognitive social psychology to the author's model of interpersonal therapy will be more fully developed in subsequent chapters of this book. At this point, I will briefly outline the primary assumptions underlying an integrative model for the conjoint therapy of marital discord.

Both psychoanalytic and social psychological theory has hypothesized that the human infant develops psychologically by gradually evolving an inner representational world reflective of external reality. This inner representational world is necessary to organize perceptions and to reliably predict external events. Gross distortions in this inner representational world are felt to signify psychopathology and to underlie interpersonal difficulties. Psychoanalytic theorists have observed that faulty interpersonal assumptions often cause many interpersonal difficulties. In the psychoanalytic literature, these schemas are labeled transference phenomena (Kaplan, 1976). Cognitive social psychologists, such as Stotland and Canon (1972), have elaborated similar hypotheses. They have postulated that because of the quantity and complexity of interpersonal stimuli and because of the limited information-processing capacity of the human nervous system, man develops interpersonal schemas or templates to organize his interpersonal perceptions. These schemas influence the manner in which new information about people is perceived and assimilated. This means that a certain perceptual bias is present in most or all interpersonal contexts.

The author's integrative theoretical framework for the treatment of marital discord rests on three primary assumptions. The first is that faulty interpersonal schemas for the perception of intimate members of the opposite sex are of primary importance in both the genesis and maintenance of chronic marital discord. I am specifically postulating that fixated misperceptions of the mate's character and motives by one or both spouses are involved in all cases of chronic discord and that these misperceptions can be documented by standard psychological testing instruments. This hypothesis bears a resemblance to speculations by psychoanalytically oriented marital therapists, such as Martin (1976) and Dicks (1967). Such therapists have suggested that transference distortions (perceptions of current interpersonal relationships as if they were identical to previous relationships) and projective identification (misperception of the mate as having certain personality characteristics denied by the perceiver) are etiologically related to marital discord.

The social psychological construct of interpersonal schema is preferentially chosen over the psychoanalytic concept of transference for several important reasons. The term *schema* is closer to a description of the observed phenomena and is more readily incorporated into the language systems of alternative approaches to therapy. It allows the eclectic clinician and theorist to utilize observational data from skilled psychoanalytically oriented clinicians without becoming entangled in concerns about the validity of related psychoanalytic concepts. The term *schemas* is more precisely defined and a technology exists for the measurement of interpersonal schemas (Kelly, 1955). A considerable research literature exists on the conditions under which such schemas are modifiable (Stotland and Canon, 1972). Use of the psychoanalytic term *transference*, with its associated theoretical assumptions, logically leads to the conclusion that fixed interpersonal misperceptions can be modified by insight alone. The term *schemas* has no such associated assumptions.

A second key concept in the author's model of marital therapy concerns the relationship of inner psychological events to the disturbed behavior patterns observed in distressed couples. This concept also relates to the presence of similar types of observable patient behavior in both individual and marital therapy as well as to the question of why faulty interpersonal schemas are not modified by usual life experiences in many patients. The hypothesis is that individuals have inner representational models for significant others and tend to behave toward other people in such a way as to invite behaviors that are congruent with that inner representational model. This hypothesis clearly implies that patients partially create their own interpersonal universes by the effects of their behavior on significant others. Similar hypotheses has been entertained by individual psychotherapists of varying theoretical orientations. Analytically oriented therapists, such as Offenkrantz and Tobin (1975), have written of the self-fulfilling interpersonal prophesies of the neurotic. Kaplan (1976) remarked on the tendency of patients "to repeatedly provoke the analyst to react in a manner similar to past object relations." Social psychologists have made similar observations and outlined similar explanatory mechanisms. Carson (1969) proposed a mechanism by which patients continually create their own misery: "One of the most important processes involved is the encouragement of self-confirmatory (complementary) reactions in others" (p. 150). More recently, the social learning theorist Albert Bandura (1977) proposed a similar explanation for how certain individuals continually recreate an unsatisfactory interpersonal environment. Leary (1957) developed the most thorough explanation of this process. He elaborated a matrix of eliciting interpersonal behaviors and the most probably induced responses in others. Using this matrix, Leary was able to demonstrate how certain personality styles (preferred forms of interpersonal behavior) have a self-sustaining function because of their impact on significant others in the current environment. This self-sustaining aspect could be comprehended independently of whatever early life events theoretically originally led to this personality predisposition.

Thus, I am suggesting that similar patterns of maladaptive behavior will be observed if the same patient is treated in individual therapy or in conjoint marital therapy. In both cases, these behavior patterns are predominantly the result of faulty interpersonal schemas for the perception of intimate others. In marital therapy, as contrasted to individual psychotherapy, most patients are highly effective in eliciting reciprocal behavior from their spouses. In a different terminology, marital therapy differs from individual psychotherapy in that each spouse arrives in therapy with a full-blown transference reaction. However, the transference reaction involves the spouse rather than the therapist (Gurman, 1978). Marital therapy is more complex than individual psychotherapy in that the "transference" relations are often bilateral and the therapist encounters a highly complex interactional system evolved over years of intimate interaction. The difference of my hypothesis from hypotheses proposed by psychoanalytically oriented marital therapists is my assumption that the behavior of marital partners is in large part the result of behavior-change maneuvers employed by the other spouse and only partly the manifestation of enduring personality traits in each. I am assuming a much greater degree of social reactivity in intimate relationship than most analytic therapists. This assumption leads to quite different therapeutic considerations.

A third key concept in the author's model is the assumption that the interactional patterns observed in couples with severe discord play a crucial role in maintaining the individual psychopathology of each of the spouses. The actual behavior of the spouse is all too often confirmatory to the other spouse's distorted view of reality and contributes to its permanence. As long as the second spouse acts in a manner confirmatory to the first spouse's view of reality, the first spouse is denied disconfirmatory life experiences and thus the opportunity for change. The repetitive maladaptive behavior patterns in distressed couples have been noted by therapists of varying theoretical orientations (Martin, 1976). Psychoanalytically oriented therapists have hypothesized that this situation is a manifestation of unconscious collusion between the marital partners (Dicks, 1967). According to this framework, the collusion is necessary to keep destructive inner forces at bay within each of the spouses. Therefore, the suggested intervention is to interpret the hypothetical feared consequences of a different sort of relationship and the past unconscious origins of such fears. In contrast, general system theorists such as Haley (1963) and Jackson (1965) have stressed that the pathology consists solely of the disturbed interaction. Thus, the therapeutic intervention is behavior change. I am hypothesizing that there is a reciprocal linkage between inner representational reality and observable behavior and that the recurring maladaptive interactional patterns are largely responsible for maintaining individual psychopathology in each of the spouses. According to my model, the goal of the therapist is to provide an interactional context that is disconfirmatory to each spouse's distorted image of the other. My model overlaps to a significant degree with the clinical observations of other theorists. It differs primarily in terms of my specifically acknowledging the interrelationship between behavior change and inner representational reality. I believe that this characteristic of my model gives the clinician a greater range of effective therapeutic options.

## CLINICAL RAMIFICATIONS

From the skeletal outline of the author's cognitive model of marital therapy, it is obvious that this model is a hybrid of contributions from general system theory, behavioral, and psychodynamic approaches to marital therapy. From the outset, I have assumed that experienced clinicians of all three schools are keen observers of human interaction, albeit from different vantage points and from different theoretical biases. I believe that an important advantage of my proposed theoretical model is that it can encompass these disparate observations within a unified framework. The advantage of a unified framework such as I am proposing is that it allows the clinician to be technically eclectic, while proceeding in a unified manner conceptually.

Practicing clinicians of the various partial schools of therapy may have various legitimate criticisms of my proposed formulation. Psychodynamically oriented therapists may hesitantly agree that certain psychoanalytic concepts can be retranslated into the language of cognitive social psychology and that this retranslation aids in defining these concepts with a different sort of explicitness and precision. They quite correctly can counter with the statement that my model neglects much of the complexity of the forces involved in marital discord. Therapists influenced by behaviorism and "social learning" may well be upset by the degree of emphasis this model places on internal psychological events. General system theorists can justifiably object that the proposed model, as elaborated so far, does not do justice to the complexity of interactional systems. What I am proposing is a beginning synthesis that I feel has clinical utility at present. It is indeed oversimplified. However, "If we begin by considering all the complexities involved in real-life events, we will never arrive at a scientific theory; if we are willing to over-simplify, we are at least enabled to make a beginning and thus to correct our errors" (Eysenck and Beech, 1971, p. 603). The system I am proposing provides a common language system whereby clinicians of varying orientations can have a means of at least minimal communication and possibly cross-fertilization. I believe that this system allows the practicing clinician to utilize the observational power provided by his current theoretical orientation without being unduly shackled by its theoretical constructs.

For example, marital therapists of dissimilar theoretical orientations are faced with a common clinical situation. Most often, when they are confronted with a couple in chronic discord, they will observe repetitive interlocking behavioral sequences that recur with great tenacity. These sequences have been described by therapists of all of the major theoretical orientations (e.g., Lederer and Jackson, 1968; Liberman, 1975; Dicks, 1967). Each school of therapy observes the same phenomenon, then identifies and labels certain hypothetical variables as of etiologic significance, and devises a therapeutic intervention based on those assumptions. General system theorists will observe the stabilizing forces maintaining the equilibrium in the system and devise interventions to disrupt this equilibrium. These interventions will ignore individual characteristics in the units (people) constituting the interactional system. Analytic therapists observe the same phenomenon and assume that the principal pathology resides in the units (individuals) constituting the interactional systems, and their interventions are focused on correcting individual psychopathology. Behavior therapists observing the same phenomenon posit that the recurring maladaptive patterns of interaction are the result of faulty reinforcement exchange maneuvers and poor negotiation skills and plan their intervention accordingly. There is reason to believe that none of these interventions are maximally effective. The systems intervention approaches neglect the role of individual psychopathology. Likewise, analysts may correctly intuit the transference reactions involved, but this information is of limited usefulness during the early stages of therapy. A correct interpretation of each spouse's perceptual distortion is of little use when the actual behavior of the spouse is confirmatory to the distortion.

According to my proposed model, the observable recurring maladaptive behavior patterns are the result of each spouse's attempt to influence the other to act in accord with the inner representational model for the opposite sex. Thus, the recurring maladaptive behavior patterns appear stable because they are confirmatory to both inner representational models. The primary goal of therapy is to dislodge these fixated perceptions, i.e., to disprove the transference distortions. A variety of technical procedures can be employed within this conceptual framework. In most cases, the initial thrust of therapy is to attempt to reduce the congruence between inner representational systems and the actual behavior of the spouses. Thus, the first therapeutic maneuver has to be to disrupt the recurring behavior patterns. In this regard, techniques and concepts employed by general systems theorists can be an ideal level of first intervention. The confirmatory interaction patterns can be further disrupted by the use of behavioral reciprocity counseling procedures to induce positive interchanges between spouses, on the assumption that this resulting new behavior will be discrepant with the negative representational models. Techniques from the communication training approaches to marital discord can be selectively borrowed, on the assumption that discrepant verbal feedback will similarly facilitate cognitive change. After a behavior change has occurred, the therapists can employ interpretations and redirection of perceptions to emphasize the contrast between the actual behavior of the spouses and previous models of the opposite sex. It is assumed that observed behavior, verbal information from the spouse, and cognitive relabeling all contribute to a cognitive shift in the perception of the spouse. This model also allows a conceptual linkage between individual and conjoint approaches to the treatment of marital discord. The proposed model hypothesizes that individual psychopathology can be related to interpersonal difficulties by emphasizing the role of interpersonal misperceptions in eliciting and maintaining disturbed behavior patterns among intimates. Whereas, in individual psychotherapy in neurotic or personality disorders, "transference reactions" of varying sorts might be involved, it is hypothesized that within the context of marital discord, fixated misperceptions of the opposite sex are primary in maintaining the disturbed behavior patterns. These cognitive schemas for the perception of intimate members of the opposite sex appear to be more readily elicited by interpersonal stimuli associated with emotionally dependent relationships. These eliciting relationships can be either marital or long-term psychotherapy.

Theoretically, the "transference reactions" should be modifiable in either individual psychotherapy or conjoint marital therapy. In individual psychotherapy, the transference reaction usually develops more slowly, and ideally the patient is unsuccessful in provoking the therapist to act in accord (collusion) with the inner representational model for emotional significant members of the opposite sex. In psychoànalysis, insight as it relates to transference can be viewed as a special type of discrimination learning. The patient begins to discriminate between inner representational models and external reality. Similar phenomena occur in conjoint marital therapy, although differences between the two types of therapy necessitate differing levels of explanation for the observed phenomena and differing therapeutic techniques.

## OVERVIEW

This book will proceed by developing in greater detail the ideas and concepts presented in skeletal form in this introductory chapter. This chapter was included to provide the reader with a framework from which to evaluate subsequent sections. As a goal of this text is to integrate contributions from various theoretical perspectives, many readers may prefer to skim lightly over certain sections.

The next chapter will be devoted to a review of the empirical evidence linking marital discord and disruption to the use of mental health services. This evidence is reviewed here because it is not readily accessible elsewhere and relates to the problem of assigning a low priority to training in marital therapy in overall mental health training programs. The available evidence suggests that such training warrants higher priority. Practicing clinicians may prefer to skip this chapter, although it will be of interest to mental health administrators and trainees.

Chapters Three through Five will review developments in the three major contemporary approaches to marital therapy. One chapter each will be devoted to psychoanalytic, behavioral, and general system approaches. Basic concepts, the clinical application, and relevant research for each viewpoint will be reviewed.

Chapter Six is a transition chapter between the review of others' work and the presentation of the author's model. This chapter will review and examine conceptual linkages between inner psychological events and external reality. This chapter is included because one of the principal dichotomies between theoretical schools in the treatment of marital discord is between the interpretative and behavioral approaches.

The last three chapters will present at integrative model of marital therapy. In the first of these chapters, the formal postulates and their empirical support will be summarized. In the second, the clinical application of this model will be elaborated. In the third, the model will be illustrated in clinical use by case examples.

## REFERENCES

Adams, C. R. The prediction of adjustment in marriage. *Educational and Psychological Measurements*, 1946, *6*, 185–193.

Bandura, A. *Social learning theory*. Englewood Cliffs, New Jersey: Prentice Hall, 1977.

Bentler, P. M., and Newcomb, M. D. Longitudinal study of marital success and failure. *Journal of Consulting and Clinical Psychology*, 1978, *46*, 1053–1070.

Birk, L., and Brinkley-Birk, A. W. Psychoanalysis and behavior therapy. *American Journal of Psychiatry*, 1974, *131*, 499–510.

Bloom, B. L., Asher, S. J., and White, S. W. Marital disruption as a stressor: a review and analysis. *Psychological Bulletin* 1978 *85*, 867–894.

Bradburn, N. M. *The structure of psychological well-being*. Chicago: Aldine, 1969.

Brady, J. P. A behavioral approach to the treatment of stuttering. *American Journal of Psychiatry*, *125*, 843–848, 1969.

Breger, L., and McGaugh, J. L. Critique and reformulation of learning theory approaches to psychotherapy and neurosis. *Psychological Bulletin*, 1965, *63*, 338–358.

Brody, S. Simultaneous psychotherapy of married couples: Preliminary observations. *Psychoanalytic Review*, 1961, *48*, 94–107.

Carson, R. C. *Interaction concepts of personality*. Chicago: Aldine, 1969.

Burgess, E. W., and Wallin, P. *Engagement and marriage*. Chicago: Lippincott, 1953.

Carson, R. C. *Interaction concepts of personality*. Chicago: Aldine, 1969.

Dicks, H. U. *Marital tensions*. New York: Basic Books, 1967.

Eysenck, J. H., and Beech, R. Counter conditioning and related methods. In A. E. Bergin and S. L. Garfield (Eds.) *Handbook of psychotherapy and behavior change*. New York: Wiley, 1971.

Eysenck, H. J., and Rackman, S. *The causes and cures of neurosis*. San Diego: Knapp, 1965.

Feather, B. W., and Rhoads, J. M. Psychodynamic behavior therapy. Theory and rationale. *Archives of General Psychiatry*, 1972, *26*, 496–502.

Fitzgerald, R. V. *Conjoint marital therapy*. New York: Jason Aronson, 1973.

Goldiamond, I. Self-control procedures in personal behavior problems. *Psychological Reports*, *17*, 851–868, 1965.

Greer, S. W., and D'Zurilla, T. J. Behavioral approaches to marital discord and conflict. In C. M. Franks and G. T. Wilson (Eds.), *Annual review of behavior therapy theory and practice: 1976*. New York: Brunner/Mazel, 1976.

Gurman, A. S. Contemporary marital therapies: a critique and comparative analysis of psychoanalytic, behavioral and systems theory approaches. In T. J. Paolino and B. S. McCrady (Eds.) *Marriage and Marital Therapy*. New York: Brunner/Mazel, 1978.

Gurman, A. S., and Knudson, R. M. Behavioral marriage therapy. 1. A psychodynamic systems analysis and critique. *Family Process*, 1978, *17*: 121–138.

Haley, J. Marriage therapy. *Archives of General Psychiatry*, 1963, *8*, 213–234.

Hunt, H. F., and Dyrud, J. E. Commentary: Perspective in behavior therapy. *Research in Psychotherapy*, 1968, *3*, 140–152.

Jackson, D. D. The study of the family. *Family Process*, 1965, *4*, 1–2.

Jacobson, N. S. Problem solving and contingency contracting in the treatment of marital discord. *Journal of Consulting and Clinical Psychology*, 1972, *45*, 92–100.

Jacobson, N. S., and Martin, B. Behavioral marriage therapy: current status. *Psychological Bulletin*, 1976, *83*, 540–556.

Jacobson, N. S., and Weiss, R. L. Behavioral marriage therapy, (Vol. 3) Critique: The contents of Gurman *et al.* may be hazardous to your health. *Family Process*, 1978, *17*, 149–164.

Kaplan, S. M. The analyst, the transference, and the representational world. *Comprehensive Psychiatry*, 1976, *17*, 47–54.

Kelly, E. L. Concerning the validity of Terman's weights for predicting marital happiness. *Psychological Bulletin*, 1939, *139*, 202–203.

Kelly, G. A. *The psychology of personal constructs*. New York: Norton, 1955.

Lazarus, A. *Behavior therapy and beyond*. New York: McGraw-Hill, 1971.

Liberman, R. Behavioral principles in family and couple therapy. In A. S. Gurman, D. G. Rice (Eds.) *Couples in conflict*. New York: Jason Aronson, 1975.

Leary, T. *Interpersonal diagnosis of personality*. New York: Ronald Press, 1957.

Lederer, W. J., and Jackson, D. D. *The mirages of marriage*. New York: Norton, 1968.

London, P. The end of ideology in behavior modification. *American Psychologist*, 1972, *27*, 913–920.

Mahoney, M. J. Cognition and behavior modification. Cambridge, Massachusetts: Ballinger, 1974.

Manus, G. L. Marriage counseling: A technique in search of a theory. *Journal of Marriage and the Family*, 1966, *28*, 449–453.

Marks, I. M., and Gelden, M. G. Transvestism and Fetishism: clinical and psychological changes during faradic aversion. *British Journal of Psychiatry*, 1967, *113*, 711–729.

Martin, P. A. *A marital therapy manual*. New York: Brunner/Mazel, 1976.

Meichenbaum, D. *Cognitive-behavior modification*. New York: Plenum, 1977.

Minuchin, S., Rosman, B. L., and Baker, L. *Psychosomatic families, anorexia nervosa in context*. Cambridge, Massachusetts: Harvard University Press, 1978.

Nadelson, C. C. Marital therapy from a psychoanalytic perspective. In T. J. Paolino and B. S. McCrady (Eds.) *Marriage and marital therapy*. New York: Brunner/Mazel, 1978.

Offenkrantz, W., and Tobin, A. Psychoanalytic Psychotherapy. In D. X. Freedman and J. E. Dyrud (Eds.) *American handbook of psychiatry*, Vol. 5. New York: Basic Books, 1978.

O'Leary, K. D., and Turkewitz, H. Marital therapy from a behavioral perspective. In
    T. J. Paolino and B. S. McCrady (Eds.), *Marriage and marital therapy*. New York: Brun-
    ner/Mazel, 1978.
Olson, D. H. A critical overview. In A. S. Gurman and D. G. Rice (Eds.), *Couples in conflict*.
    New York: Jason Aronson, 1975.
Prochaska, J., and Prochaska, J. Twentieth century trends in marriage and marital therapy.
    In T. J. Paolino and B. S. McGrady (Eds.), *Marriage and marital therapy*. New York:
    Brunner/Mazel, 1978.
Sager, C. J. *Marriage contracts and couple therapy*. New York: Brunner/Mazel, 1976.
Sager, C. J., Grundlach, R., Kremer, M., Lenz, R., and Royce, J. R. The married in
    treatment. *Archives of General Psychiatry*, 1968, *19*, 206–217.
Satir, V. *Conjoint family therapy*. Palo Alto: Science and Behavior Books, 1967.
Segraves, R. T. Concurrent psychotherapy and behavior therapy. *Archives of General Psy-
    chiatry*, 1976, *33*, 756–763.
Segraves, R. T. Conjoint Marital Therapy: A cognitive behavioral model. *Archives of General
    Psychiatry*, 1978, *35*, 450–455.
Segraves, R. T., and Smith, R. C. Concurrent psychotherapy and behavior therapy. *Ar-
    chives of General Psychiatry*, 1976, *33*, 756–763.
Stotland, E., and Cannon L. K. *Social psychology: a cognitive approach*. Philadelphia:
    W. B. Saunders, 1972.

# CHAPTER TWO

# The Relationship of Marriage to Psychological Well-being

As mentioned in the previous chapter, mental health professionals have been predominantly concerned with the treatment of psychiatrically impaired individuals. Similarly, most theoretical systems of psychiatric intervention have tended to stress individual psychopathology. This chapter is included to question whether this emphasis on treatment of individual psychopathology is warranted and to specifically question whether there shouldn't be more emphasis on the intervention in marital and family systems. My purpose is not to negate the importance of studying individual psychopathology but to suggest that it might be more profitable to think of mental disturbance as the result of individual liabilities reacting with social influences, particularly relationships with emotional intimates. Psychopathology conceptualized in this manner gives equal weight to individual and social systems levels of intervention.

This chapter will examine the relationship of marital status to mental health service usage and to various estimates of psychological impairment in the general population. Evidence relating divorce and marital discord to the development of psychopathology in the children will also be examined, and various explanatory hypotheses about these relationships will be reviewed. It may appear somewhat unusual to include a survey of epidemiological research in what is essentially a text on the treatment of marital discord. In the author's view, research and clinical activities should be complementary. All too often, research and clinical activities appear to be artificially dichotomized into separate activities.

The clinician frequently possesses a depth of vision impossible for the researcher to achieve; however, this perceptiveness is often limited to a selective view of part of the influences on emotional suffering. A clinician who treats individuals and who was trained in the school of individual psychopathology may quite perceptively understand how individual demons cause interpersonal discord, but he by the nature of his experience may underestimate the impact of interpersonal demons on individual psychological functioning. The school of social psychiatry and the clinical activities of the marital therapist have a natural complementariness, as both are concerned with the interaction of the social environment and the individual.

## MARITAL STATUS AND MENTAL HEALTH SERVICE USAGE

In the following sections, a trend will be observed in which divorced and separated individuals are consistently overrepresented in various surveys of admissions to mental hospitals, psychiatric wards of general hospitals, and psychiatric outpatient services. To help the reader appreciate these sections, some of the methodological problems involved in interpreting these data and some of the explanatory hypotheses generated to explain these observations will be briefly discussed.

To have a basic understanding of the environmental impact of a disease process, most epidemiologists need at least two basic types of information. They need to know the frequency with which new cases of the disease occur (incidence) and the extent to which the population at a given moment suffers from the disease (prevalence). For mental disorders, approximations to incidence and prevalence rates are possible. Incidence statistics can be approximated by first admission rates, i.e., the annual number of first admissions for a diagnostic entity in relationship to the population of the catchment area served by that facility. Prevalence can be estimated by the resident patient rate, i.e., the count of patients resident in a mental facility at a given time relative to the population served by that facility. These rates can be used to provide measures of the relative differences in incidence and prevalence of specific disorders among different demographic subgroups, with the reservation that a number of social attitudinal, administrative, and economic factors will also influence admission to psychiatric facilities (Kramer et al., 1972).

There are numerous difficulties in simply obtaining reliable and comprehensive data about psychiatric usage by various marital status groups. The National Institute of Mental Health annually requests data from psychiatric facilities about populations served. However, the reporting system is voluntary, and different facilities employ different methods for classifying and recording data. Information from the private sector, particularly from general hospitals that admit psychiatric patients, is frequently incomplete. The Veterans Administration hospitals don't separate first admissions from readmissions, and some facilities report discharge rates rather than admission rates. Only comparatively recently have most facilities reported standardized information on the marital status of the population served. Currently, most facilities report patients' marital status as single, married, widowed, divorced, or separated. Previously, marital status was often reported simply as single, married, or other. It is still doubtful that reliable information is available on separated individuals. In United States census data, more females than males report their marital status as separated, whereas clearly the percentages of the two sexes should be equivalent. The discrepancy may represent the wish of separated males to remain undetected by their wives and the wish of unwed mothers to obscure their marital status (Carter and Glick, 1976). In spite of these reservations, most investigators would agree that fairly reliable data are available on psychiatric service usage by marital status groups, with the possible exception of the maritally separated.

Four basic hypotheses have been generated to explain the differential usage of psychiatric facilities by different marital status groups. These hypotheses will be discussed in greater detail later in this chapter. However, they will be briefly summarized at this point to orient the reader to the discussion to follow. The correct interpretation of these data is crucial to the author's purpose. These hypotheses can be classified as the hospitalization, selection, protection, and stress hypotheses. The hospitalization hypothesis posits that certain factors independent of psychiatric impairment predispose certain marital status subgroups toward hospitalization. This hypothesis can in all probability be dismissed, as investigations of the prevalence of emotional disturbance in the untreated general population find degrees of impairment in various marital status groups to parallel the psychiatric hospitalization rates of those same groups. The selection hypothesis states that the psychiatrically impaired have greater difficulty becoming and staying married. In further discussion, it will become apparent that the selection hypothesis may account for the higher psychiatric impairment in singles but appears insufficient to explain the same in divorced and separated populations. The protection hypothesis postulates that marriage in some way protects against psychiatric impairment. This hypothesis is closely related to theories about social integration suggesting that close interpersonal ties give purpose to life and protect against emotional despair. The stress hypothesis posits that marital disruption is a significant life stress of some magnitude that may elicit psychiatric impairment in the otherwise normal population. It is of note that psychiatric facility usage by the divorced may underrepresent the significance of the stress of marital disruption, as marital separation appears to be a greater stress and frequently precedes divorce by 1 to 2 years (Bloom *et al.*, 1977).

## MARITAL STATUS AND PSYCHIATRIC HOSPITALIZATION

A number of studies have reported married individuals to have lower rates of mental hospital usage than other marital status groups. This has been a remarkably consistent finding in different types of institutions, in differing localities within the United States at different time periods, and in other countries. Studies of institutional residence rates have found single individuals to be overrepresented in psychiatric hospitals. Most studies have reported that institutional residence rates decrease for different marital status groups from highest to lowest in the following order: single, separated, divorced, widowed, and married (Carter and Glick, 1976; Brooke, 1967). The high residence rates for singles is probably due in part to the socially isolated single psychotics who become chronically institutionalized. Hospital admission rates, which are probably a better index of the incidence of mental disorder, present a slightly different picture. Hospital admission rates are generally highest for divorced and separated individuals, intermediate for widowed and single, and lowest for married individuals (Bachrach, 1975a, b, c).

This finding of highest admission rates for divorced and separated individuals has been replicated in several national surveys at different time periods both in this country and abroad. Pugh and MacMahon (1962) analyzed incidence of first admissions to mental hospitals in the United States in 1922, with admission rates for divorced followed by single, widowed, and married, in that order. Kramer (1967, 1969) analyzed data on first hospital admissions with a diagnosis of functional psychosis, derived from a collaborative study of the Office of Biometry of the National Institute of Mental Health. This represented 22,205 first admissions in 1960 for 13 states in the Model Reporting Area. Again, highest admission rates to psychiatric facilities were for divorced and separated, followed by single, widowed, and married. The admission rates for divorced individuals were approximately six times higher than for the married. Similar findings have been reported by Bachrach (1973a, b, c) in her analysis of discharges from psychiatric inpatient units of general hospitals in 1970–1971. Age-adjusted discharge rates per 100,000 population again document the highest discharges for separated and divorced, followed by never married, widowed, and married. Milazzo-Sayre (1977) reported on admission rates to state and county psychiatric facilities. Age-adjusted admission rates per 100,000 population by sex and marital status were reported for 1975. Again, the separated and divorced had admission rates approximately 10 times greater than the rate for the married group. The highest rates were for separated and divorced, followed by widowed, never married, and married. The widowed group was especially high in admissions for females. Odegard (1953) presented data on all first psychiatric hospital admissions in Norway from 1931 to 1945, a total of 23,115 admissions, and reported the divorced to have the highest admission rates of any marital status group. Somewhat similar data have been reported by Krupinski and Stoller (1962) on admissions to mental hospitals in Victoria, Australia, suggesting that these findings are not limited to the United States.

Various other studies have presented data on rates of admission to psychiatric facilities by marital status for individual states and localities. These studies are consistent in finding highest rates among the divorced and separated, intermediate rates for the single and widowed, and lowest rates for the married. These reports include studies in Ohio (Frumkin, 1955; Locke et al., 1958, 1960a), Texas (Jaco, 1960), New York (Malzberg, 1964; Thomas and Locke, 1963), Arkansas (Adler, 1953), Louisiana and Maryland (Kramer et al., 1972), and Baltimore, Maryland (Klee et al., 1967). The fact that consistent findings are reported in local, national, and foreign surveys suggests that this is a highly reliable observation.

Many investigators have attempted to examine differential admission rates by marital status for different diagnostic subgroups. These data are questionable because of poor reliability in making psychiatric diagnoses across different centers. To summarize these studies, it would appear that the divorced are overrepresented in all diagnostic categories. A possible exception is that of manic-depressive disease (Dube and Kumar, 1973; Gershon and Liebowitz, 1975; Frumkin, 1955). Numerous investigators agree that the divorced have highest rates among all marital status groups for psychiatric hospitalization with alcoholic psychosis (Klee et al., 1967; Kramer et al., 1972; Frumkin, 1955; Bachrach, 1973b; Malzberg, 1964), syphilitic psychosis (Malzberg, 1964; Odegard, 1953; Carter and Glick, 1976; Frumkin, 1955), senile psychosis (Locke et al., 1960b; Odegard, 1953; Kramer et al., 1972), and schizophrenia (Thomas and Locke, 1963; Malzberg, 1964; Pugh and MacMahon, 1962). There is also some evidence that the divorced may be overrepresented among those suffering from reactive and neurotic depressive disorders (Bachrach, 1973b; Weeke et al., 1975).

In summary, divorced and separated individuals are an extremely high-risk group for psychiatric hospitalization. This has been repeatedly found for various types of psychiatric facilities in this and other countries at different times. This is probably true for most psychiatric diagnostic subgroups, although data on this are probably less reliable. As there has been a trend in the last 15–20 years to shift psychiatric care to outpatient facilities, it is important to ascertain if similar patterns of differential usage by marital status subgroups occur in such clinics.

## MARITAL STATUS AND OUTPATIENT CLINIC USAGE

The available data on psychiatric outpatient clinic usage by different marital status group parallel the findings of surveys on inpatient psychiatric facilities. Again, the divorced and separated are overrepresented relative to their proportions in the general population as users of mental health services. Different investigators have consistently found highest rates of psychiatric clinic usage by the divorced and separated, intermediate rates for the widowed and never married, and lowest rates for the married. One group of investigators was so impressed with these data as to suggest that much greater emphasis should be placed on the provision of family and marital therapy: "One of our most interesting findings is the marked variation in outpatient rates by marital status. The rank order of these rates coincides generally with hospital findings and emphasizes the importance of marital and familial variables in determining entrance into treatment. Both the role of clinics in treating persons in 'marital crisis' and the interrelationship of psychopathology and marital status require further investigation" (Rosen et al., 1964, p. 466).

This finding has been replicated in national surveys in this country at different time periods as well as in surveys in other countries. Rosen et al. (1964) analyzed psychiatric outpatient clinic termination rates for the year ending June 30, 1961. Rosen analyzed data collected by the National Institute of Mental Health and used 1960 census data to determine rates of clinic utilization. It is of note that many clinics don't report statistics on the marital status of users. However, there is no reason to suspect that this should bias estimates of utilization by differing marital status groups. A familiar pattern of utilization was found: "Throughout virtually all adult ages, and for each sex, rates were highest for the separated, followed by those for the divorced, the never married, and the widowed, with rates for the married being the lowest" (Rosen et al., 1964, p. 460). A slightly different analysis of 1960 clinic utilization data by the Biometrics Branch of the National Institute of Mental Health produced similar results, with the exception that the clinic admission rates for the widowed group were lower (Biometrics Branch, 1963).

Similar findings were reported in 1969 and 1970 surveys. A 1969 survey of outpatient clinics, excluding federally funded community mental health centers and Veterans Administration clinics, included data from 2,088 clinics covering 1,109,081 admissions (Biometrics Branch, 1971). The age-adjusted admission rate to outpatient services for the divorced and separated was over five times as high as for the married. It is of note that this survey also included data on the diagnostic breakdown of clinic users. Among users receiving a diagnosis of conditions without manifest psychiatric disorder, marital maladjustment was the most frequent presenting complaint.

Similar data were found in 1970 surveys of outpatient clinic utilization (Meyer, 1973; Redick and Johnson, 1974). As in the previous surveys, clinic admission rates are highest for the divorced and separated. To help the reader appreciate the magnitude of the difference in utilization rates, the age-adjusted rates per 100,000 population are: (1) married, 365.3; (2) never married, 971.6; (3) widowed, 1,326.4; (4) separated, divorced, 1,750.8.

Comparable data have been reported by surveys completed by independent clinics (McKnight et al., 1966) and localities (Miles et al., 1964) in the United States as well as surveys in other countries (Robertson, 1974; Innes and Sharp, 1962). It is of interest that one survey of clinic utilization by the aged population also found highest rates for the divorced (Rosen et al., 1968). This is of particular interest, as one might expect the widowed to have the highest rates in this age group.

At this point, one can be reasonably assured of higher psychiatric usage rates in both psychiatric hospitals and outpatient clinics by the divorced and separated. Another source of psychiatric care frequently utilized is the general practitioner; surveys have indicated that many individuals turn first to their family physician in times of emotional crisis (Gurin et al., 1960). Reliable information on the psychiatric services provided by primary physicians is difficult to obtain. However, two well-conducted studies suggest that the divorced and separated are also overrepresented among this population of medical service users.

In this country, Locke and associates (1967) obtained the cooperation of 74% of general practitioners and internists in Prince George's County, Maryland. Each physician was asked to record and report on all clinic visits for 1 week during the period from February through July 1964. Of the 7,814 patients seen during this survey, 548 (7%) were diagnosed by their physician as having a psychiatric condition. Highest rates of psychiatric conditions were observed for the divorced and separated and for the widowed.

A similar survey was made of patient visits to doctors on the London Executive Council Medical List from October 1, 1961, to September 30, 1962 (Shepherd *et al.*, 1966; Cooper, 1966). Forty-six separate practitioners recorded every eighth consultation over a 1-year period for their adult practice population. Each physician was asked to formally diagnose psychiatric conditions when present in their patients. Approximately 1/7 of the patients consulted their general practitioners for symptoms that were diagnosed as psychiatric in nature. For both sexes, divorced and separated had the highest frequency of psychiatric problems when the rates were standardized for age. It is of note that psychiatric patients consulted their doctors more frequently than other patients and that marital problems were an extremely frequent reason for consultation.

Gurin and associates (1960) in a study on life adjustment and help-seeking behavior sponsored by the Joint Commission on Mental Illness and Health reported complementary findings. A cross-sectional sample of Americans over the age of 21 were personally interviewed by trained interviewers. Among those who admitted to having sought help in a time of personal crisis, 42% reported that the crisis situation was a marital problem. General physicians and clergymen were the most frequent professionals consulted for counseling and support.

## PSYCHOLOGICAL WELL-BEING AND MARITAL STATUS

From data presented in previous sections, it can be assumed with a reasonable degree of confidence that the divorced and separated are high-risk groups for psychiatric hospitalization and are more frequent users of psychiatric outpatient services than other marital status groups. This group also appears to use general medical services for nonorganic conditions more frequently than other marital status groups. It is an understatement to say that this group utilizes a significant portion of government and private financing of medical services. However, these data cannot be used to assert confidently that psychiatric impairment is greater in this group of individuals. One could argue that this group is simply a greater user of services, and that data on service utilization are not necessarily reflective of the prevalence of disorder in the general population. There have been numerous population surveys attempting to estimate the prevalence of mental disorder in the general population. Some of these studies have included data on marital status subgroups. These studies have used many different indices of mental health, and it is sometimes questionable to what degree these surveys of prevalence measure entities approximating psychiatric diagnostic categories. For the purposes of this text, this difficulty is not relevant, as numerous studies employing a wide variety of measuring instruments are consistent in finding emotional impairment, however measured, to be highest in divorced and separated individuals.

The Midtown Manhattan study (Srole et al., 1962) is one of the most well-known studies in psychiatric epidemiology. In this study, a home interview survey of residents aged 20–59 was performed. A sample of 1,660 were interviewed in their homes by trained interviewers. This sample represented a stratified probability sample of a population of 110,000. The interview materials were then rated by psychiatrists for degree of psychiatric impairment. The findings of this study parallel the findings previously surveyed, in that "the Midtown divorced of both sexes have the highest mental morbidity rates of all four marital status categories. In fact, these are the highest rates of any demographic groups reviewed to this point. The differences between the married and divorced in both Impaired and Well frequencies are well within the limits of statistical confidence. The ratio of Impaired to Well is roughly 1:1 among the married people of both sexes, is 6:1 among divorced women and 10:1 among divorced men" (Srole et al., 1962, p. 185).

Briscoe and associates (Briscoe et al., 1973; Briscoe and Smith, 1974) utilized a different research design to investigate the relationship of divorce to psychiatric impairment. Divorce decrees issued by the St. Louis County Court of Domestic Relations during December 1969 were used to obtain a population of divorced subjects. Control subjects were obtained by locating individuals living on the same street block as the divorced subjects. All control and divorced subjects were then personally interviewed and diagnosed by a psychiatrist or a psychiatry resident. For both sexes, divorced probands were more likely to be diagnosed as suffering from psychiatric impairment. The most frequent diagnoses were unipolar depression and antisocial personality. It is of particular interest that of the 40 divorced patients who had seen a psychiatrist during their lifetimes, 30 had seen a psychiatrist within 1 year of their divorce decree.

Three other interview studies of the general population should be briefly mentioned. Blumenthal (1967) conducted a mental health survey of 192 families containing children with a chronic illness—phenylketonuria, mental retardation, or cystic fibrosis. An incidental finding of this study was that divorced individuals differed highly significantly from nondivorced individuals on mental health indices. Similar findings were reported in an interview study of a representative sample of the Chicago area for the presence of depression (Pearlin and Johnson, 1977). The separated were found to be most susceptible to depression, the widowed and divorced to be intermediate, followed by the single, with marrieds being most free of depression. Weissman and Myers (1978) similarly found depression to be more frequent in persons not currently married.

Two studies attempted to evaluate the relationship of marital status to mental disorder in the aged. Lowenthal *et al.* (1967) found highest rates of psychiatric impairment in the single, widowed, and divorced elderly in a community survey in San Francisco. In a survey of people aged 65 and over residing in six census tracts in an upstate New York urban community, Bellin and Hardt (1958) found that the divorced and separated were more frequently rated as having poor mental health. Single and widowed subjects had intermediate values, and the married had the highest ratings of mental health.

One objection to the interview assessment studies just reviewed is that assessment of psychiatric impairment is a highly subjective evaluation. It is difficult for an independent investigator to be certain of the actual criteria used in the assessment by other investigators. Studies employing questionnaires are not subject to this same criticism. Uhlenhuth *et al.* (1974) reported their investigation of psychiatric symptoms and life stress in a probability sample of all households in the city of Oakland, California. Subjects' symptom levels were assessed by asking about 54 specific symptoms extracted from the Hopkins Symptom Checklist, and life stress was assessed by inquiring about 41 life events extracted from a modification of the Holmes Social Readjustment Scale. On both symptom intensity and life stress, the separated group had the highest scores, followed by the divorced, widowed, single, and married, in that order. Mellinger *et al.* (1978) reported a similar study employing similar instruments in a nationwide cross-sectional study of noninstitutionalized adults. They reported highest stress and symptom levels in the divorced of both sexes. The relative magnitude of stress and symptoms differed between the sexes for the other marital status groups.

Studies conducted by the National Opinion Research Center on the relationship of demographic characteristics to self-reported happiness have yielded similar results (Bradburn and Caplovitz, 1965; Bradburn, 1969). Representative samples of 14 different communities were interviewed by trained National Opinion Research Center personnel and were asked, among other questions, "Taken altogether, how would you say things are these days, would you say you are very happy, pretty happy, or not too happy?" It is of interest that in all of the samples, about one-third reported being very happy and about 5 to 15% reported being not too happy. Bradburn's findings, using this rather novel approach of asking people to self-rate their personal happiness, parallel those of investigators using more conventional assessments of psychological well-being: "As seen in Table 9.1, people who are married are much more likely than people who are not currently married to report that they are very happy, and much less likely to report that they are not too happy. Among the not-currently married, those who have been married but are now separated, divorced, or widowed are by far the unhappiest, while those who have never been married fall between the two" (Bradburn, 1969, p. 148). It is also of note that Bradburn analyzed data for late and early marrieds and found evidence that the reactive hypothesis fits these data better than the selection hypothesis.

## MARITAL STATUS AND ALCOHOLISM

Epidemiological studies of alcoholism have consistently found higher rates of alcoholism for males than for females. However, within both sexes, the divorced and separated have rates of alcoholism greatly exceeding their proportions in the general population. The married population has the lowest rates for alcoholism. Findings regarding the widowed and single are less consistent, although single men are usually overrepresented among alcoholics. Some studies have found higher rates' for the widowed of both sexes, whereas other studies have found that only widowed males have higher rates of alcoholism.

Bachrach (1975a, b, c) surveyed first admissions with a diagnosis of alcoholic disorders in inpatient services of state and county hospitals in October 1972. Her analysis of admission data by marital status was limited to male admissions, as female admissions were too infrequent to allow reliable estimates of the total population. Patients with a primary diagnosis of alcoholic disorders represented 38% of all male admissions. Divorced and separated males were greatly overrepresented among alcoholics, having admission rates for this diagnosis 18 times higher than their married peers. Widowed and never-married males had intermediate rates between the divorced and the married.

Locke and associates (1960a) analyzed first admissions with a diagnosis of alcoholic psychosis to Ohio State mental hospitals for a 4½-year period between 1948 and 1952. For both sexes, the divorced and separated had highest admission rates, followed by the single and married, in that order. They did not report separate data for the widowed. Similar data were reported by Malzberg (1947) for admissions to New York State hospitals in 1943–1944. Gorwitz et al. (1970) reported data on admissions in Maryland with a diagnosis of alcoholism for a 3-year period ending June 30, 1964. For males and females of both white and nonwhite racial groups, the divorced and separated were overrepresented. Rates for the single and widowed differed by sex for each racial group.

Investigators using more novel indices of alcoholism have reported similar findings. Wechsler *et al.* (1972) reported the results of performing Breathalyzer tests on 6,266 consecutive admissions to the emergency service at the Massachusetts General Hospital in Boston: "In both sexes, the divorced or separated had the highest proportion with positive Breathalyzer readings as well as the highest percentage of persons with BACS [blood alcohol concentrations] at or above 0.05%" (Wechsler *et al.*, 1972, p. 138). Similar findings had been previously reported by Bacon (1944) on the marital status of arrested inebriates. Gove (1973) reported on deaths due to cirrhosis of the liver, frequently attributed to alcoholism, for the United States in 1959–1961. Mortality rates for both sexes were highest for the divorced, followed by the widowed, the single, and then the married, in that order. Rosenblatt *et al.* (1969, 1971) have also reported that the divorced are overrepresented among multiple admissions for alcoholism.

## SUICIDE AND MARITAL STATUS

As one might expect, after reading the preceding sections of this chapter, suicide rates are higher for divorced, widowed, and separated individuals than for their same-aged counterparts in society. This is not surprising, as suicide is frequently associated with psychiatric disease, and most diagnostic categories of psychiatric disorder appear to have higher incidence rates for these marital status groups. One has to review these findings with certain reservations. Undoubtedly, suicide is grossly underreported in most societies because of the social stigma and legal difficulties associated with suicide. Interpretation of demographic variables associated with suicide rates is difficult unless the rates are corrected for the age and marital status of the general population. Youthful persons are usually overrepresented among suicide attempts, and the majority of the members of most populations are married. It is also probably important to distinguish between suicide attempts and completed suicides, as these may represent two entirely different populations. Suicide attempts are frequently conceptualized as "pleas for help," whereas the most seriously ill psychiatrically and medically might be expected to be overrepresented in the "completed" suicide group. In spite of these reservations, somewhat consistent findings have been reported by most investigators. As these findings have been reviewed extensively by others, this section will not attempt to be comprehensive.

Several authors (Kramer *et al.*, 1972, Carter and Glick, 1976; Gove, 1973) have reviewed the information on suicide in the United States collected by the National Center for Health Statistics for the 3-year period of 1959–1961. This represents data on completed suicides by race, sex, and marital status. For both races, age-specific mortality rates for death by suicide are highest for the widowed. The divorced have rates slightly lower than the widowed, followed by single and then married. This trend is true for both sexes, with the exception that the rate for the divorced is higher in white females than the rate for the widowed. Kramer and his associates (1972) also reviewed suicide rates for populations aged 15 years and older from 14 other countries for this same time period. These data were remarkably consistent in finding greatly elevated suicide rates for the divorced and widowed, as compared to the single and married in every country studied. These data were slightly different from those of the United States in that the divorced clearly had higher suicide rates than the widowed in all 14 countries. More recent studies have confirmed the tendency of the divorced and widowed to be overrepresented among completed suicides (Wenz, 1977; Modan *et al.*, 1970). In summary, these data are uniform in finding highest suicide rates among the divorced and widowed, intermediate rates for the never married, and lowest rates for the married. In other countries, the divorced clearly have the highest suicide rates. In the United States, the widowed appear to exceed the divorced in suicide rates, although the rates for the two groups are close.

It would appear that the divorced are also clearly overrepresented among suicide attempts. Weissman (1974) reviewed all studies on the epidemiology of suicide attempts published in the English language between 1960 and 1971. She concluded that studies using age-standardized population comparisons found an excess of divorced persons among suicide attempters: "The high number of divorcees is consistent with clinical observations that attempts take place in the context of interpersonal disorganization and a breakdown of personal resources" (Weissman, 1974, p. 740). Studies of admissions to psychiatric facilities for suicide attempts in other countries have also reported high rates for the divorced. Such studies have been reported from Edinburgh, Scotland (Kessel, 1965a, b; Aitken *et al.*, 1969), Newcastle, England (Smith and Davison, 1971), Australia (Krupinski *et al.*, 1967; Edwards and Whitlock, 1968), and Jerusalem (Modan *et al.*, 1970).

There are also other sources of evidence linking marital turmoil to suicide attempts. Numerous investigators have sought to identify the precipitating events for the suicide attempt. Kessel (1965a, b) was so impressed with the excess frequency of the divorced among self-poisoning cases admitted to the Incidental Delirium Ward of the Royal Infirmary in Edinburgh that he more closely examined the marriages of his married self-poisoning cases. In these marriages, separations and excess hostility were frequently noted. Troubled marital relationships were identified as a frequent precipitant of suicide attempts among his married admissions. Edwards and Whitlock (1968) attempted to interview all cases of attempted suicide in the Brisbane, Australia, metropolitan area for a 12-month period between February 1965 and February 1966. For cases in the care of a private psychiatrist, information about precipitating events was obtained from that psychiatrist without a personal interview by one of the authors. "Interpersonal disputes, social trauma and rejections accounted for 64% of all precipitating factors in the cases of attempted suicide" (Edwards and Whitlock, 1968, p. 935). Of the interpersonal disputes, problems with the spouse were by far the most frequent precipitating event. Similar findings were reported by Oliver *et al.* (1971) from their study of all patients admitted to the casualty department of Alfred Hospital in Melbourne, Australia, from May to August 1969. In 50% of cases, the precipitating events were classified as interpersonal conflict, marital discord, and family disharmony. In their study of admissions for suicide at Newcastle General Hospital from 1966 to 1969, Smith and Davison (1971) found marital conflict to be the most frequently identifiable precipitant for suicide attempts. Sclare and Hamilton (1963) studied all cases of attempted suicide referred to the Department of Psychological Medicine at the Eastern District Hospital in Glasgow between August 1960 and July 1962. They reported conflict with members of the opposite sex to be the most frequently identifiable precipitant: "The marital and romance difficulties accounted for 37.2 percent of the total cases. In many instances of marital discord, the self-assault occurred as a final act of exasperated abdication from what the patient regarded as an intolerable situation" (Sclare and Hamilton, 1963, p. 612).

## MARITAL STATUS AND MORTALITY

It is well known that mortality rates by marital status between the ages of 15 and 64 are higher for the unmarried than for the married (Kobrin and Hendershot, 1977). For both sexes, a similar pattern is observed. Mortality rates are highest for the divorced, followed by the widowed, single, and married, in that order. For males, the divorced have mortality rates approximately three times that of the married. For females, the corresponding rate is approximately two times. As might be expected, various theories have been proposed to explain these relationships between mortality rates and marital status. The explanatory hypotheses are similar to those proposed to explain the relationship between marital status and psychiatric illness, and they can be roughly classified into selection and interaction hypotheses. Carter and Glick (1976) are proponents of the selection hypotheses: "This material tends to support the thesis that a relatively large proportion of people who have serious trouble with their health are likely to have serious trouble in becoming married, maintaining a viable marriage, or becoming remarried" (Carter and Glick, 1976, p. 324). Gove (1973) is a leading exponent of the interactional school and postulates that close interpersonal ties are necessary for a sense of meaning and purpose in life. Thus, the high mortality rates for the unmarried may represent a tendency for the unmarried to be more careless or reckless about personal safety and health care.

Although current evidence does not allow a definitive test of either hypothesis, Gove attempted to answer this question by examining mortality rates by cause of death. He hypothesized that certain causes of deaths are largely unaffected by social factors, whereas others are more strongly affected by interpersonal influences. If he is correct, differential death rates by marital status should be stronger for one type of death than for the other. He analyzed data on causes of death compiled by the National Center for Health Statistics. Because of age and racial differences in death rates, he restricted his analysis to the white race between the ages of 25 and 64. An interesting pattern emerged. For both sexes, with one exception, death rates for automobile accidents, homicides, pedestrian accidents, and other accidental causes were highest for the divorced, followed by the widowed and the single, in that order. The one exception is that widowed females had a slightly higher automobile accident death rate than divorced females. Gove postulated that homicide victims in many instances may have precipitated the act, and that the more reckless and careless may have higher accidental death rates. A similar pattern of death rates by marital status was observed for cancer of the respiratory tract. In this instance, the general public is well aware of the relationship between smoking and lung cancer. The demoralized and reckless might be expected not to heed this warning, and there is evidence that the divorced and widowed smoke more than the married. For diseases requiring chronic medical care, such as tuberculosis and diabetes, divorced males also had the highest death rates. However, a different pattern was observed for females. Single females had the highest death rates.

For diseases such as leukemia and aleukemia, for which social factors are presumed to have minimal impact, death rates were roughly comparable for all marital status groups. Neoplastic disease of other types likewise did not show a convincing excess of mortality for the divorced.

## MARITAL DISCORD, PSYCHIATRIC IMPAIRMENT, AND MENTAL HEALTH SERVICE USAGE

The preceding sections make it clear that the divorced and maritally separated are greatly overrepresented relative to their proportions in the general population as users of mental health services. Population surveys have similarly indicated elevated psychopathology in these groups. There is evidence of analogous links between marital discord and psychopathology and usage of mental health services. The research in this area is less conclusive, as methodological problems abound. The linkage of marital status to psychiatric service usage can be studied because marital status is a demographic variable frequently indexed. Clearly, most mental health service providers do not record data on the degree of marital discord present in recipients of service. Similarly, when marital discord is noted by a service provider, it is difficult to assess the significance of this variable in relationship to the presenting psychological complaint, as most couples experience transient discord in their marriages at one time or another (Lederer and Jackson, 1968). Data by diagnosis or type of service provided is of limited usefulness because of the influence of prevailing theoretical systems on diagnosis and treatment. Clearly, a psychoanalytically oriented service provider will record more individual psychopathology and render more individual psychotherapy than would a family-systems-oriented facility, given the same population. Another factor possibly contributing to underreporting of family and marital therapy is that many health insurance policies do not cover marital therapy.

A recent study by Renne (1971) suggests that marital adjustment may be more closely related than marital status to psychopathology. In her study, the unhappily married appeared to be in worse physical and psychological health than the divorced, and marriage appeared to exert a "protective" function only if the marriage was a happy one. Her study is particularly of interest in that she examined various health indices by both marital status and marital adjustment. A probability sample of 4,452 households in Alameda County, California, completed questionnaires about their marriages, individual psychological functioning, social networks, and general health. From these questions, indices of marital adjustment, ego resiliency, depression, and social isolation were computed. If data were analyzed by marital status alone, her findings were comparable to those of many previous reports in that the divorced group appeared to be in poorer psychological and physical health than the married group. However, when the data were reanalyzed by degree of marital adjustment, a totally different picture emerged. Marriage was associated with better health only among the happily married, and the divorced population appeared equivalent to the unhappily still-married group. On indices of neuroticism, depression, and social isolation, the separated and divorced did not differ significantly from the unhappily married. There were no significant differences between the never-divorced married couples and the previously divorced but currently married couples on any of the indices. In many ways, the divorced population appeared better off than the unhappily marrieds. On all indices, the happily married fared best. Numerous other studies (Dean, 1966; Murstein and Glaudin, 1968; Kelly, 1941; Barry, 1970; Burchinal *et al.*, 1957; Karlsson, 1951; Locke and Karlsson, 1952) have replicated this finding of a close relationship between individual psychopathology and marital discord.

The relationship between marital status and psychopathology, is subject to various theoretical interpretations. As might be expected, the relationship between marital discord and psychological impairment is likewise subject to various explanatory hypotheses. The two main explanatory hypotheses can be summarized as the individual psychopathology hypothesis and the interaction hypothesis. The individual psychopathology hypothesis is similar to the selection hypothesis (which posits that the relationship between marriage and psychological health is due to marriage selecting the healthiest individuals). The individual psychopathology model hypothesizes that individuals with significant psychopathology will, as a result of that psychopathology, have difficulty with close interpersonal relationships such as marriage. From that framework, poor marital adjustment would be simply another manifestation of individual psychopathology. The interaction hypothesis (which is similar to the protection hypothesis) stresses the extremely important role of the marital relationship for individual emotional security. The marital relationship helps define one's role in life, complementing one's role as parent, friend, colleague, and kinsman (Renne, 1971). Similarly, because marriage represents a unique form of intimate relationship, the marital relationship also contributes to one's self-definition in a more basic way.

Clearly, the relationship between marital discord and psychopathology is not fully explainable by either theoretical system, and the picture emerges of a possibly circular relationship between these two variables (Bachrach, 1975a, b, c). It is possible that bad relations with a spouse may aggravate any preexisting psychopathology an individual possessed prior to marriage, or may create impairment in an otherwise "normal" person, and that preexisting psychopathology, when present, also may contribute in part to the bad marital relationship.

The available evidence strongly suggests that the individual psychopathology model is insufficient by itself to explain the relationship between marital discord and psychopathology. This evidence consists of prospective studies of the influence of premarital personality traits on subsequent marital adjustment, studies of concordance rates between marital partners for mental illness, and clinical reports of the effects of individual psychotherapy of one spouse on the marriage.

Prospective studies of the relationship between neurotic personality traits existing prior to marriage and the subsequent development of marital discord suggest that only approximately 9–10% of the variance in marital adjustment can be accounted for by personality difficulties preceding marriage. As might be expected, four separate studies have reported that individuals with neurotic traits preceding marriage were more likely to be unhappily married on follow-up investigation. Kelly (1939) interviewed and tested 300 couples prior to marriage and then correlated this information with measures of marital adjustment obtained 2 years later. Questions reflecting personality traits and historical information combined into a single index correlated .26 with subsequent marital adjustment in men and .30 for females. Adams (1946) administered a 143-item personality test, composed of items from the Bernreuter Personality Inventory, the Strong Vocational Interest Blank, and other instruments, to 100 engaged students and then gave the same students a marital adjustment battery, composed of the Terman, Hamilton, and Burgess-Cottrell scales, 2 years after marriage. Premarital personality measures correlated between .24 and .38 with subsequent measures of marital adjustment. The happily married had premarital personality profiles indicative of lower neuroticism. Terman (1950) reported a follow-up on 643 married couples from his gifted subject population. His testing instruments were similar to those used by Adams. The follow-up period after marriage was 8 years, and the criterion of marital success was intact or separated. He reported a biserial correlation of .47 between premarital questionnaire scores and marital outcome. Burgess and Wallin (1953) reported a follow-up of 666 couples after 3–5 years of marriage. Although they employed a variety of predictive tests, personality measures correlated between .18 and .25 with subsequent measures of marital adjustment. One more recent study (Bentler and Newcomb, 1978) reported substantially higher correlations between premarital personality and subsequent marital adjustment. This study, however, needs to be interpreted with caution. Of 162 newly married couples in the Los Angeles area, only 77 (48%) were available at follow-up 4 years later. A multiple correlation of .74 was obtained using 10 predictor variables. A multiple correlation using this many predictor variables with such a small sample size is suspect. This study is questionably relevant, as most of the predictor variables did not appear to be related to psychopathology. These variables included previous children (for the female), less female ambition, more female objectivity, more female clothes-consciousness, more female masculinity, less female intelligence, more male deliberateness, less male orderliness, more male thriftiness, and more male flexibility.

Numerous investigators have reported that the concordance of mental illness in married couples greatly exceeds the expected frequency calculated from the prevalence rates of such disorders in the general population (Gregory, 1959; Slater, 1951; Penrose, 1944; Kreitman, 1968; Nelson *et al.*, 1970). A recent review of this literature concluded: "That psychopathology occurs with greater frequency in the spouses of mental patients than in the spouses of 'normal' individuals seems unquestionable" (Crago, 1972). As might be anticipated, many hypotheses have been put forth to explain this concordance (Bachrach, 1975). The two principal hypotheses are the assortive mating and pathological interaction hypotheses. These hypotheses are similar in rationale to hypotheses previously encountered. The assortive mating hypothesis posits that psychiatrically impaired individuals tend to select other psychiatrically impaired individuals as marital partners. The pathologenic interaction hypothesis states that life with a mentally impaired spouse increases the risk of mental impairment in an otherwise well spouse. The mechanism for this might range from simple stress to the more complex and subtle interactional sequences described by family therapists (Jackson, 1965; Haley, 1963). Kreitman and his associates (1962, 1968, 1970) have devoted considerable effort to explaining the sources of concordance. From their research, they have rejected the assortive mating hypothesis as an explanation for concordance of neurotic disturbances in marital pairs. They find correlations in patient–spouse psychopathology to be nonexistent in the early years of marriage but to increase significantly in magnitude as the length of marriage increases. Control couples demonstrated declining interspouse correlations in pathology with the passage of time. Nelson *et al.* (1970) found that the concordance of psychopathology in certain married couples tends to be related to the quantity and patterns of shared activities with the spouse.

Additional evidence supporting the interactional hypothesis, particularly for neurotic disorders, is the frequently reported clinical finding that symptomatic improvement in one spouse is sometimes associated with psychological decompensation in the "well" partner (Kohl, 1962; Kaplan and Kohl, 1972) or with the eruption of marital discord (Milton and Hafner, 1978; Marshall and Neill, 1977). These reports have been interpreted as demonstrating that the symptoms of the "identified patients" serve a protective function for the "well spouse" and also serve to maintain homeostatis in the relationship.

Although the association between marital discord and individual psychological distress appears well established, the actual impact of marital discord, short of marital separation, on mental health service usage is unclear and essentially uninvestigated. It is clear that marital adjustment and individual happiness are highly interrelated (Bradburn, 1969) and that marital discord is one of the most frequent life stresses for which individuals seek professional counsel (Gurin *et al.*, 1960). However, most of these individuals appear to turn to nonpsychiatric physicians (Shepherd *et al.*, 1966) and clergymen for counseling (Gurin *et al.*, 1960). The actual impact of marital discord on the usage of mental health professional service time is unclear.

Part of the difficulty in assessing the impact of relationship disturbances on the usage of mental health services is the overlapping boundary between individual and relationship disturbances (Martin, 1976). It appears highly probable that many individuals present in mental health facilities with individual complaints and are treated in an individual psychotherapy context, when the complaint in all likelihood has an interactional origin. For example, Sager *et al.* (1968) surveyed patients in individual psychotherapy who had entered therapy because of individual complaints. In 50% of these patients, serious marital problems were later uncovered during the course of therapy.

## DIVORCE, MARITAL DISCORD, AND CHILDREN

Divorce and marital discord have a psychological impact on children as well as on adults. The potential significance of the rising divorce rate for childhood developmental abnormalities can be appreciated by realizing that there were approximately 1 million divorces in the United States in 1976, and each divorce involved an average of 1.08 children.

Thus, in 1 year alone, 1 million children were affected by divorce in this country (Bloom *et al.*, 1977). The lasting psychological impact of divorce on a child's psychosocial development is not clear and the exact mechanisms by which divorce affects children are also unclear. Some authors have stressed the role of parental separation itself in producing childhood psychopathology (Bowlby, 1958), whereas other authors have emphasized that chronic parental marital discord may be more disruptive to normal childhood development than the act of divorce itself (Rutter, 1971). In any event, it is clear that divorce results in a rather drastic change in the child's interpersonal world and that many children of divorce grow up in atypical family settings. For many children, the divorce itself is only the beginning of an intensified struggle between their parents that may last for years to come. Cline and Westman (1971) investigated 105 consecutive divorces involving children in Dale County, Wisconsin, for a 2-year period and found that in over one-half of the cases, continued hostile parental interaction required further court intervention. The postdivorce climate observed in these couples was clearly not conducive to healthy childhood development: "Manifestations of post-divorce turbulence range from hostile, bitter ambivalent feelings between divorced spouses, and between children and their divorced parents, to post-divorce assault and battery, murder, and child abduction" (Cline and Westman, 1971, p. 79). For children whose remaining parent does not remarry, psychosocial development is dependent to a large degree on the psychosocial resources of the remaining parent. The transition from married life to being a single parent is beset with numerous stumbling blocks, including financial difficulties and the disruption of extended kinship systems and social networks (Weiss, 1975). The single parent is often faced with providing both emotional and physical support for the children, with minimal aid from other adults. This can be a lonely struggle in many instances. Kellam and associates (1977) in the Woodlawn study reported clear evidence that mother-alone families are at much higher risk for having children with poor psychological well-being and social maladjustment. Family arrangements allowing for a sharing of responsibilities among adults were clearly associated with healthier children.

Numerous studies have documented that divorce has severe short-term psychological effects on children (Kelly and Wallerstein, 1975a, b, 1976; McDermott, 1968; Tolley, 1976). The significance of these reactions on the long-term psychological development of children is difficult to evaluate, as studies have indicated that children react adversely to parent–child separations of various causes (Bowlby, 1969). Other studies have indicated that parent–child separations are quite common (Munro,

1966) and that most children do not show signs of permanent psychological harm because of these separations (Rutter, 1971).

However, still other studies have reported evidence that children of divorce differ from children of intact families in certain ways. One consistent finding is that children from families with severe marital discord and/or divorce are more likely as adults to experience severe marital discord and/or divorce in their own marriages (Henry and Overall, 1975; Overall, Henry, and Woodward, 1974; Mueller and Pope, 1977; Terman, 1938; Locke, 1951; Gay and Tonge, 1967; Frommer and O'Shea, 1973; Gurin et al., 1960; Terman and Butterwiesser, 1935; Hamilton and MacGowan, 1929; Bentler and Newcomb, 1978). The most likely explanation for this finding is that children from disturbed marriages have learned to expect adult conflict to be unresolvable and possess inadequate problem-solving skills because of poor role-modeling: "This finding is viewed as supporting the hypothesis that patterns of marital interaction are the result, at least in part, of role relationships and expectations learned in childhood through observation of parental marital interaction" (Overall et al., 1974, p. 449).

Evidence exists that children from divorces are characterized by more overt signs of psychopathology at different stages in the life cycle. Gregory (1965) examined health records completed by students applying to Carleton College prior to admission for a 5-year period ending in 1960. From this sample, 127 students were identified who had lost a parent by death or divorce. A control sample of students was obtained by selecting students in the same class in alphabetical sequence who had parents still living together. There was a much higher frequency of parental divorce among those consulting the school psychiatrist, $p <$ .005. Brill and Liston (1966) examined the records of all patients 16 years or older admitted to the inpatient and outpatient psychiatry services of the University of California for a 4-year period ending in 1964 for instances of parental separation in the past due to death or divorce. Control samples were obtained from statistics on divorce and separation reported by the Metropolitan Life Insurance Company and a national survey conducted by Gurin and associates (1960). Although the control group had a higher incidence of parental death, the patient group was characterized by a greatly increased incidence of parental divorce or separation. This difference was significant at the .001 level of confidence.

Alkon (1971) investigated the incidence and type of parental separation in all inpatient admissions to the Payne Whitney Psychiatric Clinic from July 1963 to March 1969, as well as all outpatients currently seen with records of treatment for 5 years or longer. The control group consisted of respondents in the Midtown Manhattan Study (Srole et al.,

1962) who at the time of interview had never been psychiatric patients. In all, Alkon studied the backgrounds of 1,267 psychiatric patients as compared to 1,660 control subjects. Psychiatric inpatients as compared to controls were found to have a much higher incidence of parental separation and divorce. Also, an increased incidence of early deprivation due to separation and divorce before the age of 6 was noted among psychiatric inpatients and in subgroups of patients with a diagnosis of personality and neurotic disorders. Psychiatric patients did not have an increased incidence of parental death as compared to controls.

Rutter (1971) reported similar findings in his investigation of the families of 9- to 12-year-old children living in the Isle of Wight. Ratings of antisocial behavior were significantly higher in those children whose parents had separated because of family discord. Other forms of separation experiences were unrelated to childhood behavior disturbances. The finding of elevated deliquency rates for boys from homes whose parents had separated is consistent with that of other investigators (Gregory, 1965; Douglass et al., 1968; Gibson, 1969).

In summary, investigations of various indices of mental deviance in relation to childhood history of parental divorce or separation have reported evidence that parental divorce or separation in childhood has adverse psychological sequelae in these children when they become adults. Although many investigators for theoretical reasons have expected adult psychopathology to be strongly related to childhood parental death, the relationship between parental death and adult psychopathology appears much weaker than the relationship of adult psychiatric disturbance and childhoods spent in homes with severe marital discord (Rutter, 1971). These findings would suggest that the relationship of childhood experience of parental divorce to adult psychopathology may be due to the experience of growing up in a home of continual turmoil rather than to the trauma of divorce and subsequent parental separation.

Fewer studies have been conducted investigating the relationship of parental marital discord to childhood development. The few studies available suggest that this is a strong relationship. Rutter (1971) has reported the most extensive analysis of the relationship between parental marital discord and childhood disorders. In the Isle of Wight study, families were interviewed and various aspects of family life and childhood psychopathology were rated by trained interviewers. The main finding of this study was the presence of an extremely strong relationship between poor marital adjustment and childhood deviance. The extent of this relationship can be appreciated by realizing that in good marriages, the frequency of childhood antisocial behavior disorders was zero. In marriages rated fair, 22% of the children had antisocial behavior. In marriages rated poor, the corresponding percentage for antisocial disorder in children was 39%. The parental marriages most destructive to childhood development were those rated as having high tension and low warmth between spouses. The extent of childhood deviance appeared related to the duration of exposure to marital discord. Children whose mothers had previously been in poor marriages and who subsequently remarried and established good marriages fared better than those raised in continual marital discord. Evidence in this study suggested that the determining variable in normal childhood development was the marital relationship rather than parental character disorder or parenting skills. Childhood psychopathology was related much more strongly to rating of marital adjustment than to rating of personality disorder in the parents. In good marriages, the presence of parental character disorder had no detectable influence of childhood behavior disorder. The presence of a good parent somewhat mitigated a poor marital relationship, but the nature of the marital relationship was the stronger predictor of childhood behavior disorder.

Other investigators have reported findings comparable to those of Rutter. However, to my knowledge, no other investigator has conducted such detailed research. Lo (1969) investigated various etiological factors in 49 consecutive childhood admissions to the Yaumatei Psychiatric Center in Hong Kong. The control group consisted of 54 children of the same age attending a pediatric clinic in the same hospital. The neurotic children came significantly more often from families rated as having poor marital adjustment. Wolff and Acton (1968) reported on an investigation of 100 consecutive admissions of primary school children to the psychiatric department of the Royal Hospital for Sick Children in Edinburgh. The control group consisted of 100 children attending the same school classes. The clinic and control samples were matched for age, sex, and occupation of the father. Each mother was subjected to a standardized 3-hour interview. Mothers of disturbed children were much more often rated as having poor marital adjustment than mothers of well children ($p < .00001$). Oltmanns et al. (1977) compared marital adjustment scores on the Locke-Wallace Marital Adjustment Test of parents of 62 children treated at the Psychological Center of the State University of New York with a community control sample of the parents of 37 children. The parents of disturbed children had significantly poorer marital adjustment than those of the control sample. There was also significant negative relationship between parents' marital adjustment and the extent of their children's behavioral deviance.

Two studies suggest that the adverse effects of childhoods spent in marital discord may extent into adult life. Landis (1962) collected questionnaires giving information about self-esteem, dating histories, and family backgrounds from 3,000 college students. Students from self-rated happy parental marriages rated themselves higher in general competence than students from unhappy parental marriages. Abrahams and Whitlock (1969) investigated childhood histories of 152 admissions to two general hospitals in Brisbane, Australia, with a primary diagnosis of depression. A control group consisted of 152 medical and surgical outpatients at the Royal Brisbane Hospital, matched for migrant status, sex, marital status, ethnic group, age, and socioeconomic status. The patients were significantly more often rated as having bad or unsatisfactory childhood family relationships.

The little research available on the relationship between parental marital discord and psychosocial development of children is consistent in finding that marital discord and divorce have an adverse effect on children. There is suggestive evidence that these adverse effects may persist into the adult lives of some children. The available research is compatible with the hypothesis that marital discord is of etiological significance for childhood psychopathology.

## SEX AND MARITAL STATUS DIFFERENCES
## IN PSYCHOPATHOLOGY

In recent years, there has been considerable theoretical interest in differences in sex-specific disability rates for the married and the never married (Bernard, 1976; Gove, 1973). In particular, analysis of psychiatric hospital admission rates by sex and marital status appeared to indicate that among married persons, women had higher admission rates than men and that among single persons, men had higher admission rates than women. This finding was used to posit that males find single marital status more stressful and that women find being married more stressful. Women are hypothesized to find marriage more stressful because of role conflict—i.e., traditional marriage roles are in conflict with psychosocial health. This area will be briefly discussed, as it is of relevance to the explanatory hypotheses for the relationship between marital status and psychopathology. Current evidence suggests that the sex by marital status difference is extremely small, if present at all. Bachrach (1975) noted that this is an inconsistent finding. Bloom et al. (1977) analyzed more recent data on psychiatric service utilization and found that admission rates among married patients are no longer appreciably higher for women than for men. Although marriage has different role meanings for men and women, the evidence linking differential marriage role definitions to psychiatric service usage appears questionable at present.

## EXPLANATORY HYPOTHESES

As outlined earlier in this chapter, a number of explanatory hypotheses have been put forth to explain the consistent findings of strong associations between marital status and psychiatric disability. The primary dichotomy appears to be between the premarital disability (selection) hypothesis and the postmarital disability (protection, stress) hypotheses. The selection hypothesis posits that because of the incipient nature of psychopathology, seriously disturbed individuals are less likely to marry, and that the appearance of manifest psychiatric pathology increases the likelihood of divorce and separation. This particular explanatory framework tends to be favored by biologically oriented psychiatrists and views man as having limited plasticity of response capabilities. The primary determinants of behavior are viewed to be fixed by genetic and early environmental events.

The postmarital disability hypotheses posit that the relationship between psychiatric morbidity and marital status is secondary to different social influences associated with each marital status. Elevated disability in the single, divorced, and widowed groups would be viewed as secondary to the absence of certain protective influences in marriage or to abrupt changes in life circumstances. These hypotheses tend to be favored by social psychiatrists, family therapists, and psychologists, as these viewpoints often characterize man as a social animal, extremely responsive to his social environment. The postmarital disability position consists of two submodels—the stress and protection hypotheses. The stress model is most applicable to the increased disability in divorced and widowed subgroups. This model is borrowed from the research that found increased physical and psychiatric morbidity around times of significant life change. Divorce and widowhood are viewed to be significant life stresses, involving abrupt changes in social roles and social networks. The increased morbidity is viewed as secondary to the stress of overwhelming life change. The protection hypothesis is a somewhat similar model and suggests that marriage protects against mental disease by the provision of clear role definitions and norms and by the establishment of social and kinship networks.

Clearly, neither the premarital disability nor the postmarital disability hypothesis is sufficient alone to explain the complex relationships observed. The primary concern of this chapter is whether psychiatric interventions might decrease the high morbidity associated with divorce, separation, and severe marital discord. For this purpose, it is sufficient to demonstrate that the premarital disability hypothesis is insufficient to explain the available data. I believe that it can be stated with some confidence that the premarital disability hypothesis is insufficient and that postmarital events have to be considered.

The selection hypothesis may account for the association between single marital status and early-onset psychosis. There is clearly a large population of poor premorbid schizophrenics who are chronically socially handicapped and who end up in psychiatric institutions at an early age. It is doubtful, however, that the selection hypothesis completely explains the relationship between late-onset psychiatric disturbance and marital status. Surprisingly little is known of the impact of major psychiatric disorder on marriage. Several authors (*e.g.*, Clausen, 1959; Dupont *et al.*, 1971) have even reported that mental disorder, in certain circumstances, may strengthen the marital relationship.

The selection hypothesis has difficulty accounting for the ordering of psychiatric morbidity among different marital status groups. The selection hypothesis states that "a relatively large proportion of people who have serious trouble with their health are likely to have serious trouble in becoming married, maintaining a viable marriage, or becoming remarried" (Carter and Glick, 1976, p. 324). If marriageability is to be thus construed as an index of good mental and physical health, one would expect psychiatric and physical disability to be highest in the single, followed by the divorced, the widowed, and the married. The observed ordering finds highest disability rates in the divorced and separated, intermediate rates for the widowed and single, and lowest rates for the married. Something other than preexisting handicap is needed to explain why individuals healthy enough to obtain marital partners in the first place have a higher risk of emotional disturbance upon divorce than individuals supposedly too handicapped ever to become married. The selection hypothesis similarly has difficulty accounting for the disability associated with widowhood. Presumably, these individuals were biologically and psychologically similar to same-aged still-married couples prior to the event of spouse death. Selection theorists attempt to account for this by a remarriageability hypothesis. In particular, it is argued that the increased morbidity in widowed groups relative to marrieds is due to the widowed groups at the time of sampling continuing to comprise impaired individuals incapable of remarriage. The healthy widows are presumed to have already remarried and thus be counted as married rather than as widowed. This hypothesis seems unlikely. Renne (1971) found that remarriages don't select the healthiest among the divorced. There is no reason to suspect that a different process operates among the widowed. Wenz (1977), in an investigation of high suicide rates among the widowed, concluded that the remarriageability hypothesis was incompatible with the observation that suicidal deaths tend to cluster around the time of bereavement.

There is minimal evidence to support the notion that the divorced are inherently more disturbed characterologically than the nondivorced. This notion may have applied in earlier parts of this century, when divorce was a more socially deviant act. In current times, divorce has become increasingly prevalent and presumably is less reflective of pre-marital psychiatric disability. Renne (1971) reported evidence that previously divorced, currently married individuals are not identifiable as more handicapped physically or emotionally than never-divorced populations. Similarly, Glenn and Weaver (1977), in a study of the adjustment of ever-divorced and never-divorced couples, found minimal differences between the groups.

Another finding that disagrees with the selection hypothesis is the repetitive finding of better adjustment among married students than among single students (Busselen and Busselen, 1975). This finding is true for undergraduates, a population consisting predominantly of un-marrieds for whom the selection hypothesis presumably would not be operative. It is also of note that this finding of better adjustment among married students was reported as early as the 1920s (Watson, 1930), when marrying while still a student was a more socially deviant act. Several investigators have attempted to test specifically whether the selection hypothesis can account for the obtained data relating marital status to mental disability. Adler (1953) was intrigued with the different admission rates by marital status to the Arkansas State Hospital. To attempt to decipher if this was due to mental illness causing marital separation, he interviewed a 50% random sample of admissions to this hospital from Jefferson County, Arkansas, and attempted to determine the time of onset of mental illness as well as the time of admission. For singles, admission rates computed for the time of onset of mental illness were lower than comparable rates computed for time of admission. This difference is compatible with the hypothesis of reduced marriageability among this group. However, for the divorced and separated groups, a different phenomenon was observed. For this group, admission rates by marital status at time of onset of disturbance were higher than admission rates by marital status at time of admission. This finding is

Gorwitz, K., Bahn, A., Warthen, F. J., and Cooper, M. Some epidemiological data on alcoholism in Maryland. *Quarterly Journal of Studies on Alcohol*, 1970, *31*, 423–443.

Gove, W. R. Sex, marital status, and mortality. *American Journal of Sociology*, 1973, *79*, 45–67.

Gregory, I. Husbands and wives admitted to mental hospital. *Journal of Mental Science*, 1959, *105*, 457–462.

Gregory, I. Anterospective data following childhood loss of a parent. *Archives of General Psychiatry*, 1965, *13*, 110–112.

Gurin, G., Veroff, J., and Feld, S. *Americans view their mental health*. New York: Basic Books, 1960.

Hagnell, O., Kreitman, N., and Duffy, J. Mental illness in married pairs in a total population. *British Journal of Psychiatry*, 1974, *125*, 293–302.

Haley, J. Marriage therapy. *Archives of General Psychiatry*, 1963, *8*, 213–234.

Hamilton, G. W., and MacGowan, K. *What is wrong with marriage*. New York: Albert and Charles Boni, 1929.

Henry, B. W., and Overall, J. E. Epidemiology of marital problems in a psychiatric population. *Social Psychiatry*, 1975, *10*, 139–144.

Innes, G., and Sharp, G. A. A study of psychiatric patients in North-East Scotland. *Journal of Mental Science*, 1962, *108*, 447–456.

Jackson, D. D. Family rules. *Archives of General Psychiatry*, 1965, *12*, 589–594.

Jaco, E. G. The social epidemiology of mental disorders. New York: Russell Sage, 1960.

Karlsson, G. *Adaptability and communication in marriage; a Swedish predictive study of marital satisfaction*. Uppsala: Almquist and Wiksells, 1951.

Kellam, S. G., Ensminger, M. E., and Turner, R. J. Family structure and the mental health of children. *Archives of General Psychiatry*, 1977, *34*, 1012–1022.

Kelly, E. L. Concerning the validity of Terman's weights for predicting marital happiness. *Psychological Bulletin*, 1939, *139*, 202–203.

Kelly, E. L. Marital compatibility as related to personality traits of husbands and wives as rated by self and spouse. *Journal of Social Psychology*, 1941, *13*, 193–198.

Kelly, J. B., and Wallerstein, J. S. The effects of parental divorce: The experience of the child in late latency. *American Journal of Orthopsychiatry*, 1975, *45*, 253–258.

Kelly, J. B., and Wallerstein, J. S. The effects of parental divorce: Experiences of the child in early latency. *American Journal of Orthopsychiatry*, 1976, *46*, 20–32.

Kessel, N. Self poisoning, part 1. *British Medical Journal*, 1965, *2*, 1265–1270. (a)

Kessel, N. Self poisoning, part 2. *British Medical Journal*, 1965, *2*, 1336–1340.

Klee, G. D., Spiro, E., Bahn, A. K., and Gorwitz, K. An ecological analysis of diagnosed mental illness in Baltimore. *Psychiatric Research Reports*, 1967, *22*, 107–148.

Kobrin, F. E., and Hendershot, G. E. Do family ties reduce mortality? Evidence from the United States, 1966–1968. *Journal of Marriage and the Family*, 1977, *39*, 737–745.

Kohl, R. N. Pathological reactions of marital partners to improvement of patients. *American Journal of Psychiatry*, 1962, *118*, 1036–1041.

Kramer, M. Epidemiology, biostatistics, and mental health planning. *Psychiatric Research Reports*, 1967, *22*, 1–63.

Kramer, M. Statistic of mental disorders in the United States: Current status, some urgent needs and suggested solutions. *Journal of the Royal Statistical Society*, 1969, *132*, 353–397.

Kramer, M., Pollack, E. S., Redick, R. W., and Locke, B. Z. *Mental disorders/suicide*. Cambridge, Mass.: Harvard University Press, 1972.

Kreitman, N. Mental disorder in married couples. *Journal of Mental Science*, 1962, *108*, 438–446.

Kreitman, N. Married couples admitted to mental hospitals. *British Journal of Psychiatry*, 1968, *114*, 699–718.

Kreitman, N., Collins, J., Nelson, B., and Troop, J. Neurosis and marital interaction. 1: Personality and symptoms. *British Journal of Psychiatry*, 1970, *117*, 33–46.

Krupinski, J., and Stoller, A. Survey of institutionalized mental patients in Victoria, Australia, 1882 to 1959: I Admissions to and residents in mental hospitals. *Medical Journal of Australia*, 1962, *49*, 269–276.

Krupinski, J., Stoller, A., and Polke, P. Attempted suicides admitted to the mental health department, Victoria, Australia: A socio- epidemiological study. *International Journal of Social Psychiatry*, 1967, *13*, 5–13.

Landis, J. T. A comparison of children from divorced and non-divorced unhappy marriages. *Family Life Coord*, 1962, *11*, 61–65.

Lederer, W., and Jackson, D. D. *The mirages of marriage*. New York: W. W. Norton, 1968.

Lo, W. H. Aetiological factors in childhood neurosis. *British Journal of Psychiatry*, 1969, *115*, 889–894.

Locke, B. Z., Finucane, D. L., and Hassler, F. Emotionally disturbed patients under care of private non-psychiatric physicians. *Psychiatric Research Reports*, 1967, *22*, 235–248.

Locke, H. J., and Karlsson, G. Marital adjustment and prediction in Sweden and the United States. *American Social Review*, 1952, *17*, 10–17.

Locke, B. Z., Kramer, M., and Pasamanick, B. Alcoholic psychoses among first admissions to public mental hospitals in Ohio. *Quarterly Journal of Studies on Alcohol*, 1960, *21*, 457–474. (a)

Locke, B. Z., Kramer, M., and Pasamanick, B. Mental diseases of the senile at mid-century: First admissions to Ohio State public mental hospitals. *American Journal of Public Health*, 1960, *50*, 998–1012. (b)

Locke, B. Z., Kramer, M., Timberlake, C. E., Pasamanick, B., and Smeltzer, O. Problems in interpretation of patterns of first admissions to Ohio State Public Mental Hospitals for patients with schizophrenic reactions. *Psychiatric Research Reports*, 1958, *10*, 172–208.

Lowenthal, M. F., Berkman, P. L., Brissette, G. G., Buehler, J. A., Pierce, R. C., Robinson, B. C., and Trier, M. L. *Aging and mental disorder San Francisco*. San Francisco: Jossey-Bass, 1967.

Malzberg, B. A study of first admissions with alcoholic psychosis in New York State, 1943–1944. *Quarterly Journal of Studies on Alcohol*, 1947, *8*, 274–295.

Malzberg, B. Marital status and the incidence of mental disease. *International Journal of Social Psychiatry*, 1964, *10*, 19–26.

Marshall, J. R., and Neill, J. The removal of a psychosomatic symptom: effects on the marriage. *Family Process*, 1977, *16*, 273–280.

Martin, P. A. *A marital therapy manual*. New York: Brunner/Mazel, 1976.

Martin, P. A., and Lief, H. I. Resistance to innovation in psychiatric training as exemplified by marital therapy. In G. Usdin (Ed.), *Psychiatry: Education and image*. New York: Brunner/Mazel, 1973.

McDermott, J. F. Parental divorce in early childhood. *American Journal of Psychiatry*, 1968, *124*, 118–126.

McKnight, R. S., Reznikoff, M., Mulligan, R., and Giger, M. F. Characteristics of patients in an adult outpatient clinic: A survey and evaluation. *American Journal of Orthopsychiatry*, 1966, *36*, 636–642.

Mellinger, G. D., Blater, M. B., Manheimer, D. I., Cisin, I. H., and Parry, H. J. Psychic distress, life crisis, and use of psychotherapeutic medications. *Archives of General Psychiatry*, 1978, *35*, 1045–1052.

Meyer, N. G. *Admissions to outpatient psychiatric services by age, sex, color and marital status,*

*June 1970–May 1971* (Statistical Note 79). Washington, D. C.: U. S. Government Printing Office, 1973.

Milazzo-Sayre, L. *Admission rates to state and county psychiatric hospitals by age, sex, and marital status, United States, 1975* (Statistical Note 142, NIMH). Washington, D. C.: U. S. Government Printing Office, 1977.

Miles, H. C., Gardner, E. A., Bodian, C., and Romano, J. A cumulative survey of all psychiatric experiences in Monroe County, N.Y. *Psychiatric Quarterly*, 1964, *38*, 458–487.

Milton, F., and Hafner, J. The outcome of behavior therapy for agoraphobia in relation to marital adjustment. *Archives of General Psychiatry*, 1979, *36*, 807–811.

Modan, B., Nissenkorn, I., and Lewkowski, S. R. Comparative epidemiologic aspects of suicide and attempted suicide in Israel. *American Journal of Epidemiology*, 1970, *91*, 393–399.

Mueller, C. W., and Pope, H. Marital instability: a study of its transmission between generations. *Journal of Marriage and the Family*, 1977, *39*, 83–93.

Munro, A. Parental deprivation in depressive patients. *British Journal of Psychiatry*, 1966, *112*, 443–457.

Murstein, B. I., and Glaudin, V. The use of the MMPI in the determination of marital adjustment. *Journal of Marriage and the Family*, 1968, *30*, 651–655.

Nelson, B., Collins, N., Kreitman, N., and Troop, J. Neurosis and marital interaction II Time sharing and social activity. *British Journal of Psychiatry*, 1970, *117*, 47–58.

Nielsen, J. Mental disorders in married couples. *British Journal of Psychiatry*, 1964, *110*, 683–697.

Odegard, O. New data on marriage and mental disease: The incidence of psychosis in the widowed and the divorced. *Journal of Mental Science*, 1953, *99*, 778–785.

Oliver, R. G., Kaminski, Z., Tudor, K., and Hetzel, B. S. The epidemiology of attempted suicide as seen in the casualty department, Alfred Hospital, Melbourne. *Medical Journal of Australia*, 1971, *58*, 833–839.

Oltman, T. F., Broderick, J. E., and O'Leary, K. D. Marital adjustment and the efficacy of behavior therapy with children. *Journal of Consulting and Clinical Psychology*, 1977, *45*, 724–729.

Overall, J. E., Henry, B. W., and Woodward, A. Dependence of marital problems on parental family history. *Journal of Abnormal Psychology*, 1974, *83*, 446–450.

Pearlin, L. I., and Johnson, J. S. Marital status, life-strains and depression. *Americal Social Review*, 1977, *42*, 704–715.

Penrose, L. S. Mental illness in husband and wife. *Psychiatric Quarterly Supplement*, 1944, *18*, 161–166.

Prochaska, J., and Prochaska, J. Twentieth century trends in marriage and marital therapy. In T. J. Paoline and B. S. McGrody (Eds.), *Marriage and marital therapy*. New York: Brunner/Mazel, 1978.

Pugh, T. F., and MacMahon, B. *Epidemiologic findings in United States mental hospital data*. Boston: Little, Brown, 1962.

Redick, R. W., and Johnson, C. *Marital status, living arrangements and family characteristics of admissions to state and county mental hospitals and outpatient psychiatric clinics, United States, 1970* (Statistical Note 100). Washington, D. C.: U.S. Government Printing Office, 1974.

Renne, K. S. Health and marital experience in an urban population. *Journal of Marriage and the Family*, 1971, *33*, 338–350.

Robertson, N. C. The relationship between marital status and the risk of psychiatric referral. *British Journal of Psychiatry*, 1974, *124*, 191–202.

Rosen, B. M., Anderson, T. E., and Bahn, A. K. Psychiatric services for the aged: A nationwide survey of patterns of utilization. *Journal of Chronic Diseases*, 1968, *21*, 167–177.

Rosen, B. M., Bahn, A. K., and Kramer, M. Demographic and diagnostic characteristics of psychiatric clinic outpatients in the U.S.A., 1961. *American Journal of Orthopsychiatry*, 1964, *34*, 455–568.

Rosenblatt, S. M., Gross, M. M., and Chartoff, S. Marital status and multiple psychiatric admissions for alcoholism. *Quarterly Journal of Studies on Alcohol*, 1969, *30*, 445–447.

Rosenblatt, S. M., Gross, M. M., Malenowski, B., Broman, M., and Lewis, E. Marital status and multiple psychiatric admissions for alcoholism: A cross validation. *Quarterly Journal of Studies on Alcohol*, 1971, *32*, 1092–1096.

Rutter, M. Parent–child separation: psychological effects on children. *Journal of Child Psychology and Psychiatry*, 1971, *12*, 233–260.

Ryle, A., and Hamilton, M. Neurosis in fifty married couples. *Journal of Mental Science*, 1962, *108*, 265–273.

Sager, C. J., Grundlack, R., Kremer, M., Lenz, R., and Royce, J. R. The married in treatment. *Archives of General Psychiatry*, 1968, *19*, 206–215.

Sclare, A. B., and Hamilton, C. M. Attempted suicide in Glascow. *British Journal of Psychiatry*, 1963, *109*, 609–615.

Shepherd, M., Cooper, B., Broun, A. C., and Kalton, G. *Psychiatric illness in general practices*. London: Oxford University, 1966.

Slater, E., and Woodside, M. *Patterns in marriage*. London: Cassell, 1951.

Smith, J. S., and Davison, K. Changes in the pattern of admissions for attempted suicide in Newcastle Upon Tyne during the 1960's. *British Medical Journal*, 1971, *4*, 412–415.

Srole, L., Langner, T. S., Michael, S. T., Opler, M. K., and Rennie, T. A. C. *Mental health in the metropolis. The midtown Manhattan study*. New York: McGraw-Hill, 1962.

Terman, L. M. *Psychological factors in marital happiness*. New York: McGraw-Hill, 1938.

Terman, L. M. Prediction data, predicting marriage failure from test scores. *Marriage and Family Living*, 1950, *12*, 51–54.

Terman, L. M., and Butterwiesser, P. Personality factors in marital compatibility. *Journal of Social Psychology*, 1935, *6*, 143–171.

Thomas, D. S., and Locke, B. Z. Marital status, education and occupational differentials in mental disease. *Milbank Memorial Fund Quarterly*, 1963, *41*, 145–160.

Tolley, K. Antisocial behavior and social alienation post divorce. The man of the house and his mother. *American Journal of Orthopsychiatry*, 1976, *46*, 33–43.

Uhlenhuth, E. H., Lipman, R. S., Balter, M. B., and Stern, M. Symptom intensity and life stress in the city. *Archives of General Psychiatry*, 1974, *31*, 759–764.

U.S. Bureau of the Census, Current Population Reports, Series P-20, No. 297. *Number, timing and duration of marriages and divorces in the United States, June 1975*. Washington, D. C.: U.S. Government Printing Office, 1976.

U. S. Bureau of the Census, Current Population Reports, Series P-20, No. 323, *Marital status and living arrangements, March 1977*. Washington, D. C.: U.S. Government Printing Office, 1978.

Wallerstein, J. S., and Kelly, J. B. The effects of parental divorce. Experiences of the preschool child. *Journal of the American Academy of Child Psychiatry*, 1975, *14*, 600–616.

Watson, G. Happiness among adult students of education. *Journal of Educational Psychology*, 1930, *21*, 79–109.

Wechsler, H., Thum, D., Demone, H. W., and Dwinnell, J. Social characteristics and blood alcohol. *Quarterly Journal of Studies on Alcohol*, 1972, *23*, 132–147.

Weeke, A., Bille, M., Videbeck, T. H., DuPont, A., and Juel-Nielsen, N. Incidence of depressive syndromes in a Danish county. *Acta Psychiatrica Scandinavica*, 1975, *51*, 28–41.

Weissman, M. M. The epidemiology of suicide attempts, 1960 to 1971. *Archives of General Psychiatry*, 1974, *30*, 737–746.

Weissman, M. M., and Meyers, J. K. Affective disorders in a U.S. urban community. *Archives of General Psychiatry*, 1978, *35*, 1304–1311.

Wenz, F. V. Marital status, anomie, and forms of social isolation: A case of high suicide rate among the widowed in an urban sub-area. *Diseases of the Nervous System*, 1977, *38*, 891–895.

Weiss, R. S. *Marital separation*. New York: Basic Books, 1975.

Wolff, S., Acton, W. P. Characteristics of parents of disturbed children. *British Journal of Psychiatry*, 1968, *114*, 593–601.

# CHAPTER THREE

# Psychoanalytic Theory and Marriage

Of the major treatment orientations, psychoanalysis has shown the least interest in the study and treatment of marital discord. There is considerable ambivalence within that therapeutic community about the extent to which practitioners should be concerned with current interpersonal relationships of patients. Paradoxically, in spite of this ambivalence, psychoanalytic theory is probably the most influential contemporary theoretical system affecting the treatment of interpersonal difficulties. This is because of the pervasiveness of psychoanalytic concepts among mental health practitioners, particularly among psychiatrists and psychiatric social workers.

There is divided opinion within the analytic community as to the extent to which analytic practitioners should concern themselves with marital therapy. This ambivalence toward marital therapy is a logical outgrowth of that theoretical orientation which stresses the study and treatment of the individual. The bulk of analytic writing concerns intrapsychic forces within the individual patient and events within the patient–therapist dyad (Gedo and Goldberg, 1973). From the orthodox analytic position, marital discord is most often viewed as a symptom reflecting individual psychopathology in one or both partners. The ultimate cause of the discord would be viewed as greatly removed in time and quite different substantively from the presenting complaint: "People coming for marriage consultation are not affected by their marriages, but have deep-seated neurotic difficulties" (Lussheimer, 1966, p. 128). Thus, orthodox analytic treatment of marital discord focuses on the treatment of the individual in distress. It is assumed that resolution of individual psychopathology through individual psychotherapy or psychoanalysis will then free the patient to adapt to current reality. As the major therapeutic focus is on events occurring between the therapist and the identified patient, contact with the spouse or other family members is usually kept to a minimum (Glover, 1955; Saul, 1958; Menninger, 1958) or even considered to be contraindicated (Greenacre, 1954). Avoidance of family contact is advised, as it may interfere with the patient's development of trust in the therapist and because it may contaminate the development of transference to the therapist. This avoidance of family contact can be traced to some of Freud's statements about the difficulty of dealing with troublesome family members (Freud, 1912/1959), although it is of note that Freud did not always adhere to his own prohibitions, as his treatment of Little Hans (Freud, 1909/1959) involved therapeutic interventions primarily through the patient's father.

It would be unfair to characterize all psychoanalytically oriented clinicians as wholly concerned with the treatment of the individual patient and impervious to the impact of current interpersonal forces on the individual . Numerous clinicians have recognized that resistance on the part of family members can sometimes impede or prevent change in the analysand. Freud noted that resistance from relatives occasionally made psychotherapeutic change impossible: "Because when the husband's resistance is added to that of the sick wife, efforts are made fruitless and therapy is prematurely broken off" (Freud, 1953). His daughter made similar observations about the psychoanalytic treatment of children: "When the neurotic symptom, the conflict, or the regression of a child is anchored not only in the young patient's own personality, but held in place further by powerful emotional forces in the parent to whom the child, in his turn, is tied, the therapeutic action of analysis may be slowed up or, in extreme cases, made impossible." (A. Freud, 1960). Similar observations have been made by other child analysts (Johnson and Szurek, 1954; Burlingham, 1951) and by adult therapists treating married individuals (Mittelmann, 1944, 1948; Martin, 1976). This realization that current interpersonal forces may impede treatment in the analysand has led to a variety of differing therapeutic maneuvers. Some traditional analysts regard current reality problems with family members as an interference in the investigation of intrapsychic material and routinely refer such parents and spouses to other therapists (Giovacchini, 1965). Other therapists have experimented with modification of the basic analytic technique (Sager, 1966). In retrospect, some of these modifications, such as concurrent analysis of the husband and wife by the same therapist (Greene and Solomon, 1963), appear quite conservative by contemporary standards, although such modifications were, at the time, a subject of concern and debate. It was felt that concurrent therapy of this sort would distort the transference situation. It is of note in this regard that Freud treated at least one couple by simultaneous psychoanalysis of both spouses (Stone, 1971). Other therapists began to deviate more from orthodox procedure and began experimenting with conjoint therapy sessions.

It would appear that as therapists have modified their procedures to deal with troublesome current interpersonal forces in a patient's life, there has occurred a gradual shift in theoretical orientation. Also, the basic observational unit has shifted from the patient–therapist dyad to the spouse–spouse dyad. This different class of observational events has naturally led to a different type of exploratory concept. This shift from traditional theory appears to have occurred gradually and in barely perceptible units until many of the theoretical assumptions of contemporary analytically oriented family and marital therapists appear quite different from those of their more orthodox colleagues. Between these extremes is a continuum of minor modifications of analytic technique and theory by individual practitioners. The unsystematic nature of this evolution of theory and thought makes it difficult to discuss coherently the "psychoanalytic approach" to marital discord, as there are many different approaches.

The continuum ranges from the orthodox analyst who treats individuals alone and dislikes family contact to the contemporary family and marital therapist who regards the family or marital unit as the basic observational and treatment unit. Within this continuum, there appears to be a gradual shifting of certain therapeutic concepts. Current interpersonal forces are increasingly regarded as equal to or even more important than past reality (Martin, 1976). Change in actual interpersonal behavior is increasingly considered to be as important as insight (Ackerman, 1971), and transference distortions are observed to occur between spouses as well as between patient and therapist (Sager, 1967). In summary, the therapy becomes less purely psychoanalytic and begins to resemble the concepts and procedures of other theoretical orientation. This shift in emphasis is not always easy to detect, as many of these therapists continue to use the language system ot psychoanalysis even though their interventions might be better explained by concepts from general system theory or social learning theory. In spite of this, there is a treatment orientation toward marital discord that can be identifiable as basically psychoanalytic. The more the basic analytic treatment paradigm is modified, the more the boundaries between analytic marital therapy and other forms of marital therapy are blurred.

The next several sections of this chapter will review the orthodox analytic position regarding marital discord and then trace some of the technical and conceptional revisions of that orientation by other clinical theorists.

## CLASSICAL PSYCHOANALYTIC THEORY AND PRACTICE

It is difficult to discuss analytic theory and practice, as a unified analytic theory does not exist. Analytic theory and thought are peculiar in the sense that new concepts are added to explain the same observational data but are not regarded as replacing or superseding the older concepts relating to the same data. The new concepts are viewed as alternative ways of viewing and understanding the same phenomena. This trend started with Freud, as he developed differing conceptualizations of psychic functioning during his career without discarding his prior formulations. This trend has clearly continued since his death: "The principle of several concurrent and valid avenues for organizing the data of observation we shall call 'theoretical complementarity'" (Gedo and Goldberg, 1973, p. 4). However, the various alternative vantage points in analytic theory, such as the psychology of the self (Kohut, 1971), object-relations theory (Kernberg, 1976), and ego-psychology (Hartmann, 1939), can be regarded as having many things in common that contrast them with other theoretical perspectives. All of these psychoanalytic perspectives emphasize that psychopathology resides within the individual and is based on that individual's past experience. All would emphasize the role of past determinants of current behavioral difficulties and utilize higher level abstractions as explanatory concepts.

Classical analytic theory still determines the predominant analytic treatment orientation within this country (Nemiah, 1975). Classical analytic theory points out that marital difficulties are the result of individual psychopathology in one or both of the spouses (Kubie, 1956) and can be conceptualized as an "acting out" of internal conflicts within an interpersonal context. These internal conflicts would be considered as a sequelae of earlier developmental events in each individual's past life, especially early childhood. From this theoretical perspective, individual psychoanalysis is the treatment of choice for patients with interpersonal difficulties.

"The fundamental aim of psychoanalysis is to bring into conscious awareness, the unconscious elements of the psychological conflicts that underlie symptoms and character problems, and to trace these roots to their genesis in the childhood distortions of the normal process of growth and development. The two basic strategical operations employed to achieve this ultimate goal are the analysis of resistances and of transference" (Nemiah, 1975, p. 170). This process can be better understood by stating that the aim of analytic therapy is to enable the patient to consciously experience his emotional conflicts. These conflicts are assumed to underlie his current behavioral difficulties. The patient usually avoids this experience by various defense mechanisms because the conscious experience of these impulses is frightening or threatening in some respect. The frightening impulses defended against are usually related to sexuality and anger, two motivational forces that encounter considerable societal prohibition (Offenkrantz and Tobin, 1975). Thus, conflict in psychoanalytic terminology can be understood as a triad: the defense, the anxiety, and the hidden impulse (Malan, 1976). The aim of analytic therapy is to clarify all three elements of the conflict. The defense and anxiety are interpreted first, and this helps to bring into awareness the hidden and feared impulse. This triad of impulse, defense, and anxiety would be clarified in three crucial interpersonal relationships in which the conflict is presumably experienced (Menninger, 1958). These three areas are the current therapeutic context (transference interpretations), the distant past (the relationship in which the conflict arose, usually in relationship to parents), and current relationships. It is assumed that there are repetitive sequences of behavior in a patient's life that can be shown to recur predictably and that certain intrapsychic forces can be identified as responsible for these repetitions. A conscious understanding and experience of these relationships should enable the patient to recognize and self-correct such forces in the future, after analysis is terminated.

Resistance to modification of the orthodox treatment situation has often centered around concern that this may modify the transference situation. The concept of transference has been used differently by different analytic writers; analysis of the transference is presumed to be one of the major curative mechanisms in psychoanalysis, and transference as a concept has remained confusing to nonanalytic therapists. In clinical usage, transference refers to a social misperception, most often to the patient's misperception of the therapist (Sandler et al., 1970). Most typically, a patient falsely attributes motives or feelings to the therapist. Further investigation will reveal that similar attributes were attributed to parental figures and are attributed to peers in other settings. This social misperception presumably underlies the patient's recurring maladaptive behavior patterns.

Thus, a crucial element in analytic therapy is to allow the transference to the therapist to develop fully. The transference neurosis, once fully elicited in that setting, should be capable of being clarified and understood by both patient and therapist. This understanding should enable the patient to avoid the repetitive maladaptive behavior patterns of the past and thus adapt to current reality. The key element in understanding resistance to conjoint marital therapy sessions by orthodox analysts is the assumption that clear elicitation and clarification of the transference neurosis can occur only in the therapist–patient dyad.

## RETRANSLATION

The clinical practice of psychoanalysts has remained mysterious to other mental health professionals partly because it is described in a language system that is alien to most other social scientists. Psychoanalysis as a theoretical system contains serious flaws (Bandura, 1969). It is often impossible to disentangle observation from inference, and most analytic theorists employ higher level explanatory concepts that are poorly defined operationally. In spite of these obvious flaws in that theoretical orientation, psychoanalytically oriented clinicians are frequently highly astute observers of human behavior, albeit from their somewhat narrow frame of reference. Without doing serious injustice to the complexity of that theoretical system, numerous analytic concepts can be retranslated into the language of cognitive social psychology. Such a retranslation is worthwhile, as it helps to narrow the seemingly huge gap between differing theoretical systems and can prevent a large pool of clinical wisdom from being lost to other professionals.

For a nonanalytic therapist from the "behavioral" or "social learning" schools of therapy to appreciate analytic conceptualization of human behavior, it is crucial that he realize that analysts approach the understanding of behavior at a molar rather than a molecular level and that they are concerned much more with subtle interpersonal events. With that preamble, I will attempt to retranslate the previous section into social psychological terminology.

Most neurotic and character disorders can be understood as repetitive sequences of maladaptive interpersonal behavior. Underlying most of these maladaptive behavioral sequences are unrealistic fears and expectations of significant others. These fears were learned in previous relationships and then carried over to new relationships, where they are inappropriate (transference reactions). Many of these interpersonal expectations were learned primarily from parents when the child was young. Because of the child's level of developmental sophistication, he reached conclusions (unconscious fantasies) from these learning experiences different from those of an adult. Because of the fearful nature of many of these interpersonal expectations, the child avoided new interpersonal situations that might disconfirm these early fears. These interpersonal fears can be conceptualized as cognitive schemas for the perceptions of significant others in given emotional contexts. Resistance can be understood as avoidance of anxiety-eliciting stimuli, both external and internal. These interpersonal schemas, which are instrumental in causing maladaptive interpersonal situations, can be elicited with greater clarity in a therapeutic context where real consequences and interpersonal cues are kept to a minimum. This learning can then transfer to other interpersonal situations and thus free the patient to adapt to current reality without the burden of faulty past learning. One could thus describe psychoanalysis as a unique form of remedial training about intimate interpersonal relationships.

## MINOR MODIFICATIONS OF ORTHODOX ANALYTIC TREATMENT

Repetitive observations on the effect of current family pathology on the life of patients led many orthodox analysts to consider minor variations of the traditional analytic procedure. Earlier workers such as LaForque (1937) and Mittlemann (1944, 1948) noted the interlocking of husband's and wife's pathologies in some marriages, a finding repeated by more contemporary therapists as well (Ostow and Cholst, 1970; Dicks, 1964). Not only did this interlocking pattern occasionally block therapeutic change in the primary patient, it was also noted that the untreated spouse frequently deteriorated psychologically as treatment progressed for his mate (Kohl, 1962; Sager et al., 1968). In some cases, it appeared that the unsymptomatic spouse was more disturbed than the symptomatic spouse in treatment.

One initial modification of orthodox technique to accommodate for this difficulty was for both spouses to be in consecutive psychoanalysis by the same analyst. The advantage of this approach is that the second spouse could benefit from the work of the first spouse's analysis. The analyst would start this analysis with a larger pool of knowledge about the second spouse, much of which has been gathered during the first analysis. A potential theoretical objection to this method is that competition between the spouses for the analyst can be an issue, although Oberndorf (1938) claimed that this was seldom a problem. The practical disadvantage of such an approach is time. Few couples in severe marital discord are willing to wait patiently for their turns at psychoanalysis.

Other analysts (Martin and Bird, 1953) suggested a collaborative approach, with each spouse in a separate analysis by different analysts, and with the analysts meeting regularly to compare notes. Such an approach necessitates a good working relationship between the analysts.

A third minor variation of the traditional approach was concurrent but separate analyses of each spouse by the same analyst. This approach was favored by many therapists (Brody, 1961; LaForque, 1937; Miller, 1966; Greene and Solomon, 1963; Mittlemann, 1948; Greene, 1960), as it provided a more complete understanding of the complementary nature of the individual pathologies involved and provided the analyst with more complete information about the current reality of each of the spouses. Although the therapeutic approach and conceptualization remained conventional, it was noted by Greene and Solomon (1963) that this approach complicated the transference situation by adding a dimension to the transference of both spouses in relation to the therapists.

Two other therapists warrant mention in that, although their therapy procedures and conceptualization can be seen as bridging steps in the move ahead to conjoint psychoanalytically oriented marital therapy. Thomas (1956) reported a shift in thinking about marital therapy. Although his approach was simultaneous psychotherapy with both of the spouses, he modified the usual analytic technique by focusing his interpretations on the relationships between the spouses rather than on the patient–therapist relationship. Grotjahn (1960) combined traditional psychoanalysis with a unique comprehension of family interaction. When a patient presented for therapy with a history of significant family pathology, Grotjahn would interview various members of the family and choose one for analysis. His choice depended less on overt symptomatology than on the role that person played within the family and that person's amenability to treatment. The primary patient chosen would in essence then be responsible for the health of the family: "Sometimes, the mental health of an entire family improves through the analysis of the primary patient; although he may be the last one to show the results of treatment in his overt behaviors, unconsciously, he may have sparked changes in his environment" (Grotjahn, 1960, p. 173).

## PSYCHOANALYTICALLY ORIENTED CONJOINT MARITAL THERAPY

In more recent years, there has been a shift toward conjoint marital therapy as the predominant modality for marital discord (Nadelson, 1978). This has changed the basic observational unit from the therapist–

patient dyad to the couple dyad. As this shift has occurred, therapists have noted that the transference occurs primarily between spouses rather than to the therapist (Meissner, 1978; Sager, 1967). Similarly, there has been a gradual diminution in the relative emphasis on past influences as compared to present reality (Martin, 1976). The treatment focus also has tended to shift to the couple as opposed to the individuals (Watson, 1963; Sager, 1966), and therapists have become more active (Alger, 1967; Shynner, 1976). Theory is noted in different therapists.

Offenkrantz and Tobin (1975) define the essential characteristics of analytic schools of therapy: "First, it represents a strictly deterministic view of all human behavior; second, this determination is manifested by the significant effect that early life experiences have upon adult behavior, attitudes, and feelings; third, the fact of unconscious mental activity can be inferred; and fourth, consciousness produces cure" (p. 183). Paolino (1978) lists similar factors as defining the terms *psychoanalytic* and *psychodynamic*. Freud (1914/1959) defined psychoanalysis as a technique that focused on transference and resistance. Various marital therapies currently practiced meet most of the above-mentioned criteria.

Nadelson (1978) describes a form of conjoint marital therapy that fits the criteria for being called psychoanalytic. From her perspective, unconscious intrapsychic factors determine mate selection and the types of conflicts experienced. Early emotional conflicts are reactivated by the intimacy of marriage and activate defensive processes to help these conflicts from awareness. She hypothesizes that marital conflict is not based on current reality and thus is minimally influenced by current reality. She urges interpretation as a primary therapy tool: "The ultimate aim of interpretation and working through in psychoanalytically oriented marital therapy is the neutralization and integration of aggressive and libidinal needs so that behavior is motivated more in the service of the ego and less by impulse and intrapsychic conflict" (Nadelson, 1978, p. 146). She maintains that the marriage contains the "transference neurosis" and works to ally with the patient's conflict-free part of the ego to help the patients observe their pathological defensive behavior. It is of note that, despite her analytic flavor, the early portion of her therapy focuses on communication and developing problem-solving techniques. This portion of her therapy resembles that of her more behaviorally oriented colleagues.

Fitzgerald (1973) is an example of an analytically oriented therapist who has modified his technique considerably to accommodate to the therapeutic setting. In his remarkably lucid book, he provides a jargon-free description of his technique for doing couple therapy. He describes a necessary staging of interventions for this therapy to proceed. First, communication problems must be modified before the transactional problems can be identified. After the transactional problems are modified, the therapist can then focus on intrapsychic issues. At this point, his therapy focuses on the interpretation of transferences and defenses within the interpersonal context. The ultimate goal of his therapy is correction of the transference distortions between spouses: "When the treatment is successful, transferences are analyzed out, or at least modified, so that one spouse experiences the other as the real person he is, rather than through existing transference images" (Fitzgerald, 1973, p. 10). Fitzgerald achieves this goal through a variety of techniques, which resemble those of general systems theorists and even behaviorists on occasion.

Sager (1972, 1976) describes a unique form of marital therapy that is unashamedly eclectic–borrowing from systems-transsactional, psychodynamic, and learning theory. In spite of his eclecticism, his basic orientation appears psychodynamic, making use of unconscious material, interpretation of defenses, dream interpretation, and interpretation of defensive reactions. His orientation also centers around clarification of the marriage contract. The marriage contract is a metaphor for each spouse's expectation of the other in marriage. This contract is considered to exist on three levels of awareness: conscious verbalized, conscious but not verbalized, and unconscious. In congruence with the contract, the third level is hypothesized to account for most chronic marital discord. This concept overlaps considerably with transference. The goal of therapy is to help the couple to negotiate a common contract, and this is achieved, at least partially, by interpretation of the transference distortions. Martin (1976) utilizes a similar approach.

## OBJECT-RELATIONS THEORY

Another psychoanalytic movement that has influenced the treatment of marital discord is object-relations theory. This school of thought emphasizes the importance of the buildup of intrapsychic representation of the self and other by interpersonal experiences in the early mother–infant relationship. These intrapsychic representations (schemas) are hypothesized to exert considerable influence on later interpersonal relationships. This school of thought is often referred to as the British Psychoanalytic School and is frequently associated with theorists such as Melanie, Klein, Guntrip, and Fairbairn. The theoretical differences between object-relations theory and classical instinctual Freudian theory may appear trivial to the nonanalyst. The principal contribution of this school of thought is the shift in emphasis from instinctual drives and their neurotic derivatives to the study of people developing in the medium of interpersonal relationships (Guntrip, 1974).

Kernberg describes object-relations theory as a "restricted approach within psychoanalytic metapsychology stressing the buildup of dyadic or bipolar intrapsychic representations (self-and object-images) as reflections of the original infant–mother relationship." He further states that this theory "stresses the simultaneous buildup of the self (a compositive structure derived from the integration of multiple self-images) and of object-representations (or 'internal objects') derived from the integration of multiple object-images into more comprehensive representations of others" (Kernberg, 1976, p. 57). Thus, psychological health could be described as consisting of a cohesive, well-integrated sense of self and realistic, well-differentiated images of others. These self and other representations are formed by introjection. Introjection refers to the buildup of organized clusters of memory traces regarding significant others and the images of the self in relationship to that person. The concept of introjection is similar to that of vicarious learning through symbolic modeling, a concept introduced by the social learning theorist Bandura (1977). At this level of abstraction, object-relations theory has considerable overlap with social psychological theorists such as Kelly (1955), Leary (1957), and Carson (1969), who emphasized how learned expectations of significant others (or cognitive schemas for the perception of others) affect interpersonal relationships (Segraves, 1978). It is also similar in many respects to the theoretical concepts of Harry Stack Sullivan, the American interpersonalist.

Although there is an overlap among these various schools, there are indeed some quite specific differences. Whereas social psychologists have been more concerned with the study of interpersonal data in their own right, object-relations theorists are concerned more with the metapsychological description of the mind. This psychological structure is hypothesized to consist of complex relationships between self and other representations. Very early mother–infant relationships are hypothesized to play a crucial role in the determination of permanent psychological structure. If this relationship is pathological, the child is hypothesized to experience extreme vascillations of love and hate for the object (mother) and to defend against this ambivalence by the mechanism of splitting. With splitting, the introjects with positive and negative valence are kept apart. This process results in a unique distortion of self and other perceptions, such that neither is perceived as a whole being with ambivalent qualities. Projective identification is an allied concept and more often employed in marital work. Projective identification refers to the projection of inner objects onto the other, "a mechanism by which internal conflicts are translated into more concrete modes" (Greenspan and Mannino, 1974). Clinically, this would be inferred when a patient consistently misperceives or exaggerates some aspect of the spouse's (or therapist's) personality that the patient denies or minimizes in himself. The goal of therapy is the reexperience of good and bad objects during the analysis, thus allowing these states to become ego-syntonic and enabling the patient to reintegrate dissociated parts of the self (Money-Kyrle, 1974).

## OBJECT-RELATIONS MARITAL THERAPY

Main (1966) illustrated in a case example how the concept of projective identification could be used as an explanatory concept for the observable maladaptive recurring behavior patterns found in chronic marital discord. The couple presented as a henpecked husband with erectile disturbance married to a masterful, somewhat domineering wife. The marital relationship was felt to reflect the result of the projected parts of the self on the spouse by each partner. Mrs. Adams projected her weak, helpless self onto the husband and Mr. Adams projected his strength and aggression onto his wife. There appeared to be a redistribution of the selves within the relationship. Each spouse was seen in individual therapy, and the therapists met weekly with a consultant. The goal of therapy was to interpret the projection systems of each spouse. Stewart and associates (1975) reported a similar approach to the treatment of disturbed families.

Dicks (1964, 1967) has reported a therapeutic technique based on object-relations theory, primarily employing a conjoint therapy approach. This work was done at the Tavistock Clinic as a function of the National Health Service. Dicks conceptualized marital conflict as occurring on any of three levels: social and cultural norms, conscious personal expectations, and unconscious activation of self- and object-images. This primary contribution is his study of the third level of marital conflict. Dicks hypothesized that in many cases of marital discord, each spouse has defenses against "split-off ego fragments" and these defenses are needed for individual security. Marital discord is felt to result when one or both spouses do not implement, in action, the needed object-relationship for the other's inner world. Many repetitive conflicts that might be described by other theorists (e.g., Haley) as power struggles would be described by Dicks as each spouse requiring the other not to deviate from a needed internal image of the other. When internal insecurities are severe, each spouse cannot tolerate seeing in the other repressed portions of the inner object world. "The defenses, therefore, are directed to keeping the split-off ego fragments in repression, and the self image safe. This means that the partners must not act in such a way as to disturb this position. Collusion refers to a mutual acceptance of the projected images from the other spouse. The marital dyad assumes an existence as a whole and a sense of strong bonding can be observed in couples who superficially appear extremely hostile to one another" (Dicks, 1967, p. 43). The sense of belonging can be understood on the hypothesis that at a deeper level there are perceptions of the partner and consequent attitudes toward him or her as if the other were part of oneself (see Dicks, 1967, p. 69). The thrust of his therapeutic approach was the interpretation of the transference and mutual projection of images such that both spouses would no longer need to use such defenses.

Greenspan and Mannino (1974) further discussed the role of projective identification in marital and family therapy and suggested that the same phenomenon had been described by various works as trading of dissociations, externalization, pseudoidentification, and merging. Their conceptualization of marital discord is similar to that described by Dicks: "[It is] these perceptual distortions and the fear systems they maintain locked into the partners' maladaptive patterns that create a strong bond of tension between them" (Greenspan and Mannino, 1974, p. 1103). Their work is an important bridge between the more interpretive and the more active treatment approaches. They suggest that therapists can intervene in such marriages either by interpreting the unconscious fears responsible for the defense mechanisms or by directly confronting the misperceptions and helping spouses to observe behavior in each other that had not previously been perceived.

## COMMENT AND CRITIQUE

Any meaningful critique of the contribution of psychoanalytic theory to the understanding and treatment of marital discord is problematic. Most psychoanalytic theorists violate all of the cardinal rules concerning good theory construction (Ford and Urban, 1967; Maddi, 1976). Yet psychoanalytic theory is the only major theoretical orientation that stresses the influence of individual personality forces on the evolution of marital discord. Most behavioral and general systems approaches to marital discord totally neglect the contribution of individual psychopathology to marital discord and assume that the interactional problems arose *de novo* in this relationship. Prospective studies of the influences of premarital personality adjustment on subsequent marital happiness have suggested that some of the problems in marriage can be predicted from individual personality problems existing in the spouses prior to marriage (Bentler and Newcomb, 1978). A salient point in the appraisal of the contribution of psychoanalytically oriented therapists to the understanding of marital discord is that these clinicians frequently are extremely astute observers of interpersonal behavior and possess a wealth of clinical wisdom. Unfortunately, they describe their observations and inferences in a language system that precludes the verification of their assumptions and procedures. It is the author's conviction that much of this clinical wisdom can be salvaged by retranslating some of their contributions into a different language system.

There are at least two criteria that a clinical theory or language system should meet: (1) It should be clinically useful and help the clinician to organize his perceptions into a coherent framework; (2) it should be formulated in such a manner that its procedures and assumptions are publicly verifiable and thus subject to modification. In many ways, psychoanalytic theory meets the first criterion better than behavioral or general systems approaches. Psychoanalytic theory clearly enables the clinician to organize a wealth of data into a useful conceptual framework. It does justice to the complexity of the nuances of human behavior in intimate relationships. Clearly, analytic theories miserably fail the second criterion. Analytically oriented clinicians lack the tradition of scientific scrutiny of procedures and assumptions. Thus, much of psychoanalytic metapsychology consists of hypothesized relationships between higher level explanatory concepts. These concepts are seldom defined with precision, and the articulation of these concepts with a specifiable data base is frequently absent. Thus, the relative merits of various hypotheses are impossible to test because there is no agreed-upon body of observations relative to the various hypotheses. Higher level abstractions can be useful explanatory concepts if the relationship of these concepts to lower order concepts and observable data is explicitly formulated. This is seldom the case in psychoanalytic theory construction. For these and other reasons, analytic concepts are often impossible to subject to public verification.

However, certain of the lower order explanatory concepts in analytic thought about marital interventions can be retained and stated in such a way that they relate to a clear data base. Not only does such a retranslation enable consideration of verification of these concepts, it also eases the path toward a theoretical integration of the various partial schools of marital therapy.

Both classical Freudian theory and object-relations theorists postulate that at least four processes are involved in marital discord. Both theories postulate that marital discord is related in a systematic manner to a misperception of the mate's character, whether this be called transference or object representation. As indicated earlier, I prefer the term *cognitive schema*. The term *schema* is devoid of excess theoretical meanings and is more readily relatable to social psychological research on the factors influencing the changing of interpersonal schemas. In other words, a data language is available for this concept. Another concept employed by both schools is the hypothesis that these schemas or object representations are somehow related to behavior elicited in the mate. In other words, for object-relations theory, these distortions, these casual mechanisms are fairly clearly stated. For classical Freudian theory, this relationship between internal events and the required behavior of the spouse is less clear. This relationship becomes clearer when one employs the terminology of Ezriel (1952). For Ezriel, *defense, anxiety,* and *impulse* can be defined in terms of the required relationship, the feared catastrophe, and the avoided relationship. Thus, a bridge between individual neurotic behavior and observed relationship patterns is possible. For the purposes of this discussion, it is sufficient to note that both schools of thought postulate a relationship between schemas for the perception of the mate and the mate's actual behavior. Similar hypotheses have been formulated by social psychologists (e.g., Carson, 1969), and a data language is available for these concepts. Theorists of both schools tend to postulate that mate selection is involved in marital discord (Lussheimer, 1967; Dicks, 1964). This particular hypothesis has received minimal empirical support (Thorp, 1963; DeYoung and Fleischer, 1976), suggesting the need to consider postmarital factors as partially responsible for the evolution of marital discord. A fourth concept stressed by both schools of thought is the primacy of insight as a curative factor. There is no empirical support for this proposition, although it is a concept logically consistent with the other theoretical assumptions of both schools of thought. Transference and object representation were purposely redefined as cognitive schemas, as a body of evidence clearly indicated that schemas can be disproved by direct behavioral disconfirmation. This retranslation of transference, combined with the pioneering work by Greenspan and Mannino (1974), suggests a possible theoretical synthesis between the dynamic approaches and the more behaviorally oriented approaches. A vital conceptual link for this synthesis is the assumption that inner psychological events and behavior are integrally interrelated and that a change in behavior or the external environment may affect the inner psychological process. The reader is invited to keep this concept in mind as he reads the next two chapters reviewing marital therapy orientations, which utilize more active manipulation of behavior.

## REFERENCES

Ackerman, N. W., Beatman, F. L., and Sherman, S. N. (Eds.). *Expanding theory and practice in family therapy*. New York: Family Service Association, 1967.

Alger, I. Joint psychotherapy of marital problems. In J. Masserman (Ed.), *Current psychiatric therapies*. New York: Grune and Stratton, 1961.

Bandura, A. *Social learning theory*. Englewood Cliffs, New Jersey: Prentice-Hall, 1967.

Bandura, A. *Principles of behavior modification*. New York: Holt, Rinehart & Winston, 1969.

Bentler, P. M., and Newcomb, M. D. Longitudinal study of marital success and failure. *Journal of Consulting and Clinical Psychology*, 1978, *46*, 1053–1070.

Brody, S. Simultaneous psychotherapy of married couples: In J. Masserman (Ed.), *Current psychiatric therapies*. New York: Grune and Stratton, 1961.

Burlingham, D. T. Present trends in handling the mother–child relationship during the therapeutic process. *Psychoanalytic Study of the Child*, 1951, 5, 31–37.

Carson, R. C. *Interaction concepts of personality*. Chicago: Aldine, 1969.

DeYoung, G. E., and Fleischer, B. Motivational and personality trait relationships in mate selection. *Behavior Genetics*, 1976, *6*, 1–6.

Dicks, H. V. The conceptional approach to marital diagnosis and therapy developed in the Tavistock Family Psychiatric Units, London, England. In D. W. Abuse, L. Jessner, and E. M. Nash (Eds.), *Marriage counseling in medical practice*. Chapel Hill: University of North Carolina, 1964.

Dicks, H. V. *Marital tensions*. New York: Basic Books, 1967.

Ezriel, H. Notes on psychoanalytic group therapy: II Interpretation and research. *Psychiatry*, 1952, *15*, 119–129.

Fitzgerald, R. V. *Conjoint marital therapy*. New York: Jason Aronson, 1973.

Ford, D. H., and Urban, H. B. *Systems of psychotherapy: A comparative study*. New York: Wiley, 1967.

Freud, A. *The psychoanalytic study of the child* (Vol. 15). New York: International Universities Press, 1960.

Freud, S. *A general introduction to psychoanalysis*. New York: Permabooks, 1953.

Freud, S. On the history of the psychoanalytic movement. *Collected Papers, Vol. I.* New York: Basic Books, 1959. (Originally published, 1914.)

Freud, S. Recommendations for physicians on the psychoanalytic method of treatment. *Collected Papers, Vol. II.* New York: Basic Books, 1959. (Originally published, 1912.)

Freud, S. Analysis of a phobia in a five year old boy. *Standard Edition, Vol. 13.* New York: Basic Books, 1959. (Originally published, 1909.)

Gedo, J. E., and Goldberg, A. *Models of the mind*. Chicago: University of Chicago, 1973.

Giovacchini, P. L. Treatment of marital disharmonies: The classical approach. In B. Greene (Ed.), *The psychotherapies of marital disharmony*. New York: Free Press, 1965.

Glover, E. *Techniques of psychoanalysis*. New York: International Universities Press, 1955.

Greenacre, P. The role of transference: Practical considerations in relation to psychoanalytic therapy. *Journal of the American Psychoanalytic Association*, 1954, 2, 671–684.

Greene, B. L. Marital disharmony: Concurrent analysis of husband and wife. *Diseases of the Nervous System*, 1960, 21, 1–6.

Greene, B. L., and Solomon, A. P. Marital disharmony: Concurrent psychoanalytic therapy of husband and wife by the same psychiatrist. *American Journal of Psychotherapy*, 1963, *17*, 443–457. (a)

Greene, B. L., and Solomon, A. P. Marital disharmony: Concurrent psychoanalytic therapy of husband and wife by the same psychiatrist—The triangular transference transactions. *American Journal of Psychotherapy*, 1963, *17*, 443–456. (b)

Greenspan, S. I., and Mannino, F. V. A model for brief interventions with couples based on projective identification. *American Journal of Psychiatry*, 1974, *131*, 1103–1106.

Grotjahn, M. *Psychoanalysis and the family neurosis*. New York: W. W. Norton, 1960.

Guntrip, H. J. S. Psychoanalytic object relations theory: The Fairburn-Guntrip approach. In S. Arieti (Ed.). *American handbook of psychiatry, (Vol. 1)*. New York: Basic Books, 1974.

Hartmann, H. *Ego psychology and the problem of adaptation*. New York: International Universities Press, 1939.

Johnson, A. M., and Szurek, S. A. Etiology of anti-social behavior in delinquents and psychopaths. *Journal of the American Medical Association*, 1954, *154*, 814–817.

Kelly, G. A. *The psychology of personal constructs*. New York: Norton, 1955.

Kernberg, O. F. *Object-relations theory and clinical psychoanalysis*. New York: Jason Aronson, 1976.

Kohl, R. N. Pathologic reactions of marital partners to improvement of patients. *American Journal of Psychiatry*, 1962, *118*, 1036–1041.

Kohut, H. *The analysis of the self*. New York: International Universities Press, 1971.

Kubie, L. S. Psychoanalysis and marriage. In V. W. Eisenstein (Ed.), *Neurotic interaction in marriage*. New York: Basic Books, 1956.

LaForque, R. Family neurosis and the neurotic family. *Internationale Zeitschrift fuer Psychoanalysis*, 1937, *23*, 548–559.

Leary, T. *Interpersonal diagnosis of personality*. New York: Ronald Press, 1957.

Lussheimer, P. The diagnosis of marital conflicts. *American Journal of Psychoanalysis*, 1966, *26*, 127–146.

Maddi, S. R. *Personality theories: A comparative analysis*. Homewood, Ill. Dorsey Press, 1976.

Main, T. F. Mutual projection in a marriage. *Comprehensive Psychiatry*, 1966, *7*, 432–439.

Malan, D. H. *The frontier of brief psychotherapy*. New York: Plenum, 1976.

Martin, P. A. *A marital therapy manual*. New York: Brunner/Mazel, 1976.

Martin, P. A., and Bird, H. W. An approach to the psychotherapy of marriage partners—The stereoscopic technique. *Psychiatry*, 1953, *16*, 123–127.

Meissner, W. W. The conceptualization of marriage and family dynamics from a psychoanalytic perspective. In T. J. Paolino and B. S. McCrady (Eds.), *Marriage and Marital Therapy*. New York: Brunner/Mazel, 1978.

Menninger, K. *Theory of psychoanalytic technique*. New York: Basic Books, 1958.

Miller, J. Concurrent treatment of marital couples by one or two analysts. *American Journal of Psychoanalysis*, 1966, *26*, 135–139.

Mittelmann, B. Complementary neurotic reactions in intimate relationships. *Psychoanalysis Quarterly*, 1944, *18*, 479–491.

Mittelmann, B. Concurrent analysis of marital couples. *Psychoanalysis Quarterly*, 1948, *17*, 182–197.

Money-Kyrle, R. E. The Kleimian school. In S. Arievi (Ed.), *American Handbook of Psychiatry* (Volume One). New York: Basic Books, 1974.

Nadelson, C. C. Marital therapy from a psychoanalytic perspective. In T. J. Paolino and B. S. McCrady (Eds.), *Marriage and marital therapy*. New York: Brunner/Mazel, 1978.

Nemiah, J. C. Classical psychoanalysis. In D. X. Freedman and J. E. Dyrud (Eds.), *American handbook of psychiatry* (Vol. 5). New York: Basic Books, 1975.

Oberndorf, P. Psychoanalysis of married couples. *Psychoanalytic Review*, 1938, *25*, 453–475.

Offenkrantz, W., and Tobin, A. Psychoanalytic psychotherapy. In D. X. Freedman and J. E. Dyrud (Eds.), *American handbook of psychiatry* (Vol. 5). New York: Basic Books, 1975.

Ostow, M., and Cholst, B. Marital discord. *New York State Journal of Medicine*, 1970, *70*, 257–266.

Sager, C. J. The development of marriage therapy: An historical review. *American Journal of Orthopsychiatry*, 1966, *36*, 458–467.

Sager, C. J. Transference in conjoint treatment of married couples. *Archives of General Psychiatry*, 1967, *16*, 185–193.

Sager, C. J. *Marriage contracts and couple therapy*. New York: Brunner/Mazel, 1976.

Sager, C. J., Gundlack, R., Kremer, M., Lenz, R., and Royce, J. R. The married in treatment. *Archives of General Psychiatry*, 1968, *19*, 205–217.

Sager, C. J., Kaplan, H., Gundlack, R., Kremer, M., Lenz, R., and Royce, J. The marriage contract. *Family Process*, 1971, *10*, 311–326.

Sandler, J., Dare, C., and Holden, A. Basic psychoanalytic concepts: III. Transference. *British Journal of Psychiatry*, 1970, *116*, 667–672.

Saul, L. J. *Technic and practice of psychoanalyses*. Philadelphia: J. B. Lippincott, 1958.

Segraves, R. T. Conjoint marital therapy; a cognitive behavioral model. *Archives of General Psychiatry*, 1978, *35*, 450–455.

Shynner, A. C. R. *Systems of family and marital psychotherapy*. New York: Brunner/Mazel, 1976.

Stewart, R. H., Peters, T. C., March, S., and Peters, M. J. An object-relations approach to psychotherapy with marital couples, families, and children. *Family Process*, 1975, *14*, 161–178.

Stone, I. *The passions of the mind*. New York: Doubleday, 1971.

Thomas, A. Simultaneous psychotherapy with marital partners. *American Journal of Psychotherapy*, 1956, *10*, 716–727.

Thorp, R. G. Psychological patterning in marriage. *Psychological Bulletin*, 1963, *60*, 97–117.

Watson, A. S. The conjoint psychotherapy of marriage partners. *American Journal of Orthopsychiatry*, 1963, *33*, 912–922.

# General System Theory and Marriage

General system theory refers to a group of assumptions concerned with describing the formal properties of organization systems. This viewpoint assumes that certain structural characteristics of organizational systems are universal and independent of the system being studied. Thus, properties of interactional systems can be understood without necessarily considering the properties of the individual units constituting the system or even the content of the interactional data (von Bertalanffy, 1968).

This theoretical viewpoint was espoused by a relatively small group of therapists known as the Palo Alto group (Foley, 1974). This group included therapists and theoreticians loosely associated in a variety of projects and endeavors under the leadership of Don Jackson and Gregory Bateson. Don Jackson was director of the Schizophrenia Family Therapy project at the Palo Alto Veterans Administration Hospital and founder of the Mental Research Institute in Palo Alto (Watzlawick, 1977). Gregory Bateson was the director of a research project concerned with studying communication from the viewpoint of Russel and Whitehead's theory of logical types, a research project that lasted from 1952 to 1962 (Haley, 1963). Although these projects were administratively distinct, there was considerable interplay among participants in both projects. For example, Jay Haley of the Bateson group was a research associate at the Palo Alto Veterans Administration Hospital, and Don Jackson was a clinical consultant to the communication research project under Bateson's direction. This interplay involving organizational systems and professionals of differing backgrounds yielded a unique approach to the treatment of mental disturbance.

Although there are at present a relatively small number of therapists who could be identified as belonging to the "Palo Alto school" or being general system purists, the work of this group has had a marked impact on the conduct of marital and family therapy. It is an understatement to say that there are few currently practicing marital or family therapists who have not been influenced by the concepts evolved by this group. This is illustrated by a questionnaire survey of family therapists by the Group for the Advancement of Psychiatry's Committee on the Family (1970). This survey indicated that Satir, Jackson, Haley, and Bateson were listed as being among the seven most influential family theorists among practicing family therapists. As outlined in the previous chapter, most contemporary psychoanalytically oriented marital and family therapists incorporate general systems concepts in their treatment approaches. Similarly, most behavioral marital therapists employ conceptual systems and treatment approaches that overlap with those described by the Palo Alto group.

The peculiar impact of this group of clinical investigators—its pervasive influence combined with a minimal number of faithful followers—can perhaps best be understood by realizing that they did not elaborate a school of therapy. Jackson, Haley, and associates borrowed concepts from various sources such as general system theory, cybernetics, communication theory, and even formal mathematics, and these concepts were only loosely organized. Rather than a school of therapy, they espoused a peculiar orientation toward clinical data (Steinglass, 1978). They were advocating a paradigm shift in psychiatric thought (Bateson, 1972).

The significance of their attempted paradigm shift can best be appreciated by realizing that psychodynamic theory monopolized psychiatric thinking at the time that this group began publishing their early papers. Psychodynamic theorists attempted to explain complex interpersonal behavior by focusing on the individual psychodynamics of the participants in the interaction. This focus then evolved into a discussion of the interaction of hypothetical intrapsychic structures and forces. The attempted paradigm shift was away from the concern with individual psychopathology. This group suggested that complex interpersonal behavior could best be understood by analyzing the communication flow between participants. Intrapsychic events were considered basically unknowable. An alternate and preferrable approach was to focus attention on observable interactional data. Concepts borrowed from scientific disciplines concerned with communication flow in complex systems were considered better suited for this task (Watzlawick et al., 1967).

As will become clear in the next chapter, the paradigm shift advocated by this group overlaps to a considerable extent with the behavioral paradigm. In many ways, the general system paradigm, with its emphasis on observable data, laid the groundwork for behavioral marital therapy. Many of the behavioral concepts and treatment interventions appear to be rediscoveries of the work by Jackson. However, general system marital therapists differ from behavioral marital therapists in certain definite ways. The general system therapists were concerned with changing behavior at a molar rather than a molecular level, and their interventions were less content-bound than most interventions by behaviorally oriented therapists. It is also fair to say that this group of therapists tended to appreciate the subtleties of interpersonal behavior with far greater clinical wisdom than many behavior therapists.

Various authors have commented on the relationship between therapy and practice and have wondered whether theory dictates practice or whether therapists search for a theory to explain their practices (Olson, 1975). This consideration is particularly relevant for an evaluation of the relationship of general system theory to family and marital therapy. It appears that certain clinicians, such as Don Jackson, made certain clinical observations that did not fit current clinical theory (Jackson, 1957) and then looked for theoretical models to organize and explain their observations. Consistently, therapists such as Jackson loosely borrow selected concepts from other schools of thought and metaphorically apply them to clinical observations. Similarly, Bowen is often considered to be a representative of general systems theory (Foley, 1974), although Bowen evolved his theoretical orientation toward family therapy with only minimal awareness of general systems theory (Bowen, 1976).

For the purposes of this discussion, general systems theory as an approach to marital therapy will refer to treatment orientations that are mainly concerned with the analysis and modification of interaction and communication patterns between spouses. Therapists such as Jackson (1977), Haley (1976), Watzlawick (1977), and Satir (1967) will be considered in this group. These therapists were clearly influenced by a variety of conceptual schemes, only one of which could be considered general system theory.

## GENERAL SYSTEM THEORY

Although general system theory has had a marked influence on the social sciences (Grinker, 1967, 1969), it was elaborated in the biological sciences as an alternative approach to the understanding of complex biological systems (von Bertalanffy, 1968). Conventional scientific models of explanation tend to explain complex phenomena by reduction to less complex phenomena. In essence, complex phenomena are explained by a series of linear reductionistic steps. Events are explained by "a linear series of stepwise cause and effect equations, each of which is intended to unearth a fundamental precedent event assumed to be causally explanative of the final behavior under study" (Steinglass, 1978, p. 301). An extreme example of this scientific model would be to assume that the explanation of one spouse's behavior in a marital situation would ultimately be reducible to physicochemical processes at the cellular level in the central nervous system of that spouse. This particular approach to scientific understanding has led to biological science's becoming "fragmented into smaller and smaller units or disciplines that become increasingly reductionistic" (Grinker, 1975, p. 251).

General system theory maintains that complex interactional systems cannot be fully understood by extensive reductionistic scrutiny of the fragmented individual parts constituting the system, however sophisticated this study. A true understanding of complex interactional systems requires an understanding of the relationship between the parts in the system and the structure governing this relationship (von Bertalanffy, 1968). In essence, this orientation emphasizes the study of pattern at a molar level rather than the study of content at a molecular level (Foley, 1974). Von Bertalanffy (1974) maintains that traditional reductionistic scientific models cannot account for interactional phenomena in multivariable systems and that this understanding requires the introduction of new scientific models or paradigms. Interest in general system theory was accelerated by developments in applied technology in machinery. The understanding of complex electronic machinery was found to necessitate models stressing input–output relationships. In many cases, knowledge of information flow patterns among individual components in the machinery was more useful than highly specialized knowledge about the inner circuitry of the individual components.

General system theory is concerned with the study of interactional components in context, classifying systems by the way the parts are organized and deriving the laws for different types of systems and subsystems (Beavers, 1977). In other words, complex interactional phenomena are felt to be understandable only if one studies the pattern of relationships involving the components: "The system is then its own best explanation" (Watzlawick et al., 1967). General system theory is concerned with the general laws of interacting systems. In other words, this approach assumes that there are certain fundamental properties common to all interrelated systems and subsystems that can be delineated and generalized across systems irrespective of content. Von Bertalanffy makes his position on this quite explicit: "General system theory pertains to principles that apply to systems in general. A system is defined as a complex of components in mutual interaction. General system theory contends that there are principles of systems in general or in defined subclasses of systems irrespective of the nature of systems, or their components, or of the relations or 'forces' between them" (von Bertalanffy, 1974, p. 1100).

The relevance of general system theory as a perspective from which to view marriage and marital difficulties can be better appreciated by a review of some of the central concepts. A major distinction in general systems theory is whether one is dealing with a closed or an open system. Open systems allow exchange across boundaries, whereas closed systems do not. Therefore, the steady state in a closed system is always determined by the initial conditions. All living systems are open systems. The steady state is posited to be relatively independent of the initial conditions: "The steady state of open systems is characterized by the principle of equifinality; that is, in contrast to equilibrium states in closed systems which are determined by initial conditions, the open system may attain a time-independent state, independent of initial conditions and determined only by the system parameters" (von Bertalanffy, 1962, p. 7). This orientation clearly underlies the thinking of Jackson and co-workers: "So, in the analysis of how people affect each other in their interaction, we will not consider the specifics of genesis or product to be nearly so important as the ongoing organization of interaction (Watzlawick et al., 1967, pp. 127–128). This is a recurring theme in the work by Jackson (1977) and Haley (1977), and it represents a radical shift in conceptual orientation toward psychological difficulties in humans. This orientation is clearly in marked contrast to the psychoanalytic approach, which operates on a linear reductionist system and treats marriage more like a closed system determined by the initial conditions, i.e., the premarital personalities of the spouses.

The system concepts of wholeness, relationship, and nonsummativity are related concepts and refer to the concept that a system has a life and force of its own that is more than the sum of its parts. To understand an interactional system, one has to study the interrelationships among the parts. Similarly, because of this interrelationship, a change in one part of the system invariably leads to a change elsewhere. Because of this degree of interrelatedness, one has to think of causality as a circular rather than as a linear process. In other words, in close interpersonal relationships such as marriage, the behavior of spouses is so mutually reactive and interactive, one cannot say that the behavior of spouse A caused spouse B to act a certain way without also considering whether the predictable reaction of spouse B caused the behavior of

implicit assumptions about individuals. It appears that one strong implicit assumption of his is that there is a reciprocal interrelationship between self-definition and behavior in interpersonal contexts. This assumption is similar to that of many contemporary family therapists (Minuchin, 1974).

Jackson postulates that in any long-term relationship, each spouse will want to define the relationship to his or her own advantage. Thus, every communication can be viewed as an attempt to define the relationship. In every interaction, each spouse will exchange clues as to how he or she wants to define the relationship. These clues (or behavior tactics) will be modified by the other spouse. If the relationship is to persist, this relationship struggle (struggle to reach a joint agreement as to each spouse's relationship to the other) must stabilize. In other words, a "bargain" must be reached. In marital couples, this bargain is referred to as the marital quid pro quo. This term has also been used by behavior therapists (Stuart, 1969) to refer to marital negotiation over specific content issues, but it is clear that Jackson used the term quite differently. For Jackson, marital quid pro quo refers to the metaphorical bargain reached by spouses regarding their self-definitions in the other's perception.

Much of Jackson's work stresses the need to examine and modify communication patterns in disturbed marriages (Lederer and Jackson, 1968). Jackson uses the term *communication* to refer to any communication between interrelated partners. Thus, the terms "communication and behavior [are] used virtually synonymously" (Watzlawick *et al.*, 1967, p. 22). Any behavior between marital partners defines the relationship and imposes meaning.

A major contribution of Jackson's was his emphasis on the complexity of communication exchange in marital partners, "that in actual human communication a single and simple message never occurs, but that communication always and necessarily involves a multiplicity of messages, of different levels, at once" (Jackson and Weakland, 1971, p. 16). This possibility of discrepancies at multiple levels offers a possible explanation for many marital difficulties. For example, communication can be conceptualized as consisting of both a report, or content, level and a command (relationship) level. Many seeming disagreements about content in a marriage may really be difficulties at the command level that are never addressed directly. The difference may not be about the actual content in dispute but about who has the right to decide. The possible multiplicity of levels in verbal disqualification of the verbal message means that seemingly simple communications have the potential for being quite complex. This possibility of incongruence on multiple levels means that many marital disputes are never resolved, as the participants never truly understand each other's positions: "The spouses do not exchange clear, useful information. Instead, they attack each other with hypocritical messages which may mean one thing literally, but in effect mean something else" (Lederer and Jackson, 1968, p. 103). Jackson enumerated various common communication problems in couples that have later been rediscovered by behavioral marital therapists (e.g., Thomas, 1977). These problems included mind reading, incomplete transactions, cross-complaining, channel inconsistency, and subject shifts (Lederer and Jackson, 1968).

According to Jackson, the goal of family and marital therapy is to change the rules of the relationship. This is accomplished by interrupting the repetitive patterns of behavior or reframing and thus changing the assumptive world underlying the behavior patterns. In many cases, he would deduce the assumptions or rules governing a behavioral sequence and then prescribe a minor change in behavior that would lead to altered rules. For example, he described the treatment of a couple containing an alcoholic husband. His drinking allowed the wife to appear protective and stable and her behavior allowed him to be irresponsible. Therefore, the therapist instructed the man to continue drinking but only if he always drank with his wife and his wife had the first drink in each round of drinks (Watzlawick et al., 1967). Clearly, this minor change in behavior violated the basic rule of their relationship. His interventions were usually focused on interrupting the repetitive interactional sequence. For example, a common sequence in couples is excessive withholding of responses that the other spouse desires. The withholding spouse usually considers the other's requests to be limitless and insatiable. As the other spouse never receives complete gratification of his desires, he continues to make demands. Clearly, such an interaction pattern is self-sustaining. In such cases, Jackson would prescribe for each spouse to alternate meeting all of the requests for gratification that the other desired. Such forced reality testing usually interrupted the behavioral sequences (Lederer and Jackson, 1968). In other cases, he would attempt to modify the assumptive world underlying the family rules by reframing or modifying these assumptions. In this case, Jackson would interpret the couple's behavior differently from what they labeled it. The correctness of the interpretation was irrelevant. The relabeling was correct if it led to new interaction sequences.

In *The Mirages of Marriages*, Lederer and Jackson (1968) outlined various self-help programs for disturbed couples. The rationale for these programs was (1) that imposed structure would interrupt maladaptive patterns and (2) that improved communication would facilitate marital interaction. The bulk of these exercises were aimed at improving marital communication skills and consisted of listening exercises, exercises in verbal clarity, and exercises in reading nonverbal communication. These exercises in many ways are more clinically sophisticated than many communication training programs advocated by behavioral marital therapists today. Another interesting exercise was for couples to alternate being in control and later to assign areas of competence and responsibility. This was intended to interrupt escalating power struggles.

## JAY HALEY

Jay Haley's early publications on marital therapy (1963a, b) demonstrate a considerable overlap between his own and Jackson's conceptions of marriage. This is understandable, as Haley was a research associate at the Mental Research Institute founded by Don Jackson and a member of Bateson's research project on communication. In his early work, Haley differed from Jackson in that Haley emphasized marriage as a struggle of interpersonal maneuvers designed to control the other spouse's behavior. In many ways, Haley was much less a systems purist than Jackson. His work contained clear inferences about the individuals constituting the social system of marriage. In his later publications, the influence of Milton Erikson on his work is obvious (Haley, 1973, 1976). More recently, Haley was associated with the Child Guidance Clinic in Philadelphia, and the influence of Salvador Minuchin is clearly detectable. At this point, Haley begins to shift his interest from the dyadic to the triadic and then the extended-kinship network (1971a, 1971b). Similarly, Haley begins to discuss the problems of transgression of cross-generational boundaries (1971b).

Like Jackson, Haley conceptualizes marriage as necessitating the evolvement of a common set of rules. When two people decide to marry, they have to work out a set of rules for living together: "The process of working out a satisfactory marital relationship can be seen as a process of working out shared agreements, largely undiscussed between two people" (Haley, 1963, p. 123). This means that marital conflict can occur on at least three different levels: (1) the rules themselves, (2) who has the right to set the rules, and (3) enforcement of incompatible rules or ambiguous communication about the rules. Disagreement over which rules to follow is often a bitter struggle for early marriages. Part of this can be attributed to the fact that the spouses were trained in implicit and explicit rules of relationship in their families of origin. A satisfactory marriage requires a reconciliation of these conflicting long-standing expectations. This reconciliation of deeply held values entails quite a struggle for most couples. However, this level of conflict is one of the more easily resolvable. It is of note that some of the current behavioral marital therapy treatment approaches are focused on this level of intervention (Azrin *et al.*, 1973).

Conflicts about who sets the rules are some of the most intense marital struggles: "The process of defining who is to make the rules in the marriage will inevitably consist of a struggle between any couple. The tactics in this struggle are those of any conflict: threats, violent assault, withdrawal, sabotage, passive resistance, and helplessness or physical inability to do what the other wants" (Haley, 1963, p. 220). Much of Haley's original contribution to the marital therapy literature is detailing the nuances of such struggles. For example, a wife may order her husband to do something he desires to do. The husband may violently resist her instruction even though he agrees with the content of the instruction. He disagrees that his wife has the right to give him orders. He also points out how typical descriptions of domination and submission in a marital relationship may miss the complexity of the interaction. For example, "to describe a marriage as one where there is a dominating wife and a dependent husband does not include the idea that the husband might be provoking his wife to be dominating so that actually he is dominating what sort of relationship they have" (Haley, 1963, p. 222).

Haley's description of the impact of paradoxical communication is particularly useful. For example, he describes how a husband may verbally demand that his wife be sexy but nonverbally indicate that she dare not. A practical solution to this dilemma might be for the wife to say that she desires her husband but just can't respond. Of course, this interaction is seldom verbalized and usually out of consciousness. Psychosomatic symptoms can also be viewed as interpersonal ploys to circumscribe the mate's behavior as well as reactions to paradoxical communications: "The spouse of a patient with symptoms is faced with incompatible messages: his behavior is circumscribed by his mate, but at the same time it is not circumscribed by the mate because the mate's behavior is labeled as 'involuntary'" (Haley, 1963, p. 131).

In summary, Haley conceptualizes marriages as containing two interpersonal protagonists who wish to circumscribe the range of each other's behavior. This conflict involves a variety of subtle interpersonal ploys and is resolved by a compromise agreement satisfying part of each partner's behavioral requirements. This struggle is considered pathological when one partner resorts to the use of psychiatric symptoms to gain an advantage and the struggle reaches a self-perpetuating stage.

As with Jackson, Haley's work on marital therapy is concerned with interventions at the transactional rather than the individual level, wherein "a problem is defined as a type of behavior that is part of a sequence of acts between several people. The repeating sequence of behavior is the focus of therapy" (Haley, 1976, p. 2). Haley differs from Jackson in several ways. His writing is considerably less abstract and more practical. In his practicality, Haley deviates from a general systems framework by making inferences about the properties of individuals in marital and family systems. Part of Haley's genius is his description of common reactions to given interpersonal situations as the tendency to try to extend interpersonal control in incredibly subtle ways and the equally powerful tendency to resist external control. Much of interpersonal discord can be conceptualized as a conflict between these two forces.

Haley resembles Jackson in that he conceptualizes interventions as being focused on interrupting the recurring sequences of behavior in making certain strongly implicit assumptions about the people constituting the interactional networks. "He appears to be assuming that there is a reciprocal interrelationship between individuals' perceptions of each other and their behavior toward one another such that a change in this perception can occur either by a cognitive relabeling of observations or by observing behavior discrepant with the internal cognitive model" (Segraves, 1978, p. 451). Haley states this position clearly: "As a couple express themselves, the therapist comments upon what they say. His comments tend to be the following: those comments which emphasize the positive side of their interaction together, and those comments which define the situation as different from, if not opposite to, the way they are defining it. . . . He is making it difficult for the couple to continue their usual classification" (Haley, 1976, p. 139). He continues in a similar vein: "By subtly focusing upon the opposite, or a different, aspect of a relationship, the therapist undermines the couple's typical ways of labeling the relationship and they must define it in a different way and so undergo a change" (Haley, 1976, p. 140). Even Haley's often ingenious use of therapeutic directives is built on this same assumption of a link between behavior and inner representational worlds. "First the main goal of therapy is to get people to behave differently so as to have a different subjective experience. Directives are a way of making these changes happen" (Haley, 1976, p. 49). Repeatedly, in Haley's publications, the same themes appear. He emphasizes the use of behavior change or the use of cognitive relabeling. Although he describes himself as influenced by general systems theory, one could also posit that Haley was influenced by cognitive social psychology (e.g., Carson, 1969) or modern cognitive-behavioral approaches to therapy (e.g., Meichenbaum, 1977).

## VIRGINIA SATIR AND MARITAL THERAPY

Virginia Satir was cited as the most influential theorist in a poll of family therapists conducted by the Group for the Advancement of Psychiatry (1970). Her influence was particularly strong among social work family therapists and among therapists in the West Coast area. The extent of her influence is remarkable in that she has published relatively little (Foley, 1974), was associated with the Mental Research Institute in Palo Alto for a relatively small period of time (Satir *et al.*, 1975), and in more recent years has been associated with the human potential movement (Satir, 1972). The bulk of her contribution is contained in the now classic book *Conjoint Family Therapy* (Satir, 1967), although a minor sequel to this is contained in a family interview published by Haley and Hoffman (1967).

Although influenced by general system theory and frequently classified by others as a general system therapist (Foley, 1974), Satir could probably be better classified as a transactionalist. Whereas Jackson and Haley made implicit assumptions about the personalities of individuals in interpersonal systems, Satir made quite explicit assumptions about individual personalities and their contribution to interactional difficulties. Satir's conceptual system, though presented in a simplistic outline form, is quite complex in its ramifications and represents a peculiarly clinical and useful amalgamation of Sullivanian interpersonal psychology, ego psychology, and concepts preceding the development of narcissistic theory in psychoanalysis. "The essence of her theoretical position is that there is a reciprocal interrelationship between communication difficulties and individual self-concepts and self-esteem. She hypothesizes that healthy interpersonal relationships require the individuals involved to have a sense of individuality and relatedness. Stated slightly differently, she is saying that people need to learn to discriminate between internal feelings, images, and introjects and external reality (real other people), and that most of us have tendencies to project feelings and distort perceptions. She implies that a partial solution to this interpersonal difficulty is for people to learn and employ clear language that differentiates self from other and to use explicit language that limits the amount of distortion and projection possible" (Segraves, 1978, pp. 451–452). Her main contribution is the hypothesis that clear and precise verbal feedback between spouses is necessary to limit distorted perceptions and to foster emotional well-being.

She has been extremely influential: Masters and Johnson incorporated her communication skills treatment approach into their treatment package (Segraves, 1976), and numerous behavior therapists employ treatment programs quite similar to the ones she advocated (e.g., Carter and Thomas, 1973; Nunnally et al., 1975). Basically, she postulates that healthy communication requires a distinction between self and other, clarity, and congruence between levels of communication. She then gives examples of communication exchanges that violate these rules; common examples would be overgeneralization, mind reading, accusations, incomplete messages, vague referents, and indirect anger. The rationale underlying her human growth seminars appears to be that structured exercises can open the way to new experiences in relating and communicating (Satir et al., 1975). Again, her concern is the clarity of communication. Good communication in families is viewed as communication that differentiates and acknowledges self and other and is congruent with the context. This notion is similar to her earlier hypothesis that good communication is exemplified by statements like "I want this from you in this situation" (Satir, 1967, p. 87). She illustrates how certain styles of communication such as placating, blaming, being superreasonable, and irrevelance violate this model.

Satir has been influenced by general system theory in that she conceptualizes the primary thrust of therapy to be to change the communication patterns in families. Her perspective has clinical relevance, as most therapists, whether individual or family by orientation, are aware that disturbed individuals camouflage their communications for purposes of self-protection. This act itself perpuates the disturbance in many cases, as the individual prevents himself from acquiring corrective information. It is of note that Jackson emphasized the changing of interactional patterns by changing the actual behavior. Haley emphasized that this objective could be achieved by changing the assumptive world underlying the behavior. Haley achieved this by relabeling of events. Satir assumes that this assumptive world can change if proper information exchange can occur. If we transpose these orientations to the individual context, we can assume that individuals change through new experiences, or through new assumptions about these experiences.

## COMMENT AND CRITIQUE

An integral difficulty in evaluating the general systems approach to marital therapy is that there is no such school of thought or body of procedures (Steinglass, 1978). At best, it represents a new orientation toward data. At worst, it is scientism, borrowing of language, and the misuse of technical terms to simulate scientific rigor. One has to ask if Jackson, Haley, and Satir are merely pretending to theorize by borrowing concepts and applying them in a new context. Rapoport (1974) succintly outlines the danger: "On occasion some theorizers have simply borrowed the language of modern developments in the exact sciences. The more serious dangers of speculative promiscuity are rooted in this practice" (p. 1092). He continues: "It is here that the tendency to theorize by juggling words in their various contexts is greatest among those who are impressed but not disciplined by the spirit of the exact sciences."

Jackson, Haley, and Satir did introduce a new approach to the treatment of relationship disturbances and indeed a new orientation toward the data. However, the use of terms like *isomorphism*, *negative feedback*, and *family rules* could be considered as cases of metaphoric promiscuity. If one attempts to summarize some of their major contributions to the understanding of interpersonal process, the use of terms from general system theory isn't necessary to validate these contributions. Some of their major contributions are (1) the importance of current interpersonal forces in determining personality, (2) the complexity of intimate interpersonal systems necessitating considering causality as a circular process, (3) the hypothesis that certain sequences of interpersonal behavior are virtually self-sustaining, and (4) the notion that behavior change in intimate interpersonal relationship could be therapeutic. Many of these hypotheses are standard assumptions of cognitive social psychologists. For example, Stotland and Canon (1972) referred to the problem of circular causality in person–person relationships as the response-determined stimulus effect. Leary (1957) described how certain interpersonal behavior tends to invite reciprocal responses from the other person. Carson (1969) similarly described how given interpersonal styles become self-perpetuating by the encouragement of complementary reactions in others. "It would appear that all of these authors with varying degrees of explicitness are hypothesizing that individuals have representational models for significant others and tend to behave toward other people in such a way as to invite behavior from the other that is congruent with that inner representational model" (Segraves, 1978, p. 453). In 1955 Kelly had already postulated that behavior and inner representational models are reciprocally related such that behavior change in a person's immediate environment might be the way to provoke change in the person's interpersonal world. The point I'm trying to make is that the contribution of this group of therapists can be assumed under theoretical structures without metaphoric borrowing from cybernetics and general systems theory. One can assume that the recurring interactional patterns observed in couples are the product of each spouse's attempt to elicit complementary behavior in the other. An interruption of this mutually confirmatory behavioral sequence should lead to change in each by behavioral disconfirmation. On occasion, Jackson almost verbalized these assumptions about the interplay of behavior and inner representational worlds, stating that "man operates with a set of premises about the phenomena he perceives and that his interaction with reality in the modest sense . . . will be determined by these premises" (see Watzlawick *et al.*, 1967, p. 262). Thus, Jackson could be described as belonging to the school of cognitive social psychology. Similarly, there is conceptual overlap between Jackson's basic assumptions and work by current therapists who might be labeled cognitive behaviorists (e.g., Beck, 1976).

The real contribution of this group of therapists who were metaphorically influenced by general systems theory can best be understood in historical context. Their work represented a first break from the rigidly followed intrapsychic model prevalent in the 1950s. They rightly stressed that current interpersonal forces can be as important as past interpersonal forces in determining a person's behavior and that one can understand behavior best by focusing on current behavior rather than hypothesizing about internal events. They also suggested that these forces can be understood at a level of clinical sophistication above that usually employed by behavior therapists. Their approach was midway between the abstractness of psychoanalysis and the concretism of behaviorism.

## REFERENCES

Azrin, N. H., Naster, B. J., and Jones, R. Reciprocity counseling: A rapid learning based procedure for marital counseling. *Behaviour Research and Therapy*, 1973, *11*, 365–382.

Bateson, G. *Steps to an ecology of the mind*. New York: Ballantine, 1972.

Bateson, G., Jackson, D., and Haley, J. Toward a theory of schizophrenia. In D. Jackson (Ed.), *Communication, family and marriage*. Palo Alto: Science and Behavior Books, 1968.

Beavers, W. R. *Psychotherapy and growth*. New York: Brunner/Mazel, 1977.

Beck, A. *Cognitive therapy and emotional disorders*. New York: International Universities Press, 1976.

Bowen, M. Theory in the practice of psychotherapy. In P. J. Guerin (Ed.), *Family therapy: Theory and practice*. New York: Gardner Press, 1976.

Carson, R. C. *Interaction concepts of personality*. Chicago: Aldine, 1969.

Carter, R. D., and Thomas, E. J. Modification of problematic marital communication using corrective feedback and instruction. *Behavior Therapy*, 1973, *4*, 100–109.

Dicks, H. U. *Marital tensions*. New York: Basic Books, 1976.

Foley, V. D. *An introduction to family therapy*. New York: Grune and Stratton, 1974.

Grinker, R. R. Normality viewed as a system. *Archives of General Psychiatry*, 1967, *17*, 320–324.

Grinker, R. R. Symbolism and general systems theory. In W. Gray, F. Duhl, and N. Rizzo (Eds.), *General systems theory and psychiatry*. Boston: Little, Brown, 1969.

Grinker, R. R. The relevance of general systems theory to psychiatry. In D. A. Hamburg and H. K. H. Brodie (Eds.), *American handbook of psychiatry*, Vol. 6, 2nd ed., New York: Basic Books, 1975.

Group for the Advancement of Psychiatry. *Treatment of families in conflict*. New York: Jason Aronson, 1970.

Haley, J. Marriage therapy. *Archives of General Psychiatry*, 1963, *8*, 213–234. (a)

Haley, J. *Strategies of psychotherapy*. New York: Grune and Stratton, 1963. (b)

Haley, J. Approaches to family therapy. *International Journal of Psychiatry*, 1970, *9*, 233–243.

Haley, J. Family therapy: A radical change. In J. Haley (Ed.), *Changing families*. New York: Grune and Stratton, 1971. (a)

Haley, J. A review of the family therapy field. In J. Haley (Ed.), *Changing families*. New York: Grune and Stratton, 1971. (b)

Haley, J. *Uncommon therapy: The psychiatric techniques of Milton H. Erickson, M.D.* New York: Norton, 1973.

Haley, J. *Problem-solving therapy*. New York: Harper & Row, 1976.

Haley, J. Toward a theory of pathological systems. In P. Watzlawick and J. H. Weakland (Eds.), *The interactional view*. New York: W. W. Norton, 1977.

Haley, J., and Hoffman, L. *Techniques of family therapy*. New York: Basic Books, 1967.

Jackson, D. D. The question of family homeostatis. *Psychiatric Quarterly, Supplement*, 1957, *31*, 79–90.

Jackson, D. D. *The etiology of schizophrenia*. New York: Basic Books, 1960.

Jackson, D. D. The study of the family. *Family Process*, 1965, *4*, 1–2. (a)

Jackson, D. D. Family rules: Marital quid pro quo. *Archives of General Psychiatry*, 1965, *12*, 589–594. (b)

Jackson, D. D. Family practice: A comprehensive medical approach. *Comprehensive Psychiatry*, 1966, *7*, 338–344.

Jackson, D. D. They myth of normality. *Medical Opinion Review*, 1967, *3*, 28–33.

Jackson, D. D. The study of the family. In N. W. Ackerman (Ed.), *Family process*. New York: Basic Books, 1970.

Jackson, D. D., and Weakland, J. H. Conjoint family therapy: Some consideration on theory, technique, and results. *Psychiatry*, 1961, *24*, 30–45.

Jackson, D. D. The study of the family. In P. Watzlawick and J. H. Weakland (Eds.), *The interactional view*. New York: W. W. Norton, 1977.

Jackson, D. D., and Weakland, J. H. Conjoint family therapy: Some consideration on theory, technique and results. In J. Haley (Ed.), *Changing families*. New York: Grune and Stratton, 1971.

Jackson, D. D., and Yalom, I. Conjoint family therapy as an aid to intensive psychotherapy. In A. Burton (Ed.), *Modern psychotherapeutic practice: Innovations in technique*. Palo Alto: Science and Behavior Books, 1965.

Jackson, D. D., and Yalom, I. Family research on the problem of ulcerative colitis. *Archives of General Psychiatry*, 1966, *15*, 410–418.

Kelly, G. A. *The psychology of personal constructs*. New York: W. W. Norton, 1955.

Leary, T. *Interpersonal diagnosis of personality*. New York: Ronald Press, 1957.

Lederer, W. J., and Jackson, D. D. *The mirages of marriage*. New York: W. W. Norton, 1968.

Meichenbaum, D. *Cognitive-behavior modification*. New York: Plenum, 1977.

Minuchin, S. *Families and family therapy*. Cambridge, Mass.: Harvard University Press, 1974.

Nunnally, E. W., Millen, S., and Wackman, D. B. The Minnesota couples communication program. *Small Group Behavior*, 1975, *6*, 57–71.

Olson, D. H. Marital and family therapy: A critical review. In A. S. Gurman and D. G. Rice (Eds.), *Couples in conflict*. New York: Jason Aronson, 1975.

Rapoport, A. Mathematics and cybernetics. In S. Arieti (Ed.), *American handbook of psychiatry* Vol. 1, 2nd ed., New York: Basic Books, 1974.

Sager, C. J. *Marriage contracts and couple therapy*. New York: Brunner/Mazel, 1976.

Satir, V. *Conjoint family therapy*. Palo Alto: Science and Behavior Books, 1967.

Satir, V. The family as a treatment unit. In J. Haley (Ed.), *Changing families*. New York: Grune and Stratton, 1971.

Satir, V. *Peoplemaking*. Palo Alto: Science and Behavior Books, 1972.

Satir, V. Stachowiak, J., and Taschman, H. A. *Helping families to change*. New York: Jason Aronson, 1975.

Segraves, R. T. Primary orgasmic dysfunction: Essential treatment components. *Journal of Sex and Marital Therapy*, 1976, *2*, 115–123.

Segraves, R. T. Conjoint marital therapy: A cognitive behavioral model. *Archives of General Psychiatry*, 1978, *35*, 450–455.

Sluzki, C. E., Beavin, J., Tarnopolsky, A., and Vernon, E. Transactional disqualification: Research on the double bind. *Archives of General Psychiatry*, 1967, *16*, 494–504.

Sluzki, C. E., and Vernon, E. The double bind as a universal pathogenic situation. *Family Process*, 1971, *10*, 397–410.

Steinglass, P. The conceptualization of marriage from a systems theory perspective. In T. J. Paolino and B. S. McCrady (Eds.), *Marriage and marital therapy*. New York: Brunner/Mazel, 1978.

Stotland, E., and Canon, L. K. *Social psychology: A cognitive approach*. Philadelphia: W. B. Saunders, 1972.

Stuart, R. B. Operant-interpersonal treatment for marital discord. *Journal of Consulting and Clinical Psychology*, 1969, *33*, 675–682.

Thomas, E. J. *Marital communication and decision making: Analysis, assessment and change*. New York: Free Press, 1977.

von Bertalanffy, L. General systems theory—A critical review. *General Systems Yearbook*, 1962, *8*, 1–20.

von Bertalanffy, L. *General systems theory*. New York: George Braziller, 1968.

von Bertalanffy, L. General systems theory and psychiatry. In S. Arieti (Ed.), *American handbook of psychiatry*, Vol. 1, 2nd ed., New York: Basic Books, 1974.

Watzlawick, P. Introduction. In P. Watzlawick and J. H. Weakland (Eds.), *The interactional view*. New York: W. W. Norton, 1977.

Watzlawick, P., and Beavin, J. Some formal aspects of communication. *American Behavioral Sciences*, 1967, *10*, 4–8.

Watzlawick, P., Beavin, J. H., and Jackson, D. D. *Pragmatics of human communication*. New York: Norton, 1967.

Watzlawick, P., Weakland, J., and Fisch, R. *Change: Principles of problem formation and problem resolution*. New York: W. W. Norton, 1974.

Weakland, J. H. The double-bind theory by self-reflexive hindsight. *Family Process*, 1974, *13*, 269–277.

Weakland, J. Communication theory and clinical change. In P. J. Gurein (Ed.), *Family therapy*. New York: Gardner Press, 1976.

CHAPTER FIVE

# Behavioral Marital Therapy

Behavioral marital therapy is one of the most recent entries into the field of marital therapy. Behavior therapists have begun to make significant contributions to the treatment of marital discord only in the last 10–15 years. This field really began in 1965 when Goldiamond pointed out how a husband controlled his wife's behavior by stimuli he provided her. Thus, "If he wished his wife to behave differently to him, then he should provide other stimuli than the ones which produced the behavior he did not like" (Goldiamond, 1965, p. 856). Goldiamond's pioneering work was soon followed by case reports by Lazarus in 1968 and by Stuart in 1969. Shortly thereafter, the behavioral marital therapy literature burgeoned with numerous case reports, literature reviews, and treatment program descriptions (Gurman and Knudson, 1978). The rapid acceptance of this new treatment approach is especially notable among recent graduates of clinical psychology programs in this country, although it has won some psychiatrists to its ranks (e.g., Liberman, 1975; Crowe, 1973; Stern and Marks, 1973). Part of the rapid growth in popularity of this approach is its appeal to professionals who feel that treatment approaches should be firmly linked to the terminology, if not the methodology, of the stricter psychological sciences.

Behavior therapy was viewed by its founders as the first school of therapy concerned with applying scientific principles to the study and treatment of human behavioral problems (Eysenck and Beech, 1971). This approach stresses "the systematic application of experimentally derived behavior-analysis principles to effect observable and, at least in principle, measurable changes in this [person–environment] interaction process" (Birk *et al.*, 1973). This approach points out that as one analyzes the events that systematically covary with certain behaviors, one can detect the environment events that control that behavior. Thus, by modifying the controlling environment events, one should be able to design an intervention that would modify the troublesome behavior. This approach is solely or predominantly concerned with overt behavior and uses the language system of experimental psychology. As neurotic disturbance is considered to be predominantly behavioral, behavioral change is the goal of therapy. Interpersonal or marital difficulties can thus be understood by identifying the contingencies maintaining the disturbed behavior and corrected by changing these contingencies.

The behavioral approach to the treatment of marital difficulties has many conceptual and technical similarities to the interactional approach advocated by Haley, Jackson, and Satir. Both approaches arose from a dissatisfaction with the mentalism of psychoanalysis and a shared belief that therapists should focus on observable behavior rather than speculate about hypothetical mental entities (Jacobson and Weiss, 1978). The behavioral marital therapists are similar to the general system theorists on numerous other points as well. Both schools tend to view marital difficulties in an ahistorical manner and to assume that situational (environment) determinants of behavior are of primary importance. Both groups of therapists tend to be active and directive and to focus on, behavioral change. In many ways, behavioral marital therapy can be viewed as a logical extension of the broad outlines of therapy sketched by Jackson and Haley. The behaviorists precisely defined and operationalized many of the concepts introduced by the system therapists. For example, Haley described how a concerted effort to change a spouse's behavior stabilized the system because of the spouse's natural inclination to resist compulsory behavioral change (Haley, 1973). The behaviorists observe the same phenomenon and conclude that coercion (negative reinforcement and punishment) is an inefficient technique to induce behavior change (Weiss et al., 1973). There are other parallel developments. Jackson emphasized the need for clear communication in families. Current behavior therapists have developed communication training treatment packages (Gottman et al., 1976a). Whereas Lederer and Jackson emphasized the need for equality between marital partners, the behavioral marital therapists have introduced reciprocity of reinforcement exchange programs (e.g., Stuart, 1972) and formal marital quid pro quo contracts (e.g., Rapoport and Harrel, 1975). Similarly, Haley spoke of the need for couples to develop rules for resolving conflict. Modern behaviorists have developed programs to teach decision-making and conflict-resolution skills (e.g., Thomas, 1977).

However, there are certain real differences between behavioral marital therapists and general systems theorists. Strict behaviorists tend to limit their observations to blatantly observable data (Mahoney, 1974) and to dismiss nuances of interpersonal communication contained in many behavioral sequences (Gurman *et al.*, 1978). To experienced clinicians such as Jackson, the work of many behaviorists appears remarkably naïve and concrete. For example, behavior therapists prompt couples into exchanging series of desired behaviors (e.g., going to bed without hair curlers in exchange for taking out the garbage) without considering whether these discrete behaviors might be representative of general classes of behavior (e.g., power struggles). On other occasions, the choice of exchanged behaviors chosen by the therapist appear bizarre and remarkably naïve. Stuart's (1969) case example of encouraging a husband to bargain an exchange of time in conversation for sex favors from his wife exemplifies this. The point is not whether this might be an appropriate intervention for some couples. It might even be construed as a Hallian maneuver to metaphorically concretize the unspoken quid pro quo of the relationship. The point is that the therapist evidenced no awareness of this possibility or of the possibility that this intervention could be counterproductive in certain couples. The difference between the behaviorists and the general systems therapists appears to be that some behaviorists, in their rush to count and modify behavior, overlook the possibility that this behavior has a shared interpersonal meaning in an interpersonal context. In many instances, they appear to modify behavior before first appreciating the ecology of the behavioral system they are modifying.

   The main contribution of behavioral marital therapists is their effort to precisely define their interventions and to empirically test the effectiveness of their interventions. If their procedures are ineffective or if their hypotheses are incorrect, this will be discoverable. The procedures of this school are such that its basic premises can lead to its own destruction. This compliment can't be given to either of the other major schools of therapy. In fact, this approach has already generated an impressive research literature (e.g., Jacobson and Martin, 1976; Greer and D'Zurilla, 1975). If their procedures are proven valuable, they are clearly specified and thus can be taught to other therapists. The specification of procedures should minimize the importance of the artistry of the therapist. In other words, numerous therapists should be able to incorporate these procedures into treatment approaches and potentially help large numbers of disturbed marriages.

   In the earlier paragraphs of this section, it was stated that behavioral marital therapists are concerned solely with the modification of observable behavior. This is not completely true. The behavioral approach, similar to psychoanalytic marital therapy, is not a unified approach. There are considerable variations between treatment approaches and theoretical conceptions of marital therapists who identify themselves as behaviorists. This blurring of boundaries is primarily the result of changes within the field of behavior therapy as a whole. Initially, behavior therapy was advocated as the introduction of scientific principles into psychotherapy. By focusing only on observable events (behavior), it was felt that a science of stimulus–response relationships could be applied to human problems. However, many behavioral clinicians began to deviate from this paradigm by making inferences about organismic variables. Currently, many clinicians refer to their approach as mediational behaviorism (Jacobson and Margolin, 1979). Many of these clinicians make implicit and explicit assumptions about internal cognitive and emotional events.

Part of the confusion of terms is explainable by realizing that behaviorism has become a school or an ideology in the same manner as the psychoanalytic movement (Hunt and Dyrud, 1968; London, 1972). Thus, one finds behavioral authors justifying their deviations from behavioral principles by quoting Skinner (e.g., Mahoney, 1974). My criticism is not that one shouldn't consider cognitive-perceptual variables, but that one should keep one's paradigms clean. Mentalism need not be purified by attaching the label behavioral. It appears that clinicians of all three schools (behavioral, psychoanalytic, and systems) are grappling with the same issue—how to legitimately address the relationships between behavior and internal mental events. However, an appreciation of the "behavioral" approach to marital discord will necessitate a brief diversion into the history and development of behaviorism and behavior therapy. In that way, the essence of behavior therapy that doesn't overlap with analytic or systems concepts can be better appreciated.

## BEHAVIORISM AND BEHAVIOR THERAPY

Behaviorism is a philosophical orientation or a philosophy of science within the psychological sciences (Chaplin and Krawiec, 1962). This viewpoint holds that the objective study of publicly observable data is the exclusive basis for scientific investigation. Thus, psychological sciences should concern themselves solely with the study of input–output relationships, i.e., stimulus–response relationships or environment–organism relationships. Although a given environmental stimulus may undergo various modifications within the organism before a response is emitted, these processes are considered unknowable. Such covert processes are considered to be beyond the scope of scientific investigation. Concepts such as mind, conscious processes, and mental image are considered to be carry-overs from mental philosophy and to have no place in science. The behavioral metaphysical position holds that behavior should be described in "terms of stimulus and response, in terms of habit formation, habit integration and the like" (Watson, 1914, p. 9). Thus, the aim of science should be to predict the response to a given stimulus without speculating about events contained within the organism. Emotions and thoughts are relegated to the role of acquired visceral and skeletal habits.

Behaviorists have also suggested that the explanation for behavior should be at the level of observation: "That is, stimulus-response relationships should be explained in terms of stimulus and response" (Mahoney, 1974, p. 26). The reason for this is that introduction of concepts at a different level is considered to be both unnecessary and confounding (Skinner, 1950). For example, if a husband continually berates his wife, one cannot say that he does this because he is angry at her. This inference is based on certain observable behaviors and contains no more information than the observations. This type of reasoning is referred to as explanatory fictions (Ullman and Krasner, 1969). A similar phenomenon is reification (Mischel, 1971). Certain behavioral acts are summarized by a label at a different level of abstraction and this label becomes a property possessed by the organism and causing his behavior. Again, a tautology masquerades as an explanation. The husband who berates his wife is labeled as being a hostile man. Then his hostility causes his behavior. Use of inferred variables at a different level of abstraction can also result in what Skinner labels incomplete casual analysis (Skinner, 1963). If stimuli and responses occur in sequences, the use of inferred variables may circumvent the search for antecedent conditions. For example, attributing the husband's behavior to his inner hostility may obscure the search for the antecedent conditions for his hostility. His wife's behavior may be the important antecedent condition.

Mahoney (1974) points out how behaviorism in current usage refers to two separate groups of philosophical assumptions. Metaphysical behaviorism (true behaviorism) holds that the scientific study of human behavior can only concern itself with publicly observable behavior. This is the position advocated by Watson (1924). Methodological behaviorism refers to the use of scientific methodology in the study of human difficulties in living. This viewpoint advocates controlled experimentation, independent replication of results, operationism of concepts, and testability of hypotheses. Methodological behaviorism is really a misnomer. It refers simply to the use of scientific methodology. As will become obvious later in this chapter, the concept of methodological behaviorism creates conceptual confusion. Nonmetaphysical behaviorists often label themselves as behaviorists when they are concerned with mentalistic phenomena. The use of scientific methodology does not create a behaviorist.

Two basic paradigms evolved for the study of environmental–organism interactions. These paradigms are the operant and respondent conditioning paradigms. Although there is some controversy at present about the degree of overlap between the two paradigms (Kanfer and Phillips, 1970), each represents a distinctive orientation toward the study of organism–environment interactions.

Respondent conditioning is also known as classical conditioning. It is primarily concerned with elicited behavior that is involuntary or reflexive in nature and the role of antecedent stimuli (eliciting stimuli) in producing this behavior. The process by which previously neutral environment stimuli acquire the ability to elicit reflexive behavior is the result of respondent conditioning. By repeated pairing of neutral stimuli with naturally occurring eliciting stimuli, the neutral stimuli acquire the ability to elicit responses, e.g., they become conditioned stimuli. Much of the classical conditioning approach derives from Pavlov's early work. Pavlov demonstrated that dogs could be trained to salivate to previously neutral stimuli by pairing these stimuli with a natural eliciting stimulus (meat) over a series of trials (Pavlov, 1927). Thereafter, a neutral stimulus such as a bell would reliably elicit salivation in dogs. Watson and Rayner (1920) reported a similar experiment in the human. Little Albert, an 11-month-old infant, was unafraid of a laboratory rat. However, striking a steel bar behind the child's head elicited a startle response, an unconditioned response. Repeated pairings of the unconditioned stimulus (hitting the metal bar) with the conditioned stimulus (white rat) led to a conditioned response, a startle response upon seeing the white rat.

Operant conditioning (instrumental learning) is primarily concerned with the relationship between voluntary behavior and the events that follow it. In other words, behavior of the organism in relationship to its environment is determined by the presence or absence of rewards. Behavior is determined by its consequences. Operant conditioning is primarily concerned with specifying the relationship between behavior and its environmental consequences. "As organisms interact continuously with their environment, their behaviors are constantly being affected by the presence or absence of rewarding and punishing stimuli. It is possible to describe the contingencies of reinforcement in well-controlled experimental settings, that is, the exact relationships between behavior and its consequences" (Jacobson and Margolin, 1979, p. 10).

Environment consequences are classified by the way they affect the organism's behavior. Positive reinforcement refers to a stimulus that increases the probability of the behaviors it follows. Thus, it is defined empirically by its effect on behavior. Negative reinforcement refers to a stimulus whose termination leads to an increase in the frequency of the behavior that preceded its termination. If a wife nags her husband until he carries out the garbage and his taking out the garbage is increased by her stopping nagging, his behavior can be referred to as under negative reinforcement control. Punishment refers to a stimulus that decreases the likelihood of a behavior it follows. If a husband talks of divorce when his wife nags and this behavior stops her nagging, her nagging behavior can be described as partially under punishment control.

The operant model specifies another type of antecedent stimuli—discriminative stimuli. This concept helps explain how operant behavior acquires connections with the environment. Discriminative stimuli are stimuli that indicate the probable reinforcement values of various behaviors. Skinner illustrates this concept by a discussion of a pigeon whose neck-stretching is reinforced by food only when a light is on: "We describe the contingency by saying that a stimulus (the light) is the occasion upon which a response (stretching the neck) is followed by reinforcement (with food). We must specify all terms. The effect upon the pigeon is that eventually the response is more likely to occur when the light is on. The process through which this comes about is called discrimination. Its importance in a theoretical analysis, as well as in the practical control of behavior, is obvious. When a discrimination has been established, we may alter the probability of a response instantly by presenting or removing the discriminative stimulus" (Skinner, 1953, p. 108). The operant literature discriminates between stimuli ($S^D$) that signal that behavior is likely to be rewarded and those ($S^\Delta$) that signal that behavior is unlikely to be rewarded. The relevance of the discriminative stimuli metaphor for understanding marital discord is obvious. Hair curlers and yawning by a wife could serve as $S^\Delta$ that sexual advances by her husband are unlikely to be rewarded.

Response chains refer to a series of responses occurring together in a reliable sequence. "In a response chain, each response serves as a $S^D$ for the subsequent responses in the chain, and the entire chain is reinforced by the event which follows completion of the chain. Response chains appear automatic once they have been learned, yet the process of acquiring such complicated sequences of responses is often gradual and tedious" (Jacobson and Margolin, 1979, p. 11). Sexual intercourse could be construed as a response chain.

## BEHAVIOR THERAPY

Behavior therapy is unique as a therapeutic school in that its emphasis is placed on modification of *symptomatic behavior per se* without consideration of the past origins or internal meaning of the symptom. Eysenck, one of the fathers of modern behavior therapy, summarizes this viewpoint cogently: "Learning theory does not postulate any such unconscious causes, but regards neurotic symptoms as simple learned habits; there is no neurosis underlying the symptom, but merely the symptom itself. Get rid of the symptom and you have eliminated the neurosis. This notion of purely symptomatic treatment is so alien to psychoanalysis that it may be considered the crucial part of the theory here proposed" (Eysenck, 1960, p. 9). In a later work, Eysenck modified this viewpoint slightly by stating that the goal of behavior therapy was to eliminate both skeletal and autonomic features of the symptom (Eysenck and Rachman, 1965). Kanfer and Phillips similarly define the activity of behavior therapists: "Behavior therapists tend to select specific symptoms or behaviors as targets for change, to employ concrete, planned interventions to manipulate these behaviors, and to monitor progress continuously and quantitatively" (1970, p. 17). Clearly, behavior therapy represents a paradigm shift from the medical model, which posits that symptoms constitute syndromes and that appropriate treatment requires recognition of the syndrome and modification of an underlying cause. In psychoanalytic theory, the hypothetical cause is often quite remote in time and character from the presenting symptom. These symptomatic treatment approaches tend to fall into two basic treatment paradigms.

The earliest work on modifying neurotic symptoms was based on the respondent model. Much of this work was based on Mowrer's (1939) two-stage theory of anxiety. In this theory, classically conditioned fear responses served as drives to motivate instrumental escape behavior. Wolpe, Eysenck, and colleagues (Wolpe, 1958; Eysenck, 1959; Lazarus, 1963) conceptualized much neurotic behavior as being the result of classical conditioning. From fortuitous association in the natural environment, certain previously neutral stimuli were assumed to have become classically conditioned to elicit anxiety. This conditioned anxiety did not extinguish as the organism learned to avoid these now noxious stimuli. Early work by these workers focused on the treatment of phobias. The treatment approach advocated was reexposure to the conditioned stimulus under circumstances allowing for extinction to occur. Procedures based on this rationale include desensitization in imagination (Rachman, 1968), *in vivo* desensitization (Marks, 1978), and flooding (Marks, 1968). A similar treatment rationale was posited for the treatment of obsessive-compulsive rituals (Marks, 1977). Aversive conditioning was based on the rationale of conditioning emotional responses to maladaptive behaviors (Rachman and Teasdale, 1969). The only marital therapy application of behavioral therapy based on the respondent model is in the treatment of sexual dysfunction. In these cases, the sexual inhibitions are construed to be the result of conditioned anxiety responses and the treatment consists of gradual extinctions of this anxiety by *in vivo* desensitization (Segraves, 1976). However, most behavioral approaches to the treatment of sexual disorders consist of mixed models and also stress how the nonsymptomatic spouse may be reinforcing the symptomatic behavior of his or her mate (Segraves, 1980).

Behavior therapy techniques based on the operant paradigm are primarily concerned with modifying the consequences of problematic behavior. This approach assumes that problematic behavior is maintained by environmental consequences. If these consequences are rearranged, the problematic behavior should be eliminated. Similarly, desired behavior should increase in frequency if it is reinforced: "Therapeutic interventions based on the operant model primarily rearrange contingent behavioral consequences, including rewards and punishments, in order to alter undesired behaviors or to remedy behavioral deficiencies. The operant paradigm, since it does not require specification of antecedent stimulus conditions, is more convenient for conceptualizing and manipulating a wide range of responses in natural settings that do not permit clear identification of eliciting stimuli. Consequences that have effects on both the surrounding world and the behaving individual are the major objects of observation because they largely control the probability that the behavior that produced them will occur again" (Kanfer and Phillips, 1970, p. 241).

Early operant conditioning work was primarily concerned with hospitalized psychiatric patients or institutionalized children (e.g., Lindsley, 1956; Lovaas and Bucher, 1974). This is primarily because greater control of environmental contingencies was possible in these settings. This early work was the forerunner of token economy systems in institutional settings (Ayllon and Azrin, 1965). This system is based on the assumption that adaptive behavior can be increased by regularly reinforcing such behavior. Tokens are given for desired behavior, and these tokens can be exchanged for rewards. More recently, however, operant conditioning techniques have been applied to more neurotic disorders such as phobias (Agras *et al.*, 1968), depression (Seligman *et al.*, 1976), eating disorders (Stunkard and Mahoney, 1976), and other neurotic conditions (Leitenberg, 1976; Kazdin, 1978).

The essence of the operant approach to treatment can be subsumed under four major intervention strategies: use of positive reinforcement, extinction by removal of reinforcement for undesired behavior, shaping, and manipulation of discriminative stimuli. The use of positive reinforcement to increase the rate of desired behaviors is one of the main contributions of operant therapists and has the side effect of shifting the therapists' set from concern over eliminating neurotic behavior to the promotion of adaptive behavior. A classic example of this approach was reported by Allen and colleagues (1964). A nursery school child was observed to interact freely with teachers and adults but to play only seldom with other children. Her playing with other children was increased considerably by having teacher attention be contingent on playing with other children. Ingram (1967) reported a similar study on using positive reinforcement to increase peer interaction in a nursery school child. His study was interesting in that the behavior was maintained after therapeutic reinforcements were withdrawn. It is assumed that certain behaviors will be naturally reinforced by the environment once a certain threshold has been reached. Several authors have referred to the environmental maintenance of new behavior as the "behavioral trap" (Baer and Wolf, 1967). Similar techniques have been used successfully to modify eating behavior in anorexia nervosa. In these studies, certain reinforcements such as social interaction and physical activity are made contingent upon weight gain (e.g., Bachrach *et al.*, 1965; Blinder *et al.*, 1970). The demonstrated effectiveness of positive reinforcement procedures in a variety of clinical settings has clearly influenced behavioral marital therapists, who consistently work to get couples to employ positive reinforcement procedures with each other (Patterson *et al.*, 1976). If a couple can be shifted into a new style of interaction based on positive reinforcement, it is assumed that this new style of interacting will be self-sustaining. In other words, the therapists hope to modify the marital interaction such that a "marital behavioral trap" occurs.

It is of note that operant therapists seldom use punishment as a means of reducing undesired behaviors. Punishment has consistently been found to be a relatively ineffective means of suppressing behavior (Skinner, 1953). This finding partially explains the tendency of behavioral marital therapists to try to get couples to employ behavioral change maneuvers other than punishment.

Rather than use punishment to suppress undesirable behavior, operant therapists tend to employ extinction procedures. If one observes a specified behavior, one will usually find that this behavior is maintained by certain environmental contingencies. Alteration of these contingencies should lead to the extinction of the behavior in question. For example, Ayllon and Micheal (1954) noted that a psychotic patient's disruptive behavior was maintained by nurse attention. When attention for this disruptive behavior was withheld, the behavior dropped in frequency. Similarly, other behavior therapists have noted that children's temper tantrums may be reinforced unwittingly by parental responses. Modification of parental responses has led to a decrease in this behavior. Goldiamond (1965) was addressing this issue when he instructed a distraught husband to modify his wife's behavior by withdrawing his reinforcement for that behavior. In the field of sex therapy, it is quite common to observe a wife's lack of sexual responsiveness being maintained by her husband's urgent insistence that she be sexually responsive. It is a common clinical observation that if one can successfully modify the husband's behavior, his wife will progressively become more sexually responsive.

Shaping and stimulus control procedures are less commonly used in behavioral marital therapy. Shaping refers to the process by which complex new behaviors are molded by building chains of simpler responses: "An operant is not something which appears full grown in the behavior of the organism. It is the result of a continuous shaping process" (Skinner, 1953, p. 91). A classic example of shaping was reported by Goldiamond and his associates (Isaacs et al., 1960). A mute psychotic was first reinforced for looking at chewing gum, then for lip movements while looking at the gum. Later, he was given the gum only if he vocalized a sound. Eventually, the reinforcement was given only for closer and closer approximations of the sound of the word *gum*. Shaping as a concept has perhaps influenced behavioral marital therapy indirectly, as therapists instruct couples not to expect the desired behavior immediately. They have to expect to shape the desired behavior.

Stimulus control procedures have had a minimal impact on behavioral marital therapy to date. These procedures are concerned with manipulating the stimuli governing certain behaviors. These procedures are used in the control of overeating. A patient is instructed to eat in one location alone and to indulge in eating only at that time to bring eating under stimulus control (Stuart, 1967). Similar types of interventions have been used to bring studying (Fox, 1962) and smoking (Bernard and Efran, 1972) under stimulus control. It is of note that Haley could be described as using a stimulus control procedure when he instructed couples to argue only at specific times and places. Similarly, Goldiamond (1965) used this concept to decrease arguing in a couple. They were required to have conversations in a setting where arguments were unlikely to occur.

In the last 10 years, there has been a revival of interest in cognitive variables among clinical psychologists (Mahoney and Arnkoff, 1978).

Part of this interest stems from work by Bandura and his associates (Rosenthal and Bandura, 1978; Bandura, 1969, 1977) on vicarious learning. They demonstrated that learning could occur without overt practice reinforced by environmental contingencies. New skills could be acquired by observing another individual in a learning situation. This led to the conclusion that the behavioral outcome in any given situation is strongly dependent on organismic variables—i.e., thought and perceptual process. This revival of interest in cognitive process was aided by Piaget's description of the infant as an active information-seeking being, by which internal cognitive structure evolved (Murray and Jacobson, 1978). Similarly, Homme's work on covert conditioning suggested that thought processes could be scientifically studied and controlled by a coverant behavioral technology (Homme, 1965). This development laid the groundwork for a group of intervention strategies alternatively labeled mediational behaviorism or by the misnomer cognitive behaviorism. Therapists of this school are concerned with direct modification of thought process. They resemble behaviorists in their use of the language of learning theory, their emphasis on the therapist's activity, and their concern with molecular rather than molar units of behavior.

However, this approach should not be confused with behaviorism. The boundaries between behaviorism and cognitivism should be kept distinct. The social learning school of thought represents a revival of interest in cognitive processes and the study of the reciprocal relationship between the organism and his environment.

## BASIC CONCEPTS IN BEHAVIORAL MARITAL THERAPY

Many of the behavioral marital therapists have been influenced by social exchange theorists such as Thibaut and Kelley (1959) and Homans (1961). Social exchange theorists are concerned with the interdependence of persons in social relationships and attempt to define outcomes or payoffs relative to costs to participants in social interaction. Although Homans evolved a more formal and elaborate theory of social exchange than did Thibaut and Kelley (Chadwick-Jones, 1976), the work of Thibaut and Kelley appears to have had more impact on behavioral therapists.

In any dyadic relationship, according to Thibaut and Kelley, participants strive to maximize rewards while minimizing costs. Thus, social relationships are influenced by the ratio of rewards and costs for each participant, since "for a dyadic relationship to be viable it must provide rewards and/or economics in costs which compare favorably with those in other competing relationships or activities available to individuals"

(Thibaut and Kelley, 1959, p. 49). The viability of dyadic relationships is hypothesized to require this reward/cost ratio to be higher than the comparative level of alternative relationships. In other words, the relationship will survive only if the individuals receive more rewards in this relationship than in alternative possibilities. "This means that for each member adequate rewards must be provided and costs of participation in the group must be kept down to reasonable levels" (Thibaut and Kelley, 1959, p. 24). A peculiarity of dyadic situations is the independence of reinforcement. "The joint payoff matrix for couples contains an inherent confusion" (Weiss, 1978, p. 186). Thus, for a relationship to be mutually satisfying, each partner must obtain a reward/cost ratio above possible alternative relationships. This creates a difficulty in that each spouse's behavior in a relationship is partially determined by the other spouse's behavior. "The most socially significant behavior will not be repeated unless it is reinforced" (Thibaut and Kelley, 1959, p. 12).

The impact of this conceptual model is evident in the work of most marital therapists. For example, Azrin and associates (1973) described a reciprocity approach to the treatment of marital discord that they state is based on learning theory and experimentally derived principles. They state that "happiness in marriage is considered to result when the reinforcements (satisfactions) derived from marriage exceed the reinforcements derived from the nonmarital state" (p. 367). Similarly, Stuart (1969) has clearly been influenced by the model when he states that "the exact pattern of interaction which takes place between spouses at any given point in time is the most rewarding of all the available alternatives" (Stuart, 1969, p. 675). Other theorists have also been influenced by this theoretical approach (Jacobson and Margolin, 1979; Weiss, 1978).

This conceptual orientation clearly complements the operant approach, which stresses that behavior is maintained by its consequences. A consistent theme of behavioral marital therapists is that in cases of marital discord, the costs are high relative to the rewards. One of the major sources of marital discord is that "the reinforcements received from marriage are too few in number" (Azrin et al., 1973, p. 367). Stuart (1968) and others (Jacobson and Martin, 1976; Wieman et al., 1974) have made similar observations. There is some empirical support for this assumption. Birchler (1973) found that couples in distressed marriages reported fewer exchanges of rewarding behavior on a behavior checklist. Using laboratory coding of behavioral interactions in standardized problem-solving settings, distressed couples have been observed to exchange fewer positive interactions as coded by independent raters (Birchler, 1973; Vincent et al., 1975). Similarly, distressed couples have been reported to have lower rates of presumably rewarding activities such as sexual activity, conversation (Stuart, 1969), and joint recreational activities (Weiss *et al.*, 1973).

A related hypothesis is that distressed marriages are characterized by higher costs, i.e., negative interchanges between spouses. Patterson *et al.* (1976) speak of the crucial role of punishment in distressed marriages. A coercive process is hypothesized to occur when one spouse requests a behavioral change in the other and the other spouse doesn't comply. This sequence can then lead to the deliverance of an aversive stimulus. "It is assumed that when one member introduces an aversive stimulus, the interaction shifts into a coercion process. An aversive stimulus is presented in either of two ways. It can be delivered contingently following a certain response which is to be suppressed, or it can be presented prior to the behavior which is to be manipulated and then withdrawn only when the other person complies. Punishment and negative reinforcement describe the process involved in coercion." (Patterson *et al.*, 1976b, p. 244). Coercion is considered to be a high-cost behavior change mechanism in that it usually elicits reciprocal aversive behavior in the spouse. Typical aversive stimuli in marriage would include nagging and character assassination. As might be expected, there is considerable evidence that distressed marriages are characterized by more aversive stimuli, as perceived both by the participants (Gottman *et al.*, 1976) and by outside observers (Birchler *et al.*, 1975).

A closely related concept that has received less empirical support is the concept of reciprocity. This concept rests on the hypothesis that each spouse desires reinforcements from the other, and the only way this can occur is for each spouse to contingently reinforce the other spouse for reinforcing behavior. Thus, good marriages are hypothesized to be characterized by reciprocity of reinforcement exchange. Several studies have reported associations between exchanges of rewards to be higher in nondistressed marriages than in distressed marriages (Birchler, 1973; Wills *et al.*, 1974; Birchler *et al.*, 1975). However, Gottman *et al.* (1976b) have criticized these findings as being artifacts of high rates of positive responses in happy marriages. In happy marriages, if the spouses emit high rates of positive responses to each other, this may increase the probability of a positive response by one being followed by a positive response by the other. This doesn't demonstrate reciprocity of reinforcement. It only demonstrates a high base rate for positive responses. Gottman and his colleagues formally tested the reciprocity hypothesis in a standardized high-conflict task situation and found minimal support for the view that disturbed marriages are characterized by less positive and more negative reciprocity than happy marriages.

Although different behaviorally oriented marital therapists have slightly different conceptions of the genesis and maintenance of marital discord, all share the tendency to use operant principles to evaluate disturbed behavior problems in distressed marriages. In the writing of most operant conditioning therapists, the use of negative reinforcement as a behavior change mechanism in distressed marriages is stressed as a core concept (e.g., Weiss *et al.*, 1974; Knox, 1974; O'Leary and Turkewitz, 1978). A successful marriage is viewed as requiring numerous modifications of each spouse's behavior. Conflict arises when requests for change are met with noncompliance and one spouse resorts to coercive behavior change mechanisms. The use of faulty procedures to attempt to change the spouse's behavior is considered to be the crucial interpersonal error in disturbed marriages. As the whole field of operant conditioning is concerned with developing a technology of behavior control, operant therapists are attempting to transfer this technology to the marital situation. All such therapists would agree that the transfer of this technology is complicated by the fact that each spouse partially controls the behavior of the other by the contingencies he or she establishes for that behavior. Therefore, therapeutic change requires a simultaneous change in both spouses.

## TREATMENT

Two principal approaches have been taken in the behavioral treatment of marital discord. The end point of one treatment approach is some form of mutual exchange of positive reinforcements on the assumption that positive reinforcement is more effective than coercive control as a change mechanism. The procedures following this rationale would include contracting (Stuart, 1969), reciprocity counseling (Azrin *et al.*, 1973), and negotiating training (Weiss, *et al.*, 1974). In less technical terminology, the spouses are taught how to barter effectively.

The other approach emphasizes the teaching of communication skills to distressed couples. This approach tends to emphasize that distressed marriages result from faulty communication patterns (e.g., Thomas, 1977; Gottman *et al.*, 1976a). One of the reasons couples have difficulty resolving and negotiating conflicts is that their communication patterns are such that the source of the conflict and thus possible solutions are never clearly specified in communicative interactions.

Although there is considerable overlap between the two approaches and many therapists use combinations of both approaches, each approach has its respective technology and will be considered separately.

## Positive Reinforcement Exchange Procedures

Behavior marital therapy programs based on increasing the exchange of positive reinforcement between partners usually contain at least three parts: an orientation to the rationale of the program stressing operationalizing complaints, specifying desired behavioral change in the partner, and contracting for a mutual acceleration of these behaviors. "Pinpointing, negotiating, and setting-up contracts become the modus operandi" (Patterson and Hops, 1972, p. 432).

Therapists differ in the degree to which they explicitly orient patients to the theoretical rationale of their program. Stuart (1969) explicitly informs spouses that their impressions of one another are the result of observed behavior and that personality differences are not the cause of their problem. He similarly informs them that the behavior of each of them is controlled by the behavior of the other and that both must therefore change. The precise orientation offered by others is less clear. Couples are taught to operationalize their complaints and requests for change. Global complaints and vague statements are converted into specific concrete operations. In particular, molar statements are converted into molecular statements. For example, if a husband states that his wife should be more "feminine," the therapist would require the husband to pinpoint exactly what he means by that statement. This global statement might be a request for anything from more frequent sexual activities to his wife not interrupting him at social gatherings. He would further be required to specify the conditions under which he desires this behavior to occur and at what frequencies. Most therapists also tend to convert terminal hypotheses into instrumental hypotheses (Hurvitz, 1975). For example, a statement that one's husband is passive would be converted into a statement that he possesses certain behavior that the wife labels as passive. The specific behaviors could then be pinpointed as targets for change. A common problem in couples is their expectancy of clairvoyance—"she should know"—or their tendency to make vague expectational statements. These too would be converted into specific nondemanding requests.

The second stage in most programs is pinpointing specific behavioral changes desired from the other. At this point, most therapists would focus on low-frequency positive occurrences to be accelerated rather than on the elimination of aversive behavior. Patients would also be required by most therapists to record the frequency of these behaviors. The Oregon Social Learning group uses a daily list of Pleases and Displeases for this purpose. This recording of base rates serves the purpose of focusing the couple's attention on positive interchanges as well as negative ones, as well as documenting changes in the desired frequency of such behaviors. The couple would be required to set values for the desired behavioral changes in order to differentiate minor from more important requests. Through this interchange, a menu of rewards and possible penalties evolves.

The next stage involves setting up an agreement whereby behaviors may be equitably exchanged. Some therapists do this informally by simply asking spouses if they are willing to exchange certain behaviors. For example, Stern and Marks (1973) worked successfully with a couple by getting the wife to exchange 10 minutes of having her breast touched and 15 minutes of reading a sexual manual for the husband's completing various household tasks such as redecorating the kitchen. Other therapists have evolved more formal reward and punishment systems. These contracts have tended to take one of two forms: a quid pro quo model or a good faith model (Weiss et al., 1974). The quid pro quo model is based on contingent exchanges of reinforcers. An example of a quid pro quo model would be the exchange of washing dishes for a home-cooked meal. This model has tended to be used less frequently, as the behavior desired by each spouse is yoked to the behavior desired by the other. If one spouse fails to act, the system fails to operate. Stuart (1969) slightly modified this model by the exchange of tokens for desired behavior. A certain number of tokens could then be exchanged for reinforcers from the spouse. This model also has certain potential disadvantages. For example, if a husband desires sex and the wife desires household chores, the husband could accumulate enough tokens and demand immediate payment from his wife during a marital fight. The good faith contract attempts to circumvent these problems by not involving direct contingency control of problem behaviors. Each spouse agrees to accelerate certain desired behaviors, and rewards and punishments consist of separate events. For example, a husband might agree to accelerate time spent in conversation with his mate and his wife might agree to accelerate frequency of sexual initiations. The rewards and penalties for performance would consist of a different class of events. For example, the wife's reward might consist of money for a new dress. The husband's reward might be preparation of his favorite meal. Penalties might include a reduction in spending money or eating out.

In the Oregon model (e.g., Weiss et al., 1973), contracting and negotiation training is also used to communicate a particular philosophy of marriage: "Negotiation training refers to the fact that couples are taught to think in terms of behavioral utilities and the resources they are willing to offer in exchange for resources gained. Contracting refers to the use of a systematic procedure for setting forth behavior change agreements" (p. 328).

Most therapists would begin contracting with relatively minor issues first. After these conflicts are resolved, more emotionally laden issues would be addressed in the same manner.

## Communication

Most behavioral therapists employ some aspect of communication training as a basic skill element necessary before contracting can occur. For example, Azrin et al. (1973) employed a positive statement procedure in their rapid reciprocity counseling program. In this procedure, couples were taught how to communicate disagreements in a more positive way. For example, "That was a dumb thing to say" would be replaced with "That may be true, but have you thought of it this way?" Liberman (1975) and Stuart (1969) similarly emphasized the necessity of modifying communication prior to successful implementation of reinforcement exchange procedures. A component of the University of Oregon marital therapy package consists of a communication training module. It is clear that a large part of the module is geared toward facilitating negotiation. This is a consistent theme in many of the behavioral programs that are based on the social exchange model. As successful marriage is viewed to result from exchange of reinforcements, communication training is viewed as a necessary element to prepare couples for negotiating exchanges.

The Oregon social learning group (e.g., Weiss, Patterson, Hops, Reid, and colleagues) have described the most extensive communication training program, which is based on social exchange theory. Their treatment intervention begins with a standardized problem-solving task. Couples are asked to discuss current problems in their marriage. This discussion is videotaped and the videotape is coded by independent raters. This coding system, the Marital Interaction Coding System (Hops et al., 1971), is based on a modification of the Patterson et al. (1969) family interaction coding scheme. Twenty-nine interactive behaviors are coded in various categories, including problem solving, positive and negative responses, and negotiation-impending behaviors. It is of note that there is minimal external validation as to the validity of these codes (Gurman and Knudson, 1978). After this, couples are taught "correct" negotiation skills. Most often, cotherapists replay videotape segments, demonstrating faulty communicative behavior to the couple. Then the therapists model correct responses and coach the couple in rehearsing these skills. Couples are coached in basic skills such as reflecting back and paraphrasing the other's comments. A large portion of this training is focused on modifying behavior that decreases problem-solving efficiency. Couples are specifically coached to change behaviors that detract from the topic area or the problem to be solved. Negative behaviors of this sort would include digression, topic changes, irrelevancies, interruptions, countercomplaining, sidetracking, and excuses. Thus, couples are coached into choosing the topic to be resolved and maintaining that focus until the problem is indeed resolved. Anything diverging from that goal would be classified as faulty communication. A variety of practical suggestions about negotiations are offered to couples. They are instructed to choose specific times and places for negotiation, to choose the agenda in advance, and to announce their purposes (i.e., negotiations, catharsis, etc.). The list of positive behaviors includes describing the problem in neutral terms, listening to the other and paraphrasing the content heard, and focusing on the solution rather than on the other person. The list of negative behaviors includes discussing the past, lecturing, sidetracking, generalizing, and defending self.

Jacobson and Margolin (1979) have recently described a communication training package that overlaps considerably with the one described by the Oregon group. They differ slightly in that they view communication as a significant source of positive reinforcement as well as a basic skill necessary for negotiation. They are similar in utilizing feedback, modeling, coaching, and behavioral rehearsal as means to teach better communication skills. Their program differs slightly in technique from the Oregon approach. They tend to stress the learning-empathic listening skills. In this regard, they have been influenced by the conjugal relationship enhancement approach of Guerney (1977). They also stress the importance of "feeling-cause-statements." This refers to statements of the form "I feel X in situation Y when you do Z." This clearly reflects the influence of Satir (1967). Their list of practical suggestions for couples resembles the list elaborated by Patterson's group and consists of things such as be specific, be brief, discuss one problem at a time, don't make inferences, don't shift the focus.

Thomas (1977) has reported the most extensive study of marital communication to date. He views verbal behavior as operant responding to the contingencies provided by the mate as well as potent sources of positive/negative reinforcement to the mate. In other words, his theoretical orientation is similar to Stuart's (1969), except that he focuses his attention on verbal exchanges rather than exchanges of concrete behaviors. Thomas has evolved an unwieldy 49-category verbal behavior checklist. However, for clinical purposes, he has found that approximately 9 of these categories represent the most common communication problems (Thomas et al., 1974). These categories include (1) negative talk surfeit (i.e., aversive statements), (2) excessive disagreement, (3) positive talk deficit, (4) overgeneralization, (5) poor referent specification, (6) content shifting, (7) content persistence, (8) acknowledgment deficit, and (9) obtrusions. These behaviors are coded, preferably by on-line coding. However, for clinical purposes, a simpler verbal problem checklist has been developed (Thomas *et al.*, 1974). Using this checklist, the clinician rates each of the 49 categories after observing an interaction. Initially, Thomas and associates (1970) advocated the use of a special signaling system to modify communication patterns. During a couple interaction, a red light would flash until faulty communication ceased. However, for usual clinical purposes, simpler procedures are sufficient. The clinician chooses a few target responses identified from the verbal problem checklist, identifies the problems for the couple, and then gives instructions for correcting this problem and coaches them in practice sessions. Similar to the Marital Interaction Coding System evolved by the Oregon group, there is minimal evidence documenting that the codes used by Thomas and his associates actually differentiate good from bad marital situations.

Gottman and his associates at the University of Illinois (Gottman *et al.*, 1976a) recently described a communication training approach that has the potential of being the most clinically useful and sophisticated model to date. In a series of clinical studies, Gottman concluded that the available data offer minimal evidence for the reciprocity model as an explanation for marital distress. Although reciprocity differences tended to discriminate distressed from nondistressed marriages, the magnitude of this discrimination was not impressive. Differences in style of verbal interaction had much greater discriminatory power. In an earlier study (Gottman *et al.*, 1976b), he observed distressed couples to differ from nondistressed couples by the negative impact of their verbal statements. However, they did not differ in how they intended their messages to be received: "The couples . . . behaved in a way consistent with a communication deficit explanation of distressed marriages" (Gottman *et al.*, 1976b, p. 14). Similarly, he found minimal evidence for the reciprocity model of marital distress: "The data on reciprocity indicate only minimal support for the view that distressed marriage is characterized by less positive or more negative reciprocity than nondistressed marriage" (p. 14). In other words, distressed couples don't necessarily reciprocate negative interchanges more than nondistressed couples. Distressed couples are better differentiated by the frequency with which their intended messages are received differently. One probable explanation for this deficit is deficiency of communication skills. In subsequent work, Gottman *et al.* (1977) attempted to further delineate the nature of this communication deficit. The interactions of distressed and nondistressed couples were videotaped during conflictful discussions. These videotapes were then coded on both content and nonverbal coding scales. The eight content areas included agreement, disagreement, mind reading, problem solving, problem talk, general communication, summarizing self, and summarizing other. Face, voice, and body nonverbal cues were rated by a separate group of raters. It is of note that nonverbal behavior often discriminated couples better than verbal behavior and that particular combinations of verbal and nonverbal behavior were powerful discriminators. Distressed couples were more likely to express feelings, to disagree, and to mind-read with accompanying negative nonverbal behavior (e.g., frowning, sarcastic voice tone, pointing). It is also of note that distressed couples were more likely to express verbal agreement while expressing negative nonverbal behavior. This discrepancy could perhaps be a partial source of the communication deficit noted in distressed couples. It is interesting that this observation is consistent with the observations of general system therapists that distressed couples often manifest channel inconsistency. In other words, verbal content indicates one message while the content or nonverbal behavior indicates another. Gottman's approach to therapy resembles that described by others, such as Jacobson and Margolin (1979), and consists of establishing certain rules of good communication and coaching couples in their use.

## COMMENT AND CRITIQUE

The emphasis of the behavioral approach on specifying procedures, operationalizing concepts, and empirically investigating the outcome of treatment is a refreshing addition to the field. The tendency to provide a concise structure for therapy and a given time frame for therapy is also a nice counterbalance in the field. Similarly, the readiness to use concepts from learning theory tends to make it more firmly linked to the data and to serve as a counterbalance against the tendency of other schools of therapy to use abstract concepts whose data referents are obscure. However, the evidence to data cautions against "a near wholesale and exclusive endorsement of a behavioral approach to marital problems" (Gurman and Knudson, 1978, p. 122).

The evidence for the efficacy of this treatment approach and even the evidence regarding some of the basic assumptions underlying the approach are far from unequivocal. Although there have been a fair number of controlled studies concerning the efficacy of behavioral marital therapy (O'Leary and Turkewitz, 1978; Jacobson and Martin, 1976; Greer and D'Zurilla, 1975a, b), there is minimal evidence demonstrating the superiority of behavioral over other treatment approaches. Even behaviorists such as Jacobson and Weiss conceded this point in a recent review of the literature: "Although it is unclear whether behavior therapy is more effective than other types of intervention strategies with couples, it is certainly true that no single approach has accumulated as much empirical support at the present time" (Jacobson and Weiss, 1978, p. 157). In their review of the outcome studies, Gurman and Kniskern (1978) noted minimal evidence for the superiority of behavioral over nonbehavioral treatment approaches. They also noted that many of the behavioral outcome studies were conducted on nonclinical subjects who were minimally distressed. Other investigations have noted that studies of this sort have minimal relevance to clinical problems (Marks, 1978; Rosen, 1975). "Evidence of the efficacy of behavioral marriage therapy, however, is no more persuasive and may, in fact, be somewhat less persuasive than the existing research on nonbehavioral treatment because of too frequent use of nonclinical analogue demonstrations with minimally distressed couples" (Gurman and Kniskern, 1978, p. 144). They also note that some of the behavioral studies are flawed by the contamination of treatment and outcome parameters. For example, the Oregon group uses the tracking of positive and negative reinforcements both as a therapeutic tactic and as an outcome measure. In general, one can observe a tautology in much of the behavioral research. The subjects are trained toward a criterion and that same criterion is used as an outcome measure. For example, couples are trained in negotiation skills, and negotiation skill proficiency is measured as an outcome measure. This research demonstrates the trainability of negotiation skills as defined by the research group. However, the research doesn't demonstrate that this approach appreciably influences marital discord. Another problem in the behavioral outcome research is that, frequently, total packages consisting of numerous modules are evaluated (e.g., Jacobson, 1977). In such studies, it is impossible to determine whether the outcome was mediated by the whole package or by one or more of the separate modules.

Many of the basic assumptions underlying these approaches have minimal support to date. As previously mentioned, the evidence supporting reciprocity is equivocal. Similarly, the communication differences observed by Gottman were obtained in a restricted population and may not be generalizable. Strictly speaking, all that is known is that many couples in self-described good marriages tend to be nicer to one another (have higher emission rates of positive reinforcement and lower rates of negative reinforcement) than couples in self-described bad marriages. This finding doesn't offer differential support for the behavioral theoretical framework over any other framework.

The notion that therapeutic interventions should be ahistorical and, more particularly, that historical factors play a minor role in the genesis of marital discord is flatly contradicted by research data. At least five well-conducted prospective studies have demonstrated that premarital personality traits are related to marital outcome (Kelley, 1939; Terman, 1950; Adams, 1946; Burgen and Wallin, 1953; Bentler and Newcomb, 1978). In most of these studies, premarital personality traits suggestive of neuroticism were predictive of subsequent marital distress. Such findings don't mean that interventions have to be focused on past causes. Clearly, effective interventions don't always address etiological agents. However, these data imply that a theoretical system explaining the genesis of marital distress has to consider past personality tendencies and experiences. A focus on current observable data alone is not a comprehensive theory of marital distress.

A cogent criticism of the behavioral model is that if it is strictly used, it limits the productive use of an experienced clinician's other clinical skills. It is not uncommon for a couple to become deadlocked in a struggle around some seemingly minor issue and refuse all attempts at compromise. On occasion, an experienced clinician can intuit the meaning of the conflict for the participants, clarify this for the couple, and thus pave the way for an easier compromise. Strict adherence to the behavioral model would deprive the clinician and the couple of this intervention. For example, a Protestant wife and her Orthodox Jewish husband were unable to compromise about Christmas activities and were deadlocked in a counterproductive struggle. The therapist's comment that the rituals of Christmas were really a symbol of a time when, as a child, the wife felt safe was enough for the Jewish husband to be willing to compromise. Thus, clarification of personal meaning systems greatly accelerated further "reciprocity" in the marriage. Countless other examples could be cited illustrating that the struggle isn't always over exchange of desired behaviors. On numerous occasions, these behaviors appear to be external referents for internal symbols. The clinician's explication of the internal symbols can often put the meaning of the external referent in perspective. This process can tone down the emotional intensity of the struggle and generate a sense of cooperativeness that did not previously exist. For an experienced clinician to help couples to barter without using his clinical expertise to decipher the significance of the barter is similar to a professional boxer tying one arm behind his back.

It also appears that the behavioral models may be useful on occasion for reasons that behaviorists don't acknowledge. Many of the psychodynamic therapists have as a goal the establishment of clear "ego boundaries" or the interpretation and resolution of projection systems in disturbed marriages. The behavioral exchange model could be construed as a concretization of this goal. For example, this model explicitly states the responsibilities of each spouse and the ways in which goods (reinforcements) are exchanged between adults. Furthermore, these instructions are then behaviorally reinforced by reciprocity exercises. It is possible that couples enter therapy because of both unrealistic expectations and projections of needs onto each other. Part of the benefit of therapy may derive from a cognitive learning of a different set toward marriage. The "behavioral" set clearly states that each spouse is responsible for self alone and that psychological exchanges are bartered between separate entities. Although this model of marriage may not be ideal, for many couples it may be a better model than the enmeshment model with which they enter therapy.

In other couples, it appears that the bitter struggles over concrete issues occur because each is unaware of the internal referents for the behavior desired. A concrete exchange of these external behaviors may make this issue clear. For example, one wife was depressed because she had "such a lousy husband." Through a reciprocity exchange form of therapy, she was able to obtain all of the behaviors that she defined a perfect husband to have. This process enabled the woman to realize that her husband wasn't the problem. Using any other form of therapy, this stage would have taken much longer to reach. In some couples, the behaviors desired from the spouse appear to serve as a validation of self according to an idiosyncratic meaning system, unverbalizable by either spouse. An external validation of this sort can help to stabilize a marriage, although the therapist might have preferred a different solution. It appears that many of the requests for behavior changes are really requests for validation. The use of the communication training program gives the behaviorist greater freedom in addressing these issues. At least, he can address the need for verbal as well as motoric reinforcement between spouses.

Some therapists who identify themselves as behaviorists address the internal meaning systems of spouses. For example, Jacobson and Margolin (1979) stress cognitive evaluation as part of their assessment: "Spouses enter therapy with numerous assumptions about what has caused their relationship problems, with evaluations of themselves and their mates as marital partners and with attitudes about the quality of the relationship. These cognitions play an important role in determining why a couple is seeking marital counseling and how the couple might respond to behavior change activities" (pp. 70–71). Similarly, Stuart (1969) speaks of how a therapist must understand the "core symbols of a relationship," and Liberman (1975) appears on occasion to attempt directive cognitive restructuring in couples: "I actively redirected his attention from his wife, 'the unhappy depressed woman' to his wife 'the coping woman'" (Liberman, 1975, p. 113). These therapists appear to be mixing therapeutic models, an issue addressed eloquently by Eysenck and Beech: "We deplore this attitude in behavior therapists as we deplore it in psychotherapists; we believe that it results in a gigantic mish-mash of theories, methods, and outcomes that is forever beyond the capacity of scientific research to resolve. Theoretical differences should be recognized and their practical and applied consequences differentiated as clearly as possible; only in this way can the good and bad points of each theory be disentangled" (Eysenck and Beech, 1971, p. 602).

If certain variables deemed significant cannot be addressed by a given model, the model requires modification or replacement. If a clinician addresses cognitive variables, he is not a behaviorist. This need not be a mortal sin.

It appears that certain clinicians in all three theoretical camps have ventured into unorthodox waters when they have struggled to address the relationships involving internal organismic variables, behavior of the organism, and the elicited behavior of the environment. I feel that a truly useful theory of marital therapy has to address these reciprocal interrelationships. However, numerous individual therapists have struggled with this same difficulty. A brief review of their struggle and contributions might facilitate the evolvement of a coherent theory of marital therapy. This will be the content of the next chapter.

## REFERENCES

Adams, C. R. The prediction of adjustment in marriage. *Educational and Psychological Measurement*, 1946, *6*, 185–193.

Agras, W. J., Leitenberg, H., and Barlow, D. H. Social reinforcement in the modification of agoraphobia. *Archives of General Psychiatry*, 1968, *19*, 423–427.

Allen, K. E., Hart, B. M., Buell, J. S., Harris, F. R., and Wolf, M. M. Effects of social reinforcement on isolate behavior of a nursery school child. *Child Development*, 1964, *35*, 511–518.

Ayllon, T., and Azrin, N. H. The measurement and reinforcement of behavior of psychotics. *Journal of Experimental Analysis of Behavior*, 1965, *8*, 357–383.

Ayllon, T., and Michael, J. The psychiatric nurse as a behavioral engineer. *Journal of Experimental Analysis of Behavior*, 1954, *2*, 323–334.

Azrin, N. H., Naster, B. J., and Jones, R. Reciprocity counseling: A rapid learning-based procedure for marital counseling. *Behavioural Research and Therapy*, 1973, *11*, 365–382.

Baer, D. M. The entry into natural communities of reinforcement. Paper presented at the meeting of the American Psychological Association, Washington, D. C., 1967.

Bachrach, A. J., Erwin, W. J., and Mohr, P. J. The control of eating behavior in an anorexic by operant conditioning techniques. In L. P. Ullmann, L. Krasner (Eds.), *Case studies in behavior modification*. New York: Holt, Rhinehart and Winston, 1965.

Bandura, A. *Principles of behavior modification*. New York: Holt, Rinehart & Winston, 1969.

Bandura, A. *Social learning theory*. Englewood Cliffs, N.J.: Prentice-Hall, 1977.

Bentler, P. M., and Newcomb, M. D. Longitudinal study of marital success and failure. *Journal of Consulting and Clinical Psychology*, 1978, 46, 1053–1070.

Bernard, H. S., and Efran, J. S. Eliminating versus reducing smoking using pocket timers. *Behaviour Research and Therapy*, 1972, 10, 399–401.

Birchler, G. R. Differential patterns of instrumental affiliative behavior as a function of degree of marital distress and level of intimacy. *Dissertation Abstracts*, 1973, 33, 14499B–144500B.

Birchler, G. R., Weiss, R. L., and Vincent, J. P. A multimethod analysis of social reinforcement exchange between maritally distressed and non-distressed spouse and strange dyads. *Journal of Personality and Social Psychology*, 1975, 31, 349–360.

Birk, L., Stolz, S. B., Brady, J. P., Brady, J. V., Lazarus, A. A., Lynch, J. J., Rosenthal, A. J., Skelton, W. D., Stevens, J. B., and Thomas, E. J. *Task force report #5. Behavior therapy in psychiatry*. Washington, D.C.: American Psychiatric Association, 1973.

Blinder, B. J., Freeman, D. M., and Stunkard, A. J. Behavior therapy of anorexia nervosa: Effectiveness of activity as a reinforcer of weight gain. *American Journal of Psychiatry*, 1970, 126, 1093–1098.

Burchard, J. D., and Harig, P. T. Behavior modification and juvenile delinquency. In H. Leitenberg (Ed.), *Handbook of behavior modification and behavior therapy*. Englewood Cliffs, N.J.: Prentice-Hall, 1976.

Burgen, E. W., and Wallin, P. *Engagement and marriage*. Chicago: J. B. Lippincott, 1953.

Chadwick-Jones, J. K. *Social exchange theory: Its structure and influence in social psychology*. London: Academic Press, 1976.

Chaplin, J. P., and Krawiec, T. S. *Systems and theories of psychology*. New York: Holt, Rinehart & Winston, 1962.

Crowe, M. J. *Marital behavior psychotherapy*. Paper presented at the Annual Conference of the British Association of Behavioral Psychotherapists, Leicester, April 1973.

Eysenck, H. J. Learning theory and behavior therapy. *Journal of Mental Science*, 1959, 105, 61–75.

Eysenck, H. J. Learning theory and behavior therapy. In H. J. Eysenck (Ed.), *Behavior therapy and the neuroses*. London: Pergamon Press, 1960.

Eysenck, H. J., and Beech, R. Counter conditioning and related methods. In A. E. Bergin and S. L. Garfield (Eds.), *Handbook of psychotherapy and behavior change*. New York: Wiley, 1971.

Eysenck, H. J., and Rachman, S. *The causes and cures of neurosis*. San Diego: R. R. Knapp, 1965.

Fox, L. Effecting the use of efficient study habits. *Journal of Mathematics*, 1962, 1, 75–86.

Goldiamond, I. Self-control procedures in personal behavior problems. *Psychological Reports*, 1965, 17, 851–868.

Gottman, J., Markman, H., and Notarius, C. The topography of marital conflict: A sequential analysis of verbal and nonverbal behavior. *Journal of Marriage and the Family*, 1977, 39, 461–477.

Gottman, J., Notarius, C., Gonso, J., and Markman, H. *A couple's guide to communication*. Champaign, Ill.: Research Press, 1976. (a)

Gottman, J., Notarius, C., Markman, H., Bank, S., Yoppi, B., and Rubin, M. E. Behavior exchange theory and marital decision making. *Journal of Personality and Social Psychology*, 1976, *34*, 14–23. (b)

Greer, S. E., and D'Zurilla, T. J. Behavior approaches to marital discord and conflict. *Journal of Marital and Family Counseling*, 1975, *1*, 299–315. (a)

Greer, S. E., and D'Zurilla, T. J. Behavioral approaches to marital discord and conflict. *Journal of Marriage and Family Counseling*, 1975, *1*, 299–315. (b)

Guerney, B. G. *Relationship enhancement*. San Francisco: Jossey-Bass, 1977.

Gurman, A. S., and Kniskern, D. P. Behavioral marriage therapy: II. Empirical perspective. *Family Process*, 1978, *17*, 139–148.

Gurman, A. S., and Knudson, R. M. Behavioral marriage therapy. I. A psychodynamic systems analysis and critique. *Family Process*, 1978, *17*, 121–138.

Gurman, A. S., Knudson, R. M., and Kniskern, D. P. Behavioral marriage therapy. IV. Reply: Take two aspirin and call us in the morning. *Family Process*, 1978, *17*, 165–180.

Haley, J. *Strategies of psychotherapy*. New York: Grune and Stratton, 1973.

Homans, G. C. *Social behavior: Its elementary forms*. London: Routledge and Kegan Paul, 1961.

Homme, L. E. Perspective in psychology. Control of coverants, the operants of the mind. *Psychological Research*, 1965, *15*, 501–511.

Hops, H., Wills, T. A., Patterson, G. R., and Weiss, R. L. *Marital interaction coding systems*. Unpublished manuscript, 1971. (Available from Oregon Research Institute, Eugene, Oregon.)

Hunt, H. F., and Dyrud, J. E. Commentary: Perspective in behavior therapy. In J. M. Shlien (Ed.), *Research in psychotherapy*. Washington, D. C.: American Psychology Association, 1968.

Hurvitz, N. Interaction hypnothesis in marriage counseling. In A. S. Gurman and D. G. Rice (Eds.), *Couples in conflict*. New York: Jason Aronson, 1975.

Ingram, E. M. Discrimination and reinforcing functions in the experimental development of social behavior in a preschool child. Unpublished master's thesis. University of Kansas, 1967.

Isaacs, W., Thomas, J., and Goldiamond, I. Application of operant conditioning to reinstate verbal behavior in psychotics. *Journal of Speech and Hearing Disorders*, 1960, *25*, 8–12.

Jacobson, N. S. Problem solving and contingency contracting in the treatment of marital discord. *Journal of Consulting and Clinical Psychology*, 1977, *45*, 92–100.

Jacobson, N. S., and Margolin, G. *Marital therapy*. New York: Brunner/Mazel, 1979.

Jacobson, N. S., and Martin, B. Behavioral marriage therapy: Current status. *Psychological Bulletin*, 1976, *83*, 540–556.

Jacobson, N. S., and Weiss, R. L. Behavioral marriage therapy. III. Critique. The contents of Gurman *et al.* may be hazardous to our health. *Family Process*, 1978, *17*, 149–164.

Kanfer, F. H., and Phillips, J. S. *Learning foundation of behavior therapy*. New York: Wiley, 1970.

Kazdin, A. E. The application of operant techniques in treatment, rehabilitation, and education. In S. L. Garfield and A. E. Bergin (Eds.), *Handbook of psychotherapy and behavior change*. New York: Wiley, 1978.

Kelley, E. L. Concerning the validity of Terman's weights for predicting marital happiness. *Psychological Bulletin*, 1939, *139*, 202–203.

Knox, D. *Marriage happiness*. Champaign, Ill.: Research Press, 1974.

Lazarus, A. The results of behavior therapy in 126 cases of severe neurosis. *Behaviour Research and Therapy*, 1963, *1*, 65–78.

Lazarus, A. A. Behavior therapy and marriage counseling. *Journal of the American Society of Psychosomatic Dentistry and Medicine*, 1968, *15*, 49–56.

Leitenberg, H. Behavioral approaches to treatment of neuroses. In H. Leitenberg (Ed.), *Handbook of behavior modification and behavior therapy*. Englewood Cliffs, N.J.: Prentice-Hall, 1976.

Liberman, R. Behavioral principles in family and couple therapy. In A. S. Gurman and D. G. Rice (Eds.), *Couples in conflict*. New York: Jason Aronson, 1975.

Lindsley, O. R. Operant conditioning methods applied to research in chronic schizophrenia. *Psychiatric Research Reports*, 1965, *5*, 118–153.

London, P. The end of ideology in behavior modification. *American Psychologist*, 1972, *27*, 913–920.

Lovaas, O. L., and Buchner, B. D. Perspectives in behavior modification with deviant children. Englewood Cliffs, N.J.: Prentice-Hall, 1974.

Mahoney, M. J. *Cognition and behavior modification*. Cambridge, Mass.: Ballinger, 1974.

Mahoney, M. J., and Arnkoff, D. B. Cognitive and self-control therapies. In S. L. Garfield and A. E. Bergin (Eds.), *Handbook of psychotherapy and behavior change*. New York: Wiley, 1978.

Marks, I. M. Flooding (impulsion) and related treatments. In W. S. Agras (Ed.), *Behavior modification: Principles and clinical applications*. Boston: Little, Brown, 1968.

Marks, I. M. Phobias and obsessions. In J. Maser and M. Seligmen (Eds.), *Experimental psychopathology*. New York: Wiley, 1977.

Marks, I. M. Behavioral psychotherapy of adult neurosis. In S. L. Garfield and A. E. Bergin (Eds.), *Handbook of psychotherapy and behavior change*. New York: Wiley, 1978.

Meichenbaum, D. Cognitive-behavior modification. New York: Plenum, 1977.

Mischel, W. *An introduction to personality*. New York: Holt, Rinehart & Winston, 1971.

Mowrer, O. H. Stimulus-response theory of anxiety. *Psychological Review*, 1939, *46*, 553–565.

Murray, E. J., and Jacobson, L. I. Cognition and learning in traditional and behavioral therapy. In S. L. Garfield and A. E. Bergin (Eds.), *Handbook of psychotherapy and behavior change*. New York: Wiley, 1978.

O'Leary, K. D., and Turkewitz, H. Marital therapy from a behavioral perspective. In T. J. Paolino and B. S. McCrady (Eds.), *Marriage and marital therapy*. New York: Brunner/Mazel, 1978.

Patterson, G. R. *Families*. Champaign, Ill.: Research Press, 1976.

Patterson, G. R., and Hops, H. Coercion, a game for two: Intervention techniques for marital conflict. In R. E. Ulrich and P. T. Mountjoy (Eds.), *The experimental analysis of social behavior*. New York: Appleton-Century-Crofts, 1972.

Patterson, G. R., Shaw, D., and Cobb, J. *Manual for coding family interactions*. Unpublished manuscript, 1969. (Available from Oregon Research Institute, Eugene, Oregon.)

Patterson, G. R., Weiss, R. L., and Hops, H. Training of marital skills: Some problems and concepts. In H. Leitenberg (Ed.), *Handbook of behavior modification and behavior therapy*. Englewood Cliffs, N.J.: Prentice-Hall, 1976.

Pavlov, I. P. *Conditioned reflexes*. London: Oxford University Press, 1927.

Rachman, S. Phobias. *Their nature and control*. Springfield, Ill.: Charles C Thomas, 1968.

Rachman, S., and Teasdale, J. *Aversion therapy and behavior disorders: An analysis*. Coral Gables, Fl.: University of Miami Press, 1969.

Rappoport, A. E., and Harrel, J. E. A behavioral exchange model for marital counseling. In A. S. Gurman and D. G. Rice (Eds.), *Couples in conflict*. New York: Jason Aronson, 1975.

Rosen, G. M. Is it really necessary to use mildly phobic analogue subjects. *Behavior Therapy*, 1975, *6*, 68–71.

Rosenthal, T. L., and Bandura, A. Psychological modeling: Theory and practice. In S. L. Garfield and A. E. Bergin (Eds.), *Handbook of psychotherapy and behavior change*. New York: Wiley, 1978.

Satir, V. *Conjoint family therapy*. Palo Alto: Science and Behavior Press, 1967.

Segraves, R. T. Primary orgasmic dysfunction: Essential treatment components. *Journal of Sex and Marital Therapy*, 1976, *2*, 115–123.

Segraves, R. T. Female sexual inhibition. In R. J. Daitzman (Ed.), *Clinical behavior therapy and behavior modification* (Vol. 2). New York: Garland Press, 1981.

Seligman, M. E. P., Klein, D. C., and Miller, W. R. Depression. In H. Leitenberg (Ed.), *Handbook of behavior modification and behavior therapy*. Englewood Cliffs, N.J.: Prentice-Hall, 1976.

Skinner, B. F. Are theories of learning necessary? *Psychological Review*, 1950, *57*, 193–216.

Skinner, B. F. *Science and human behavior*. New York: Macmillan, 1953.

Skinner, B. F. Behaviorism at fifty. *Science*, 1963, *140*, 951–958.

Stern, R. S., and Marks, M. Contract therapy in obsessive-compulsive neurosis with marital therapy. *British Journal of Psychiatry*, 1973, *123*, 681–684.

Stuart, R. B. Behavioral control of overeating. *Behaviour Research and Therapy*, 1967, *5*, 357–365.

Stuart, R. B. *Prostitution as treatment of marital discord*. Paper presented to the Association for the Advancement of Behavior Therapy, San Francisco, August 1968.

Stuart, R. B. Operant-interpersonal treatment for marital discord. *Journal of Consulting and Clinical Psychology*, 1969, *33*, 657–682.

Stuart, R. B. Operant-interpersonal treatment for marital discord. In C. J. Sager and H. S. Kaplan (Eds.), *Progress in group and family therapy*. New York: Brunner/Mazel, 1972.

Stunkard, A. J., and Mahoney, M. J. Behavioral treatment of the eating disorders. In H. Leitenberg (Ed.), *Handbook of behavior modification and behavior therapy*. Englewood Cliffs, N.J.: Prentice-Hall, 1976.

Terman, L. M. Prediction data: Predicting marriage failure from test scores. *Marriage and Family Living*, 1950, *12*, 51–54.

Thibaut, J., and Kelley, M. *The social psychology of groups*. New York: Wiley, 1959.

Thomas, E. J. *Marital communication and decision making*. New York: Free Press, 1977.

Thomas, E. J., Carter, R. D., Gambuill, E. D., and Butterfield, W. H. A signal system for the assessment and modification of behavior (SAM). *Behavior Therapy*, 1970, *1*, 252–259.

Thomas, E. J., Walter, C., and O'Flaherty, K. A. A verbal problem checklist for use in assessing family verbal behavior. *Behavior Therapy*, 1974, *5*, 235–246.

Ullman, L. P., and Krasner, L. A. *A psychological approach to abnormal behaviors*. Englewood Cliffs, N.J.: Prentice-Hall, 1969.

Vincent, J. P., Weiss, R. L., and Birchler, G. R. A behavioral analysis of problem solving in distressed and non-distressed married and stranger dyads. *Behavior Therapy*, 1975, *6*, 475–487.

Watson, J. B. *Behavior. An introduction to comparative psychology*. New York: Holt, 1914.

Watson, J. B. *Behaviorism*. Chicago: University of Chicago Press, 1924.

Watson, J. B., and Rayner, R. Conditioned emotional reactions. *Journal of Experimental Psychology*, 1920, *3*, 1–14.

Weiss, R. L. The conceptualization of marriage from a behavioral perspective. In T. J.

Paolino and B. S. McCrady (Eds.), *Marriage and marital therapy*. New York: Brunner/ Mazel, 1978.

Weiss, R. L., Birchler, G. L., and Vincent, J. P. Contractual models for negotiation training in marital dyads. *Journal of Marriage and the Family*, 1974, 36, 321–330.

Weiss, R. L., Hops, H., and Patterson, G. R. A framework for conceptualizing marital conflict, a technology for altering it, some data for evaluating it. In L. A. Hammerlynck, L. C. Handy, and E. J. Mash (Eds.), *Behavior change methodology and practice*. Champaign, Ill.: Research Press, 1973.

Wieman, R. J., Shoulders, D. I., and Farr, J. H. Reciprocal reinforcement in marital therapy. *Behavioral Therapy and Experimental Psychiatry*, 1974, 5, 291–295.

Wills, T. A., Weiss, T. L., and Patterson, G. R. A behavioral analysis of the determinants of marital satisfaction. *Journal of Consulting and Clinical Psychology*, 1974, 42, 802–811.

Wolpe, J. *Psychotherapy by reciprocal inhibition*. Stanford: Stanford University Press, 1958.

# Inner Worlds, External Reality, and Interactional Systems

The purpose of this chapter is to lay the groundwork for an integrative conceptual model for the treatment of marital discord. It is assumed that each of the treatment models reviewed in previous chapters offers a valuable contribution to the conceptualization and treatment of marital discord. However, each model, in and of itself, is only a partial theory of treatment. What is needed is a model that integrates intrapsychic, interpersonal, and behavioral data. Such an integration will necessitate diversions into various unrelated areas in order to forge the necessary conceptual linkages.

This chapter will begin with a brief summary of the current state of knowledge about the treatment of marital discord, followed by a statement of the requirements of a good clinical theory of treatment. Subsequent sections will examine the interrelationships between inner psychological events and behavior change and interpersonal events. This discussion will be followed by a section on cognitive social psychology. From this section, a new language system will evolve that allows a more precise description of relationships between internal psychological phenomena and observable interactional data. At this point, the nature of the relationship between past psychological events and current interpersonal behavior will be addressed. In other words, this chapter will by necessity proceed by briefly considering work in seemingly unconnected areas in order to have the knowledge base for an integrative model.

## CURRENT STATUS

In a previous chapter, evidence linking marital discord with psychiatric service usage was reviewed. From this evidence, it is clear that marital discord is related to help-seeking behavior and is a potent source of emotional turmoil. There is suggestive evidence that marital dissolution may serve as a stress-precipitating psychiatric illness. In spite of the evidence linking marital discord with psychiatric impairment, marital therapy has been relatively neglected by mental health professionals. Other authors have suggested various reasons for the neglect of this area (Martin and Lief, 1973; Berman and Lief, 1975). However, it is my belief that the absence of a coherent theory has been the most significant obstacle to clinicians interested in marital therapy. The field could best be described as consisting of many partial theories. Each partial theory offers a unique vantage point for the organization of data and the making of therapeutic interventions. However, none of these theoretical approaches is a sufficient theory by itself. Polemical disputes between advocates of differing theoretical perspectives (e.g., Gurman et al., 1978; Jacobson and Weiss, 1978) and the absence of a common language system obscure the potential linkages between the opposing partial theories.

The empirically oriented clinician interested in the treatment of marital discord simply does not have an adequate conceptual model to guide his therapeutic interventions. This situation can perhaps best be appreciated by briefly reviewing the contributions and weaknesses of the three major treatment orientations. Psychoanalytic theory is unique in its emphasis on the importance of past experience in determining current interactional difficulties. This orientation also stresses that the perceived reality of the spouse may be of far greater importance than the actual behavior of the spouse. In other words, transference distortions are felt to play a major role in marital difficulties, and a major thrust of this orientation is the modification (resolution) of these perceptual distortions. This orientation aids the clinician in organizing data about how the past lives of both spouses may be contributing to the current marital difficulty. No other major orientation to the treatment of marital discord accomplishes this. However, the psychoanalytic approach has several serious limitations. Two of its most serious clinical limitations are (1) its relative neglect of the importance of current interpersonal forces in maintaining deviant behavior and (2) its emphasis on insight as a curative mechanism and its de-emphasis of the importance of behavioral change. Any clinician with clinical experience in the field of marital and family therapy realizes that there is a complex reciprocal interaction between intrapsychic phenomena and the social field (e.g., Ackerman, 1966, 1970; Bowen, 1975). Similarly, most clinicians recognize that behavioral change sometimes has to precede internal change. For example, if the maladaptive behavior patterns in a marriage confirm each spouse's distorted inner representational world, the behavioral models do achieve a degree of misfit or disequilibrium allowing for their modification. Many analytically oriented therapists have implicitly recognized this phenomenon (e.g., Fitzgerald, 1973; Nadelson, 1978), even though their theoretical orientation has difficulty accommodating the data. Another major disadvantage of the psychoanalytic approach is the absence of an empirical tradition in analytic circles and the choice of an unfortunate language system to describe their postulates and observations. The language system used by this theoretical camp emphasizes internal forces, uses higher level abstractions as explanatory concepts, confuses inference with observation, and does not allow empirical testing of basic assumptions. In fact, many of the basic assumptions employed by this theoretical orientation have never been substantiated (Olson, 1970, 1975).

The theoretical approach advocated by therapists influenced by general system theory provides a counterbalance to the psychoanalytic approach. This viewpoint emphasizes the importance of current interpersonal forces in producing psychological suffering and states that current reality is more important than past internalized experiences. Accordingly, this explanatory system tends to use explanatory concepts that are closer to observable data. Clinically, this approach appears to have two major deficiencies. First, it tends to give minimal consideration to past experiences of either spouse and almost acts as if the two spouses appeared *de novo* in the marriage without past experiences of any sort. If a clinician adhered strictly to this approach, he would have to discard much data of potential significance to the marriage. The other main fault with the general system theory approach is that it is not a theory of therapy. It is an orientation toward data and as such enlarges upon the viewpoint espoused by analytic therapists in a very useful way. However, this theory does not then lead to a series of procedures and techniques. Instead, a body of diverse procedures are employed under the guise of this theoretical orientation.

The main contribution of behavioral marital therapy is its strict focus on observable data and concern with the empirical validation of procedures and assumptions. No other theoretical orientation has yielded such a concern among practitioners as to whether their procedures and interventions are empirically valid. This precision of thought is not without its price. As with general systems theory, behavioral marital therapy cannot accommodate data about the past lives of spouses. A strict adherent of this approach could not even consider molar constructs about belief systems underlying patterns of behavior. The main fault of this approach is that if it is followed strictly, its assumptions and procedures are often so simplistic that the experienced clinician would need to forgo using many of his subtler clinical skills.

## REQUIREMENT OF A THEORY

A good theory of marital therapy needs to meet both clinical and empirical requirements. Clinically, an ideal theory would allow the experienced clinician to relate individual historical data and observable interactional data in his formulation of the difficulty. Similarly, an adequate theory would provide an organized scheme for treatment, under which both behavioral and internal cognitive-emotional change could be subsumed. Ideally, such a theory would allow a multifaceted approach, drawing on the clinician's skill and wisdom, within an organized theoretical structure.

In other words, such a theory needs to address person–environment interaction as a reciprocal process. It must address the interrelationship involving internal events, behavior, and induced environmental consequences. The theory must address how a person thinks and feels as well as how he behaves and how that in turn influences the behavior of others. If a theory includes these three areas, it allows the clinician to intervene at any of the three levels. To any individual not caught up in present polemical struggles among theoretical schools, the statements above appear so commonsensical as not to need stating. Ideas such as this were stressed by George Mead in the 1930s (Mead, 1934a, b) and are only recently being rediscovered by current theoreticians (e.g., Bandura, 1977).

Fortunately, current clinicians and theoreticians are beginning to bridge the gaps between individual and interpersonal psychotherapy and between behavioral and intrapsychic types of therapy. In subsequent sections, some of these bridges will be detailed, as they are crucial to the author's theory.

Another characteristic of a good theory of therapy is that it tends to lead to formulations and hypotheses that are capable of empirical validation or invalidation. This concern with empiricism need not take the form of radical behaviorism. Hypothetical variables, even about intrapsychic phenomena, are acceptable if they are stated in such a way that they can be verified. Only if a theory is stated with some precision can its assumptions be tested and the theory modified as knowledge progresses. Part of the difficulty with analytic theory is that its structure does not allow faulty premises to be discarded. This characteristic of analytic theory has probably been one of the main factors contributing to stagnation of thought in analytic circles and is one of the principal factors leading to the behaviorists' aversion to considering any variable even remotely similar to analytic hypotheses. However, I strongly believe that some of the contributions of analytically oriented therapists are extremely useful clinically and can be retained in a scientific theory of interpersonal discord if these hypotheses are carefully reworded in a different language form. This endeavor constitutes a major effort of the author in this text.

## BEHAVIORAL CHANGE AND INNER REPRESENTATIONAL EVENTS

The relationship between behavioral change and inner representational events has been a recurring concern among contemporary psychotherapists. This concern is perhaps best understood in a historical context. Until the last several decades, psychoanalytic theory was the uncontested dominant influence in clinical psychology and psychiatry. However, behavior therapy began exerting an increasing influence on the practice of psychotherapy. The presence of the two schools of psychotherapeutic thought and practice led to a situation that was described by some as a paradigm clash (Eysenck and Beech, 1971). Psychodynamic theory stressed the importance of subjective mental events and employed explanatory concepts that were hypothetical constructs about inner mental events and structures. On the other hand, behavior therapists stressed the importance of environmental determinants of behavior and of limiting scientific discourse to the study of observable events. Each paradigm had its group of followers, and the scientific literature was soon replete with attacks by representatives of one school of thought on the results and flaws of the opposing theoretical system (Eysenck and Rachman, 1965; Breger and McCaugh, 1965). As a brief aside, it is interesting to note that similar types of articles are now beginning to appear in the marital therapy literature (Gurman et al., 1978; Jacobson and Weiss, 1978). At any rate, behavior therapists pointed out that there was little evidence to support the basic assumption of analytic theory or even to verify the efficacy of that form of treatment (Eysenck and Rachman, 1965). Analytic therapists maintained that behavioral therapy at best achieved superficial changes in behavior and did not address the underlying difficulty causing the maladaptive behavior (Breger and McCaugh, 1965). Meaningful treatment was felt to occur only when internal structural change occurred. Internal structural change was felt to occur when the internal conflicts had been resolved through insight-oriented psychotherapy.

As the debate raged through the clinical literature, it became obvious that much of the struggle appeared to serve political as well as scientific motivations (London, 1972). Psychoanalytic theorists were predominantly psychiatrists, and behaviorists predominantly psychologists. In certain ways, the intensity of paradigm clash could be understood as a power struggle between professional groups. However, throughout this period of time, certain clinicians were able to stand outside of the power struggle and see the need for a sensible integration of approaches and basic concepts. The work of Dyrud (Hunt and Dyrud, 1968; Goldiamond and Dyrud, 1968; Dyrud, 1971) and more recently that of Marmor (1971) emphasized the futility of the struggle and the need for integrative efforts.

There have been both methodological and theoretical attempts to bridge the gap between behavioral and psychodynamic psychotherapy. One approach has been to assume that a given symptom might arise either from learning of inappropriate behavior or from internal conflict. Either psychodynamic or behavioral approaches might be used given the clinical situation. In other words, the experienced clinician would appropriately diagnose the difficulty and prescribe the appropriate intervention. Each intervention and theoretical orientation is essentially treated as equal yet independent. The theoretical orientation of H. S. Kaplan (1974, 1976) in the treatment of sexual dysfunction is a prime example of this approach. Another approach to methodological synthesis is to assume that each orientation is suited for different classes of problems. Thus, psychodynamic therapy is utilized to resolve intrapsychic conflicts and behavior therapy is used to modify problematic behavior. Numerous therapists have reported promising results using this approach (e.g., Levay et al., 1976; Woody, 1968).

The separate but equal approach is easy to accommodate intellectually and has won many advocates. However, certain clinical observations render this approach untenable. In particular, clinicians found that behavior therapy frequently elicited changes in nonbehavioral domains—that there was a significant overlap between behavioral change and intrapsychic events.

In the early literature, behaviorists noted that successful behavior therapy was occasionally marked by abreactive experiences. Brady (1966) reported that anamnesic experiences frequently occurred during the systematic desensitization of women with primary anorgasmia. Unfortunately, he provided no clinical details about these experiences. However, Jones and Park (1972) also reported that abreactive experiences sometimes occurred unexpectedly in their treatment of sexual dysfunction by systematic desensitization. They reported one case in some detail. A woman with anorgasmia was asked to visualize herself nude under the bed sheets as one scene in the imaginary hierarchy to be desensitized: "she wept quietly, then openly, and cried out repeatedly, Betty, Betty, dead, dead, under that sheet." In subsequent discussion, she recalled seeing her deceased sister, 29 years previously, lying under a sheet. The scene brought the experience back with all of its associated feelings (Jones and Park, 1972, p. 413).

Marks and co-workers (1972) also reported that some patients remembered past events connected with their phobia during behavior therapy. Under a section labeled anecdotal data, they reported one example. A woman with a fear of heights was being treated by *in vivo* flooding (having her stand on a rooftop). Treatment progressed unremarkably until the patient "suddenly screamed when she saw a man walking near the edge of a nearby roof. She then told the therapist for the first time that her phobia had begun years earlier after she saw a fireman fall to his death from a ladder. Evocation of this memory was accomplished by intensified fear" (Marks *et al.*, 1972, p. 501). Boulougouris and Bassiakos (1973) reported a case in which the abreactive experiences elicited by behavior therapy were of symbolic significance. They reported treating a 50-year-old obsessive-compulsive woman with a 25-year history of excessive washing elicited by a fear of being contaminated by objects related to death, funerals, and dirt. She also held her head in a peculiar flexed position. During the third session of flooding in imagination (forced imaginary evocation of highly anxiety-arousing fantasies), a rather dramatic change occurred: "In tears, she interrupted the fantasy session and spontaneously described the period just after her marriage . . . she recalled vividly that while she was washing her infant, her mother accused her of nearly suffocating her baby by the way she held its neck. The day after this reaction, the patient showed pronounced improvement. Her neck was again held erect. She also had disturbing dreams" (Boulougouris and Bassiakos, 1973, p. 228). The author recently encountered a similar phenomenon in a slightly different clinical context. A young woman who complained of lack of sexual interest was treated in a modified Masters and Johnson (1970) approach for primary orgasmic dysfunction. The behavioral intervention was quite successful, and the woman became increasingly sexually responsive to her husband. At this point, her husband became increasingly agitated and finally reported that as he observed his nude wife lying in bed sexually aroused, her face became like his mother's face. He spontaneously reported numerous childhood memories in which he had perceived his mother to be sexually provocative. As he habituated to his sexually aroused wife, the distorted perception gradually subsided.

Other authors have reported cases in which events occurring during symptomatic treatment suggested that the symptom was intertwined with other mental events and symbol systems. For example, Feather and Rhoads (1972b) reported several cases where changes in target behavior were associated with changes in other behavior, not related to the target symptom at an overt level. In one case, desensitization to the expression of anger led to a decrease in an airplane phobia. In another case, desensitization to anger led to improvement in a speech phobia. In a separate report, the author (Segraves and Smith, 1976) reported three cases where behavior therapy elicited events suggesting a psychodynamic etiology to the problem. The most striking case was of a young woman with a bird phobia dating from early childhood. Prior to touching a bird during *in vivo* desensitization, this woman spoke of the supposedly fear-eliciting phobic object as if it were a sexual object toward which she had ambivalent feelings: "I feel as I did in high school when I desired intercourse with my boyfriend, but felt that I shouldn't." Subsequent to this session, she spontaneously reported a series of sexual dreams, a changed attitude toward her father, and a feeling of greater sexual freedom. In a previously unreported case, the author treated a severely neurotic man with graduated assignments emphasizing assertiveness at work. This behavioral approach was successful in developing assertive behavior. In one session, the patient was relating an instance of assertive behavior the previous week when he suddenly became giddy, on the verge of laughing out of control. The author and the patient were puzzled by this event until the patient spontaneously reported, "The only other time that I remember ever feeling like this was when a high school counselor said, "Wouldn't you like to tell your father to get the hell off your back?" Other authors have also reported that behavioral therapy frequently evokes material of psychodynamic significance (Kaplan, 1976; Hafner, 1978; Scharff, 1976).

Events similar to those reported above led to the conclusion that the separate but equal doctrine was insufficient to guide the clinician in the appropriate choice of either behavioral or psychodynamic therapeutic interventions. Clearly, there is a relationship between behavior and inner cognitive-emotional events, and this relationship appears to be reciprocal. In certain cases, behavioral change may produce internal symbolic change similar to that sought by psychodynamic therapists. A useful clinical theory needs to discuss the interrelationship between behavior and inner symbolic events.

The attempt to achieve rapprochement between behavioral and psychodynamic theory has taken many forms. Dollard and Miller (1950) attempted to translate psychoanalytic concepts into learning theory terminology. Subsequent theorists have similarly attempted retranslations across theoretical boundaries (Feather and Rhoads, 1972a; Stampfl and Lewis, 1968; Hogan, 1968). More recently, theoreticians have been less concerned with retranslations across theoretical boundaries and more concerned with a description of the relationship between events subsumed by each theoretical orientation.

Numerous clinicians have noted that there is a reciprocal linkage between behavior change and intrapsychic events (Birk and Brinkley-Birk, 1974; Segraves and Smith, 1976; Marmor, 1971). Although stated slightly differently by each, it is hypothesized by all three authors that phobic and neurotic behavior can be understood as reflecting a discrepancy between a patient's cognitive-emotional inner representational world and external reality. This viewpoint was recently stressed by Birk and Brinkley-Birk (1974) in a discussion of a patient who had a mother transference reaction to his wife. His deficiency in assertiveness toward his wife was treated behaviorally: "Not only does the patient learn to change his behavior, but he is also compelled to give up the faulty assumptions, often unconscious or preconscious, about himself and about his wife, that were part of the cognitive/emotional matrix out of which his maladaptive behavior with her arose, grew, and was neurotically nourished by him in the first place. If uninterrupted, this maladaptive behavior continues to reinforce the erroneous, albeit unconscious, coalescence of wife and mother. When the old behavior is interrupted and replaced by new assertive behavior, however, the new pattern stands in direct contradiction, as a counterinstance, to the chronic unconscious equation of wife and mother. In other words, the patient is behaving as if he no longer believed in this equation. The consequent shift in cognitive set and attendant increase in self-esteem serve as internal reinforcers for the continuance and increasing adaptiveness of the new behavior patterns" (1974, p. 506).

Marmor (1971) reached similar conclusions about the impact of symptom removal on inner psychic structure: "If the conflicted elements involved in neurosis formation are assumed to be part of a closed system, it follows logically that removal of the symptomatic consequences of such an inner conflict without altering the underlying dynamics should result in some other symptom manifestation. If, however, personality dynamics are more correctly perceived with the framework of an open system, then such a consequence is not inevitable. Removal of an ego-dystonic symptom may, on the contrary, produce such satisfying feedback from the environment that it may result in major constructive shifts within the personality system, thus leading to modification of the original conflictual pattern" (p. 22). Segraves and Smith (1976) similarly reported that symptom removal by behavior therapy often produced significant internal symbolic change: "More importantly, in these three cases, the symptoms appeared to be key factors in the way the patients organized their subjective views of the world, and removal of these symptoms rather dramatically opened the way for a new subjective reorganization" (p. 762).

In summary, there is increasing agreement among eclectic therapists that useful clinical theory needs to address the interrelationship between behavior and inner symbolic events. The increasing rapprochement between behavioral and psychodynamic therapies has been hampered by the absence of a theoretical system that subsumes both behavioral and intrapsychic events. In fact, the basic elements of such a theory are contained in the works of social psychologists such as George Kelly (1955) and Robert Carson (1969). This will be pursued in a later section of this chapter, after the relationship between internal symbolic events and the behavior of social intimates is briefly discussed.


## INNER REPRESENTATIONAL EVENTS AND SOCIAL BEHAVIOR

A basic difficulty in integrating psychoanalytic concepts about psychopathology with other theoretical orientations is that the psychoanalytic orientation places an extreme emphasis on the psychology of the individual. Malan (1976) discusses that the goal of psychoanalytic psychotherapy is to help the individual patient to experience his emotional conflicts and bring them into consciousness. Symptoms are hypothesized to arise when an unacceptable impulse or feeling threatens eruption into consciousness and the patient keeps these feelings at bay by various defense mechanisms. In this way, Malan discusses the classical psychoanalytic triad: the defense, the anxiety, and the hidden impulse. The goal of therapy is to bring into awareness the hidden impulses. This is accomplished by interpreting the defense and the anxiety.

The difficulty with Malan's formulation is that it implies that all of these events are contained within the individual as a closed system. It is difficult to relate this closed system approach to interactional data. However, as Malan states, the psychoanalytic triad can be restated in Ezriel's (1952) relationship terminology. In this terminology, defense, anxiety, and impulse become required relationship, feared catastrophe, and avoided relationship. This redefinition suggests how certain interpersonal systems might be understood from a psychoanalytic viewpoint.

Thus, a passive husband who continually avoids confrontations might be understood as avoiding angry-competitive interactions with his wife (mother?) because he fears loss of the nurturing relationship. Presumably, his wife also has intrapsychic needs, which are expressed in the relationship. The resulting interaction could be understood as a compromise equilibrium that is reached, minimizing each of their imaginary feared catastrophes if the avoided relationship is realized.

Other authors have similarly attempted to link intrapsychic phenomena with interpersonal behavior. Leary (1957) emphasized how much interpersonal behavior can be understood as attempts to avoid anxiety and maintain self-esteem. He postulated that early childhood fears of destruction and abandonment are experienced by adults as fear of rejection and social disapproval. His contribution was particularly valuable in that he addressed the interpersonal impact of certain social behavior, and how certain psychopathology could be self-sustaining: "Interpersonal reflexes tend (with a probability significantly greater than change) to initiate or invite reciprocal interpersonal responses from the 'other' person in the interaction that lead to a repetition of the original reflex" (p. 123). He gave an example of a 30-year-old man who entered group therapy complaining of depression, social isolation, and that no one cared for him. The patient was placed in group therapy with complete strangers. Within eight sessions, he had reproduced his world by provoking the other group members into critical unsympathetic behavior toward him. The seemingly maladaptive behavior of this patient presumably served a function of avoiding some other form of relationship and accompanying subjective state.

Other theorists (Carson, 1969; Satir, 1967; Kelly, 1955; Stotland and Canon, 1972) have evolved theoretical systems to explain the linkage between inner symbolic events and social behavior and the elicited social behavior of others. In most of these formulations, the elicited behavior of intimate others serves an intrapsychic purpose for the person who elicited that behavior. Implicit in most of these formulations is also the possibility that repetitive refusal to participate in one's required relationship by social intimates would force one to experience the avoided relationship and thus experience intrapsychic change.

It would appear that various theorists have grappled with the issue of the interrelationship involving behavior, intrapsychic events, and behavior in intimate interactional systems. However, most of these theorists have been limited by the language system of their theoretical orientation. These language systems, by and large, are incapable of subsuming all of the necessary data.

## DESCRIPTION OF INNER REPRESENTATIONAL EVENTS

Recently, it has again become respectable to speak of cognitive events in psychological circles. As recently as 10 years ago, one was immediately suspect if one were not a behaviorist. The rebirth of cognitive psychology is in large part due to Albert Bandura's work stressing the importance of symbolic learning in the understanding of human behavior (e.g., Bandura, 1969, 1977). Bandura has made significant advances in conceptualizing the reciprocal interaction involving cognitive events, behavior, and environmental determinants of behavior. More importantly, he has made this whole area of inquiry respectable and has emphasized the need for a unified conceptual approach: "Because of the complex interdependence of antecedent, consequent, and cognitive regulatory systems, the sharp distinctions commonly drawn between behavioral and cognitive processes are more polemical than real. It has been customary in psychological theorizing to construct entire explanatory schemes around a single regulatory system, to the relative neglect of other influential determinants and processes. Some theorists have tended to concentrate upon antecedent control created principally through the association of environmental events; others have focused primarily upon regulation of behavior by external reinforcement; still others favor cognitive determinants and confine their studies largely to cognitive operations. Strong allegiances to part processes encourage intensive investigation of subfunctions, but considered independently, they do not provide a complete understanding of human behavior" (Bandura, 1977, p. 191). Bandura considers behavior to be partially under cognitive self-regulatory control and partially environmentally controlled. However, these dimensions are highly intertwined. The behavior of the organism is conceptualized to play a large role in determining the environmental consequences and the anticipated consequences in controlling behavior. Of course, anticipated consequences were learned in similar environmental interactions in the past. In spite of the significant role played by cognitive regulation of behavior, environmental disconfirmation of these expectations is considered more potent than symbolic persuasion. Similarly, social verification is considered to play a significant role in maintaining attitudes. Bandura primarily speaks of these internal cognitive regulatory functions in a molecular rather than a molar way. In most of his writing, each behavioral act is linked with a discreet cognitive variable. In fact, he specifically addresses why he dislikes the Piagetian notion of schema, a molar cognitive function. Although Bandura helps to lay the groundwork for a unified theory, his approach is deficient mainly because of the scant attention devoted to a precise description of cognitive processes.

Bandura's theoretical perspective complements the writings of a social psychologist, George Kelly. Kelly's main contributions were published in the 1950s (Kelly, 1955) and are only recently being rediscovered, primarily by English psychiatrists (Slater, 1969; Bannister and Mair, 1968). Essentially, Kelly assumed that one of man's primary tasks in life is to build an inner representational world of increasing complexity approximating external reality. He assumed that many of the phenomena in clinical psychology could be understood by assuming that man forms constructs to subsume environmental events. These constructs could be understood as templates for organizing perceptions or as abstractions of reality. Psychological growth could be understood as the gradual development of construct systems by successive approximation. These construct systems are hypothesized to be arranged in a hierarchical way such that some constructs are subsumed by others. These constructs are abstractions or deductions from life experience and usually subject to modification. Clearly, Kelly's concepts of constructs are similar to Piaget's notion of *schemata* and the processes of assimilation and accommodation (Piaget, 1948). It is also similar to the psychoanalytic concept of transference, i.e., the concept that present object relations are perceived as similar to past object relations.

"Thus construct systems can be considered as a kind of scanning pattern which a person continually projects upon his world. As he sweeps back and forth across his perceptual field he picks up blips of meaning. The more adequate his scanning pattern, the more meaningful his world becomes. The more in tune it is with the scanning patterns used by others, the more blips of meaning he can pick up from their projections. Viewed in this manner the psychology of personal constructs commits us to a projective view of all perception. All interpersonal relations are based essentially on transference relations, though they are subject to validation and revision" (Kelly, 1955, p. 145).

For clinical phenomena, interpersonal constructs are assumed to be of primary importance. Kelly attempted to operationalize these interpersonal construct systems in an ingenious way. The Role Construct Repertory Test was developed to give a reliable measure of a person's microcosm. In this test, a person is given a list of 15 role titles of people likely to be important in most people's lives. He is then asked to discriminate ways these people are similar and dissimilar to one another. The end result of this procedure is theoretically a map of the person's private interpersonal universe (object world). It is of note that the nature of the test construction is such that the person's private universe can then be represented in a matrix, which is subject to usual matrix mathematical procedures. This test can be used to measure the cognitive complexity of an individual and the discrimination between people in a person's life (i.e., mother as similar to wife). These functions of the test have made this procedure useful in a variety of clinical settings by psychodynamically oriented therapists (Ryle and Lunghi, 1969; Fransella and Joyston-Bechal, 1970).

The main contribution of Kelly was his introduction of a more precise manner of describing how past events are encoded and and then influence current interpersonal relationships. Kelly was also significant in his recommendations about how one could alter a person's construct system. Kelly assumed that all interpretations (constructions) of the universe are subject to revision, a concept he labeled constructive alternativism. By this he meant that no patient needs to be a victim of his biography. Alternative constructions can be brought to bear. Kelly recommended a novel approach for changing construct systems. Fixed role therapy consisted primarily of encouraging a patient to behave the complete opposite of the way he described himself, on the assumption that this behavioral change would free (disprove) the construct system within which he had bound himself. Fixed role therapy was clearly a forerunner of cognitive-behavior therapy.

Kelly's conception of the importance of construct systems in understanding person–environment interaction has been extended by the work of cognitive social psychologists such as Carson (1969) and Stotland and Canon (1972). This work is especially important, as it provides a language system that subsumes individual and environmental events and similarly provides a theoretical framework whereby past events can be expected to influence current behavior.

A central concept in the Stotland and Canon system is the term *schema*. This term is analogous to Kelly's use of *construct*. People are assumed to generate generalizable rules or schemas about certain regularities among environmental events. These schemas are formed via direct observation, observations of others (i.e., modeling), and communication from others. Once formed, these schemas tend to guide actions, to assimilate new information, and to be impervious to change. These schemas can also be understood to be abstractions from life experience and implicit personal theories or hidden assumptions about life.

Because of the limited information-processing capacity of the human and the danger of information overload, these schemas serve as templates by which to organize new experiences. According to this framework, few interpersonal events are ever perceived as they really are:

"The requirement that new material be efficiently integrated with old sometimes causes trouble. Thus, because unfamiliar material is not readily assimilated into memory, we are apt to retrieve what ought to have happened rather than what actually did. When we view a complex event, we may attempt to evaluate it according to previously acquired rules and memories" (Norman, 1969, p. 181). In other words, what we perceive in a given situation is partly a function of our past experience and partly a function of the current environmental stimulation. The concept of schema as it applies to interpersonal situations is clearly analogous to the analytic concept of "transference" and concepts about the "inner object world."

The advantage of the cognitive schema formulation over analytic concepts is that the language system employed allows a greater precision of description and prediction. Methodologies such as that developed by George Kelly are available to test facets of these schemas, and an experimental literature has evolved about the conditions under which schemas are most likely to be modified (Stotland and Canon, 1972). For example, new schemas are less likely to evolve in situations where the cues are equivocal or ambiguous. In such situations, the individual's perception would be strongly influenced by remnants of past experiences. Similarly, extremely complex situations offering perceptions discrepant with multiple schemas would be expected to be anxiety-provoking because of information overload and not to be conducive to the acquisition of new schemas. Personal adaptation would be postulated to be a function of cognitive complexity, or the number and complexity of available interpersonal schemas.

The main contribution of the hypothesis of cognitive schemas is that this orientation allows a precise language system for the description of how past events are encoded in such a way as to influence current perceptions and interactions. If one assumes, as does Bandura, that a person partially creates his own environment contingencies, one can then envision how certain people do become caught in their biographies. A viewpoint is offered for which to observe the repetitive maladaptive behavior sequences that analysts refer to as repetition compulsions. According to the analytic framework, such repeating sequences of behavior would be viewed as misdirected attempts to repair internal trauma experienced early in life. The same phenomena could be viewed differently from a social-psychological point of view. Thus, our hidden assumptions or schemas about certain interpersonal situations tend to guide us to act in certain ways. Our actions in turn influence the environment to react often in ways that confirm our initial assumptions: "If we respond with anxiety, indifference, defensive maneuvers, or outright hostility to someone, he is likely to react defensively or aggressively himself, no matter how benign or friendly his intentions may have been initially. Since we do not have direct access to information about these positive intentions on his part, as they are private, intrapersonal events, and, in our example, never externalized in the form of overt behavior, it is difficult for us to access the contribution our own behavior has made in shaping the other's responses. What we see instead is evidence that this person does indeed possess some highly unattractive qualities just as we'd anticipated" (Stotland and Canon, 1972, p. 28).

## PSYCHOANALYTIC CONCEPTS AND COGNITIVE THEORY

As briefly mentioned in Chapter Three, there is significant overlap between certain psychoanalytic hypotheses and concepts employed by cognitive theorists and social learning theorists. These divergent theoretical perspectives all place varying degrees of emphasis on the role of cognitive mediating events in the control of behavior. All are concerned with describing how past environmental events continue to exert an influence on current behavior. Bandura as a proponent of social learning theory tends to speak of these internal mediating events on a molecular level, as if discrete behaviors are linked to discrete cognitions. However, cognitive-social psychologists tend to speak of cognitive events on a molar level, as cognitions occur in interrelated clusters. When Stotland and Canon speak of interpersonal schemas, the phenomena they describe are similar to what psychoanalysts would label transference. It also bears a marked resemblance to Sullivan's concept of personification (Sullivan, 1953). In other words, current perceptions, cognitions, and emotions are assumed to consist in part of remnants of past similar experiences. Carson (1969) makes this point quite explicitly: "The parataxic distortions that sometimes emerge in given relationships might be due, in part, to the eliciting of emotional responses acquired at an earlier time by some analogous relation existing between the cues emanating from the other person in the contemporary relationship and those associated with an earlier significant other, or with a personification of him" (p. 62).

Classical psychoanalytic therapy employs similar concepts, although stated in different language form. Analytic theory assumes that transference distortions underlie many interpersonal difficulties, and many analytic theorists consider the resolution of the transference neurosis to be the primary goal of psychoanalysis. In clinical descriptions of the analytic process, transference appears to refer to certain interpersonal schemas elicited during this form of therapy. These schemas usually relate to some faulty assumptions about the dangerousness of certain forms of intimate relationships, and the origins of these schemas may be traced to certain real or fantasied happenings in earlier life. Through interpretation, the analysand begins to appreciate the erroneousness of these hidden assumptions and how they have affected his life, and to discriminate between these internal images and real relationships.

It appears that certain interpersonal schemas are more fully elicited by prolonged intimate relationships, whether they be marriage or psychoanalysis. Similarly, one could assume that these faulty assumptions could be unlearned in a variety of circumstances. In psychoanalysis, the unlearning may be conceptualized as a form of discrimination training. The patient begins to appreciate that all relationships are not as he had feared. In fact, it is safe to feel angry, competitive, sexual, etc., with the analyst, whereas it did not appear to be so with a parent or in the early family situation. With this discrimination, and with the knowledge of one's perceptual bias, the patient can presumably test out different forms of relationship in life outside the therapist's office.

In this discussion, I have purposely focused on the similarities among different theoretical approaches. Real dissimilarities also exist. The point that I am trying to establish is that clinicians of varying orientations have been observing similar clinical phenomena and describing their observations from their particular vantage points and in their preferred language systems. It is reasonable to assume that these clinicians from varying professional and theoretical orientations are of equal intelligence, perceptiveness, and integrity. The common ground of their observational data might be an ideal place to begin to build a comprehensive theory.

Analytic theorists have assumed that these transference distortions can be remedied only through insight-oriented psychotherapy. This conclusion is reasonable when one realizes that few analysts have experimented with alternative forms of therapy. The notions of behavioral disconfirmation of schemas would appear alien, as their theoretical structure doesn't allow for this.


## HOW SCHEMAS ARE SELF-SUSTAINING

If one agrees that transference phenomena are basically equivalent to interpersonal schemas and that both can be defined as learned expectations of significant others, the question remains as to why these faulty expectations don't modify through normal life experiences. Analytic theory can accommodate this by assuming that transference distortions are related to unconscious phenomena and are thus not subject to modification through normal events. Cognitive-social psychology doesn't have this luxury. The persistence of schemas is related to the extent that man creates his own environment or the extent to which his actions predetermine the actions of others. This class of events is the mechanism of preservation of schemas or self-fulfilling prophesies.

The mechanism whereby man creates his own environment has been discussed in similar ways by theorists as dissimilar as Albert Bandura and Harry Stack Sullivan. The basic notion is that certain preconceived expectations lead to evocation of confirming stimuli from the social environment.

Classical analysts are well aware of this phenomenon. An important source of information about a patient's inner representation would be the emotional reactions elicited in the analyst by the patient. It is almost as if the patient is trying to get the analyst to act in accordance with the patient's interpersonal schemas for similar relationships.

For example, Kaplan described this phenomenon as the tendency of patients to "repeatedly attempt to provoke the analyst to react in a manner similar to past object relations" (Kaplan, 1976, p. 51). Harry Stack Sullivan (1953) described similar phenomena. A classic example of his would be that of the malevolent transformation of the need for tenderness. According to his formulation, certain parents are unable to respond to their child's need for tenderness. The child's reaching out for tenderness is rebuffed. Therefore, the child develops a protective interpersonal sequence, consisting of transforming the need for tenderness such that its emergence elicits hostile behavior. As Carson (1969) pointed out, such a sequence of events would be self-sustaining. The original assumption that friendly dependent behavior is dangerous would forever be reconfirmed in most human situations, with the possible exception of a therapeutic setting. Paul Wachtel (1977) similarly described how certain feeling states and interpersonal behaviors could become self-sustaining independent of the original learning situation. Wachtel's purpose in doing this was to illustrate how behavior therapy modifying current maladaptive behavior might be more effective than psychoanalytic interpretation of its etiology:

"Similarly, consider the patient whose excessive niceness and gentleness is seen as defending against extreme rage and vengeful desires. If, in the traditional fashion, we look back into his history, we may well seem to find sufficient justification and understanding of his situation from that direction. We may uncover in his history the presence of violent death wishes toward a parent, which he desperately attempted to cover up; and we may be able to see a continuity in this pattern which seems to suggest that he is still defending against those same childhood wishes. We may even find images and events in his dreams that point to continuing violent urges toward the parent and may discern many other indications of warded-off rage toward that figure. If we look in detail at his day-to-day interactions, however, we see a good deal more. We may find that his meekness has led him to occupy a job that is not up to his real potential and that he silently and resentfully bears. On the job and in his other social interactions as well, he is likely to be unable to ask for what is his due, and may even volunteer to do things for others that he really doesn't want to do. One can see this excessively unassertive and self-abnegating behavior as motivated by the need to cover up his strong aggressive urges, and this would be correct as far as it goes. But it is equally the case that such a life style generates rage. Disavowed anger may be a continuing feature of his life from childhood, but the angry thoughts that disturb his dreams tonight can be understood by what he let happen to himself today. Such a person is caught in a vicious cycle" (Wachtel, 1977, p. 44).

Bandura (1977) pointed out that false belief systems are maintained by people themselves creating situations that are self-confirmatory. The person's interpersonal behavior predetermines the probable responses of his social intimates. Leary (1957) similarly noted that the purpose of certain interpersonal behavior appeared to be to induce complementary behavior from others, and that many neurotics are quite skilled at such interpersonal ploys. Carson (1969) also stated that if a person notes a discongruence between his schema for an interaction and the other person's behavior, "attempting to induce changes in the other's 'real' behavior has certain notable advantages as a method of interpersonal incongruency reduction."

## SUMMARY

Within this chapter, I have hopscotched in and out of various theories and clinical phenomena. To the author, who has struggled for 8 years of his professional career to achieve this synthesis, the overall pattern is obvious. To the reader, the clarity of the pattern may be less obvious. At this point, I will briefly summarize the main points that I have tried to establish.

1. Our patients don't tend to be as theoretically orthodox as we therapists do. They tend to experience intrapsychic change as the result of behavior modification or changes in the behavior of intimate others.

2. One way to understand this phenomenon is to assume that man forms cognitive schemas (inner representational worlds) that regulate his activities and perceptions of others. Analytically oriented therapists frequently refer to this phenomenon as transference reactions.

3. In certain cases, these schemas can be self-perpetuating. The mechanism for this is that man's actions toward others often elicit behavior in others that is confirmatory to man's original hypotheses about the interaction. In other words, we tend to create our own interpersonal universes.

4. These schemas can be disconfirmed behaviorally. The mechanism for change is for the patient to experience a discrepancy between his internal schema and life experience.

## REFERENCES

Ackerman, N. W. *Treating the troubled family.* New York: Basic Books, 1966.

Ackerman, N. W. Family psychotherapy and psychoanalyses—Implications of differences. In N. W. Ackerman (Ed.), *Family process.* New York: Basic Books, 1970.

Bandura, A. *Principles of behavior modification.* New York: Holt, Rinehart & Winston, 1969.

Bandura, A. *Social learning theory.* Englewood Cliffs: Prentice-Hall, 1977.

Bannister, D., and Mair, J. M. M. *The evaluation of personal constructs.* London: Academic Press, 1968.

Berman, E. M., and Lief, H. I. Marital therapy from a psychiatric perspective: An overview. *American Journal of Psychiatry,* 1975, *132,* 583–591.

Birk, L., and Brinkley-Birk, A. W. Psychoanalysis and behavior therapy. *American Journal of Psychiatry,* 1974, *131,* 499–510.

Borman, D. A. *Memory and attention.* New York: Wiley, 1969.

Boulougouris, J. C., and Bassiakos, L. Prolonged flooding in cases with obsessive-compulsive neurosis. *Behaviour Research and Therapy,* 1973, *11,* 227–231.

Bowen, M. Family therapy after twenty years. In D. X. Freedman and J. E. Dyrud (Eds.), *American handbook of psychiatry,* Vol. 2, *Treatment.* New York: Basic Books, 1975.

Brady, J. P. Brevital-relaxation treatment of frigidity. *Behaviour Research and Therapy,* 1966, *4,* 71–77.

Breger, L., and McCaugh, J. L. Critique and reformulation of learning theory approaches to psychotherapy and neurosis. *Psychological Bulletin,* 1965, *63,* 338–358.

Carson, R. C. *Interaction concepts of personality.* Chicago: Aldine, 1969.

Dollard, J., and Miller, N. E. Personality and psychotherapy. An analysis in terms of learning, thinking and culture. Toronto: McGraw-Hill, Canada, 1950.

Dyrud, J. E. Behavior analysis, mental events, and psychoanalysis. *Science and Psychoanalysis,* 1971, *18,* 51–62.

Eysenck, H. J., and Beech, H. R. Counter conditioning and related methods. In A. E. Bergin and S. L. Garfield (Eds.), *Handbook of psychotherapy and behavior change.* New York: Wiley, 1971.

Eysenck, H. J., and Rachman, S. *The causes and cures of neurosis.* London: Routledge and Kegan Paul, 1965.

Ezriel, H. Notes on psychoanalytic group therapy: II. Interpretation and research. *Psychiatry,* 1952, *15,* 119–127.

Feather, B. W., and Rhoads, J. M. Psychodynamic behavior therapy. Theory and rationale. *Archives of General Psychiatry*, 1972, *26*, 496–502. (a)

Feather, B. W., and Rhoads, J. M. Psychodynamic behavior therapy II. Clinical aspects. *Archives of General Psychiatry*, 1972, *26*, 503–511. (b)

Fitzgerald, R. V. *Conjoint marital therapy*. New York: Jason Aronson, 1973.

Fransella, F., and Joyston-Bechal, M. P. An investigation of conceptual process and pattern change in a psychotherapy group. *British Journal of Psychiatry*, 1970, *119*, 199–206.

Goldiamond, I., and Dyrud, J. E. Some applications and implications of behavioral analysis for psychotherapy. *Research in Psychotherapy*, 1968, *3*, 54–89.

Gurman, A. S., Knudson, R. M., and Kniskern, D. P. Behavioral marriage therapy. IV. Reply: Take two aspirins and call us in the morning. *Family Process*, 1978, *17*, 165–180.

Hafner, R. J. Catharsis during prolonged exposure for snake phobia: An agent of change? *American Journal of Psychiatry*, 1978, *135*, 247–248.

Hogan, R. A. The implosive technique. *Behaviour Research and Therapy*, 1968, *6*, 423–431.

Hunt, H. F., and Dyrud, J. E. Commentary: Perspective in behavior therapy. *Research in Psychotherapy*, 1968, *3*, 140–152.

Jacobson, N. S., and Weiss, R. L. Behavioral marriage therapy. III. Critique: The contents of Gurman *et al.* may be hazardous to your health. *Family Process*, 1978, *17*, 149–164.

Jones, W. J., and Park, P. M. Treatment of single-partner sexual dysfunction by systematic desensitization. *Obstetrics and Gynecology*, 1972, *39*, 411–417.

Kaplan, H. S. *The new sex therapy*. New York: Brunner/Mazel, 1974.

Kaplan, H. S. Psychoanalysis and the behavioral therapies. *Journal of the American Academy of Psychoanalysis*, 1976, *4*, 3–6.

Kelly, G. A. *A psychology of personal constructs* (Vol. 1). *A theory of personality*. New York: Norton, 1955.

Leary, T. *Interpersonal diagnosis of personality*. New York: Ronald Press, 1957.

Levay, A., Weissberg, J., and Blaustein, A. Concurrent sex therapy and psychoanalytic psychotherapy by separate therapists: Effectiveness and implications. *Psychiatry*, 1976, *39*, 355–363.

London, P. The end of ideology in behavior modification. *American Psychologist*, 1972, *27*, 913–920.

Malan, D. H. *The frontier of brief psychotherapy*. New York: Plenum, 1976.

Manus, G. L. Marriage counseling: A technique in search of a theory. *Journal of Marriage and the Family*, 1966, *28*, 449–453.

Marks, I. M., Viswanathan, R., Lipsedge, M. S., and Gardner, R. Enhanced relief of phobias by flooding during waring diazepam effect. *British Journal of Psychiatry*, 1972, *121*, 493–505.

Marmor, J. Dynamic psychotherapy and behavior therapy: Are they irreconcilable? *Archives of General Psychiatry*, 1971, *24*, 22–28.

Martin, P. A., and Lief, H. I. Resistance to innovations in psychiatric training as exemplified by marital therapy. In G. Usdin (Ed.), *Psychiatry, education and image*. New York: Brunner/Mazel, 1973.

Masters, W. H., and Johnson, V. E. *Human sexual inadequacy*. New York: Brunner/Mazel, 1970.

Mead, G. H. *Mind, self and society*. (C. W. Morris, Ed.) Chicago: University of Chicago Press, 1934. (a)

Mead, G. H. *On Social Psychology*. Chicago: University of Chicago Press, 1934. (b)

Nadelson, C. C. Marital therapy from a psychoanalytic perspective. In T. J. Paolino and B. S. McCrady (Eds.), *Marriage and marital therapy*. New York: Brunner/Mazel, 1978.

Norman, D. A. *Memory and Attention*. New York: Wiley, 1969.

Olson, D. H. Marital and family therapy: Integrative review and critique. *Journal of Marriage and the Family*, 1970, *32*, 501–538.

Olson, D. H. A critical overview. In A. S. Gurman and D. G. Rice (Eds.), *Couples in conflict*. New York: Jason Aronson, 1975.

Paolino, T. J. Introduction: Some basic concepts of psychoanalytic psychotherapy. In T. J. Paolino and B. S. McCrady (Eds.), *Marriage and marital therapy*. New York: Brunner/Mazel, 1978.

Piaget, J. *The moral judgment of the child*. Glencoe, Ill.: Free Press, 1948.

Ryle, A., and Lunghi, M. E. The measurement of relevant change after psychotherapy: Use of repertory grid testing. *British Journal of Psychiatry*, 1969, *115*, 1297–1304.

Satir, V. *Conjoint family therapy*. Palo Alto: Science and Behavior Books, 1967.

Scharff, D. E. Sex is a family affair: Sources of discord and harmony. *Journal of Sex and Marital Therapy*, 1976, *2*, 17–31.

Segraves, R. T., and Smith, R. C. Concurrent psychotherapy and behavior therapy. *Archives of General Psychiatry*, 1976, *33*, 756–763.

Slater, P. Theory and technique of the repertory grid. *British Journal of Psychiatry*, 1969, *115*, 1287–1296.

Stampfl, T. G., and Lewis, D. J. Implosive therapy—A behavioral therapy? *Behaviour Research and Therapy*, 1968, *6*, 31–36.

Stotland, E., and Canon, L. K. *Social psychology, a cognitive approach*. Philadelphia: W. B. Saunders, 1972.

Sullivan, H. S. *The Interpersonal Theory of Psychiatry*. New York: Norton, 1953.

Wachtel, P. L. *Psychoanalysis and Behavior Therapy*. New York: Basic Books, 1977.

Woody, R. H. Toward a rationale for psychobehavioral therapy. *Archives of General Psychiatry*, 1968, *19*, 197–204.

# An Integrative Model

The purpose of the next three chapters is to present an integrative model for the treatment of chronic marital discord. Previous chapters have documented the absence of a comprehensive model for the conduct of marital therapy. In particular, it has been argued that the formation of theoretical schools and ideologies has hampered the clinician's vision and range of permissible activities. Necessary linkages between alternative conceptual systems are absent and no clinically sophisticated theoretical model articulates with a data language. As stated previously, three principal conceptual dichotomies are felt to hinder integrative efforts within the field. Thus, the proposed model will attempt to establish linkages between present and past determinants of behavior, between observable behavior and internal psychological events, and between individual psychopathology and interpersonal behavioral systems. Such minimal linkages are necessary for the responsible treatment of marital disorders.

The aim of this chapter is to present an integrated conceptual system. As subsequent chapters will be devoted to the clinical application of this model, this chapter will focus primarily on theoretical issues. The language system chosen for the development of this model may seem alien and unnecessarily awkward to many clinicians, particularly to those of a psychodynamic orientation. The language of cognitive social psychology was purposely chosen as the most appropriate system allowing for the specification of intuited and inferred clinical phenomena in a data-based language. One of the principal reasons that behaviorally oriented therapists dismiss the writings of psychodynamically oriented therapists is that this literature tends to utilize higher level abstractions whose linkages to observable data are often unclear. Thus, these clinicians are asked to bear with the author momentarily. Many contemporary clinical theoreticians (Strupp, 1960, 1978; Olson, 1975) are beginning to emphasize the tragedy of the schism between psychotherapy research and practice. Similarly, other authors (Bowlby, 1977; Carson, 1969) have appreciated the potential usefulness of social psychological theory for bridging this schism.

The ideas developed in this chapter will appear as radical departures from standard theory to certain clinicians and as old hat to others. Most of these ideas are extensions of concepts already developed by other eclectic clinicians. For example, this model assumes that a reciprocal relationship exists between environmental events and internal events within the individual organism. Family therapists have clearly documented the influence of behavior in interpersonal systems on the individuals involved (Ackerman, 1966; Bowen, 1971; Minuchin, 1971). From another perspective, individual psychotherapists and theoreticians have advocated clinical approaches stressing both internal and external sources of psychopathology (Wolf, 1980; Birk and Brinkley-Birk, 1980), have stressed the importance of both behavioral and subjective variables in psychopathology (Strong, 1978; Bergin and Lambert, 1978), and have advocated treatment approaches emphasizing both behavioral and intrapsychic variables (Wachtel, 1977; Birk and Brinkley-Birk, 1980). All of these therapists have been concerned with the nature of the relationship between private events within the organism and events in the interpersonal environment. Most of these therapists have concluded that this relationship is reciprocal. Family therapists have tended to concentrate on the influence of variations in interpersonal events in social systems on the private lives of participants. Eclectic individual therapists have tended to focus on the influence of a change in an individual's behavior on his private universe. Implicit in both of these orientations is the assumption of a mutual interaction between private organismic events and interpersonal behavior among intimates. In other words, private events within the individual are related to his behavior toward others and thus to their reactions to him. In turn, their behavior toward him influences his behavior and private universe. Conceptually, the nature of the interactive influences becomes more complex as the number of participants increases.

The goal of this chapter is ambitious. It seeks to explicitly link individual psychopathology with interpersonal behavior in social systems. It seeks to conceptualize linkages between private organismic variables and interpersonal behavior in such a way that the practicing clinician can utilize individual, marital, behavioral, or interpretive interventions within a unified conceptual framework. It also attempts this synthesis in a data-oriented language. Understandably, this model is offered as a beginning effort in that direction. The author has no illusions that it is a complete model. He asks that this section be judged on the basis of whether it offers a new perspective from which to conceptualize the treatment of marital discord and on the basis that the major propositions are capable of being disproved if they are erroneous. The value of a beginning model such as this is mainly heuristic (Eysenck, 1960).

## BASIC ASSUMPTIONS

In order to evolve a theoretical model concerning marital therapy, it is necessary to make certain assumptions regarding psychotherapy and psychopathology in general. This basic groundwork is necessary in order to have a base from which to build a more specific therapeutic model.

### Interpersonal Consistency

From my perspective, one has to assume that individuals have predispositions to act in given ways in certain specified interpersonal contexts. One can reasonably speak of someone's personality as reflecting a certain consistency of behavior in seemingly different interpersonal situations. A reasonably skilled clinician can detect a theme of recurring behavioral disturbance in most psychiatric patients, and this recurring pattern can usually be noted in multiple interpersonal situations. The skilled clinician can usually formulate provisional hypotheses about the interpersonal contexts that will, with a high degree of probability, elicit the maladaptive behavior pattern.

Individual psychotherapists reading this text may question why a section on personal consistency is even included, as this appears to be an established fact. However, certain clinical theoreticians differ with this assumption. Theoreticians such as Bandura (1969) and Mischel (1968) have questioned the existence of general response dispositions in humans and have suggested that this belief among clinicians may represent "a tendency to construe behavioral consistencies even from variable performances" (Bandura, 1969). According to Bandura, the fiction of generalized response dispositions is maintained at a broad inferential contruct level by clinicians, whereas a high degree of behavioral specificity can be observed. Bandura suggests that several factors may account for the mistaken impression of clinicians. These include the limited stimulus conditions under which a person is observed and the broad and ambiguous descriptive categories utilized. Bandura's position is supported by the fact that considerable research reveals little evidence for consistency in behavioral patterns across different stimulus situations. Several factors may explain this divergence of viewpoints between therapists and theoreticians, and the failure of research to substantiate this common clinical assumption. First, clinicians are speaking of a specific form of personal consistency. The stimulus conditions for eliciting these forms of behavior are seldom approximated by research endeavors. The clinician is usually referring to a behavioral consistency, given a particular emotional state. For example, certain patients can be observed to consistently rebuff offers of emotional support when feeling particularly lonely or emotionally distraught. Other patients may be observed to consistently provoke a certain interpersonal distance, when they feel sexually aroused, from someone with whom they also feel an emotional closeness. From the clinician's viewpoint, these nuances of interpersonal behavior may constitute the patient's primary problem in adaptation. Understandably, these interpersonal situations can seldom be experimentally reproduced in a research context. Second, much psychological research is conducted on normal volunteers. There may well be differences in the strength of generalized response predispositions in psychiatric patients and normal volunteers. In fact, generalized response predispositions may be a characteristic differentiating psychiatric populations from normals. Part of their lack of adaptability to environmental stresses may be their limited repertoire of response capabilities: "In many cases the 'sicker' the patient, the more likely he is to have abandoned all interpersonal techniques except one—which he can handle with magnificent finesse" (Leary, 1957, p. 116). As previously reviewed, marital therapists connected with general system theory have also questioned the assumption of interpersonal consistency. These therapists have been impressed with the reactivity of humans in social settings and the power of contemporary interpersonal events in determining behavior. Although these therapists have correctly emphasized processes relatively ignored by individual therapists, it would appear that they have overstated a correct perception. The fact that numerous studies have found that premarital personality is related to subsequent marital adjustment, of course, indicates the presence of at least a minimal degree of consistency in interpersonal behavior.

The hypothesis of relative consistency in behavior is essential to many theories of personality and psychotherapy. This issue has been addressed differently by different theorists. Harry Stack Sullivan, an interpersonally oriented psychiatrist, referred to personality as "the relatively enduring patterns of recurrent interpersonal situations which characterize a human life" (1953, p. 11). A similar viewpoint has been advocated by social psychologists such as Leary (1957), Carson (1969), and Stotland and Canon (1972). Thus, Carson, in a discussion of the interaction of man with his environment, concluded: "The facts seem to require that we attribute a portion of the regularities in individual behavior to some form of relatively persistent dispositional tendencies existing 'within' persons. These dispositional tendencies, variously conceived as traits, habits, 'need' and so forth, are in the main acquired in the course of experience rather than being innately determined, and they are subject to alteration as a consequence of new experience" (Carson, 1969, p. 9). A psychoanalytic concept of some importance is the triangle of insight (Menninger, 1958; Malan, 1976). According to this formulation, the patient can be observed having a similar difficulty in three different interpersonal contexts—with the therapist, with a significant person outside of therapy, and with a significant person in the past (usually a parent). Thus, the therapist's goal is to provide linking interpretations. In these interpretations, the therapist helps the patient to realize the similarities of feelings, perceptions, and actions in these interpersonal contexts. The concept of perceptual consistency is also implicit in recent therapeutic development such as cognitive therapy (Beck, 1976; Beck et al., 1979). In this approach, the therapist works to modify certain thought processes on the assumption that these enduring, habitual patterns of thinking are linked to the patient's failure of adaptation.

It is important to emphasize that the author's assumption of interpersonal consistency emphasizes the predisposition to act in certain ways given certain interpersonal stimuli. This assumption differs from many dynamic therapists who assume that certain self-regulatory structures within the organism have a life of their own, only partially influenced by environmental events. The author's assumption is more relative and probabilistic. Although consistencies of behavior can be noted in most individuals, these individuals do change (self-regulatory structures are modified by environmental events) and they demonstrate seeming inconsistencies in behavior. Given the complexity of interpersonal stimuli, seeming inconsistencies in behavior may be the result of changes in unidentified interpersonal stimuli. In other cases, inconsistencies may be the result of other overriding environmental pressures. For example, a patient with a strong tendency to be argumentative with authority figures may be submissive and compliant with his boss when his job is at risk during a period of economic uncertainty.

The implication of this supposition for marital theory is important.

The same individual behavioral problems noted in the marital context will be noted in other interpersonal settings as well. In certain patients, the repetitive pattern will be obvious in multiple interpersonal settings, while in other patients, this abnormality may be restricted to interpersonal contexts involving enduring intimate interactions with significant members of the opposite sex.

## Person–Environment Interaction

Whereas orthodox analysts tend to stress internal organismic determinants of behavior, modern behaviorists have tended to deviate too far to the other extreme, characterizing man's behavior as totally under environmental control. Using concepts of linear causality, which have been useful in the physical sciences, behaviorists tend to view man's behavior as controlled by the stimuli that evoke it and the reinforcing stimuli that maintain it. There are two difficulties with this simplistic behavioral model. First, in complex interpersonal situations, it is difficult to attribute cause and effect. One simply observes a chain of complex alternating behavior between participants. "Punctuation" of these chains, assigning cause and effect, is always arbitrary (Bateson, 1958; Watzlawick et al., 1967).

Second, man's interpersonal behavior influences his own environment (Bandura, 1977; Carson, 1969). One needs to conceive of man's relationship with his social environment as a reciprocal process, each influencing the other. This process may be referred to as circular causality, the response-determined stimulus effect, or reciprocal determinism. This process has been aptly described by Bandura: "Personal and environmental factors do not function as independent determinants, rather they influence each other. Nor can 'persons' be considered causes independent of their behavior. It is largely through their actions that people produce the environmental conditions that affect their behavior in a reciprocal fashion" (Bandura, 1977, p. 9). Later in the same text, Bandura makes his position more explicit: "Environments have causes as do behaviors. It is true that behavior is regulated by its contingencies, but the contingencies are partly of a person's own making. . . . To the oft-repeated dictum, 'change contingencies and you change behavior,' should be added the reciprocal side, 'change behavior and you change the contingencies.' "

Stotland and Canon (1972) discuss the same topic in a manner that may be more relevant to clinicians: "On the other hand, we are probably less likely to be acutely aware of the influence our behavior has on the social stimuli with which we interact. Although the point being made here is rather obvious—that we are not just passive recipients of the information we receive from environmental stimuli but actively play a role in shaping and creating them—the ways in which this occurs are not obvious, especially to the participants. The influence our behavior may have on the social stimulus may be quite direct in that it actually alters the stimulus itself. . . . If we respond with anxiety, indifference, defensive maneuvers, or outright hostility to someone, he is likely to react defensively or aggressively himself, no matter how benign or friendly his intentions may have been initially" (p. 28).

In other words, man partially creates his own interpersonal universe by his impact on significant others, and men vary to the extent to which they are aware of the impact of their behavior on intimate others. Given the complexity and quantity of interpersonal stimuli influencing man at any given instance, it is highly improbable that any human is fully cognizant of the impact he is having on his environment. This is especially true of complex enduring relationships such as marriage. The process of person–environment interaction is highly complex in marriage, as each partner is influencing the other in ways he is unaware of. Thus, each spouse partially determines the other spouse's behavior toward himself.

## Behavior as a Function of Perceived Environment

Behavioral therapy has its roots in experimental psychology and thus emphasizes the impact of the environment on the organism. Similarly, behaviorism as a school of thought excludes unobservable organismic variables from consideration. In experiments with lower animals, it may be reasonable to assume that the experimentally manipulated stimulus (shock, light, food pellets) is the effective stimulus for the organism. From this perspective, it is not unreasonable to assume that reinforcement works by automatically strengthening stimulus–response connections.

Psychotherapists have long realized the difficulties involved in transposing this model to interpersonal contexts. Due to the complexity and multiplicity of stimuli in most interpersonal relationships, it is difficult to ascertain the effective or perceived stimulus for any given individual. It is is a common finding that different participants will give differing reports and interpretations of the same interpersonal situations (Stotland and Canon, 1972). Because of the complexity of interpersonal stimuli, some selectivity of perception is necessary to avoid information overload. Even if one ignores the possibility of motivated attention shifts (e.g., selective inattention, repression), one cannot assume a close correspondence between private experience and "objective observable environmental events."

Accordingly, numerous theorists of varying theoretical persuasions (e.g., Bandura, 1977; Carson, 1969; Beck et al., 1979; Mahoney, 1974) have stressed the importance of perceived reality as a determinant of behavior. In a review of experimental studies, Bandura (1977) concluded that the bulk of evidence suggests that behavior is governed more by its perceived consequences than by its actual consequences. This conclusion is supported by both clinical observation and experimental findings. Various studies have demonstrated that people tend to shift their behavior to anticipated consequences rather than to actual consequences (Kaufman et al., 1966; Dulany, 1968; Bandura and Barab, 1971). The assumption that behavioral disturbance is often the result of reacting to misperceived reality is, of course, a central tenet of much clinical theory.

The author feels that considerable evidence supports the assumption that perceived reality is the predominant force in interpersonal situations. Similarly, considerable evidence suggests that perceived reality is partially a function of external reality and the patient's way of construing that reality. Numerous studies suggest that a person's method or characteristic way of construing reality is related to his past experience in analogous situations. From the perspective of marriage, this suggests that one's behavior toward one's spouse is partially a function of the spouse's actual behavior and partially a function of one's perception of that spouse's behavior.

## Nature of Cognitive Events

Theorists of multiple theoretical persuasions have assumed that behavior is influenced by inner representational events (e.g., Wilson, 1978; Marmor, 1980; Meichenbaum, 1977; Mahoney, 1974), and that such cognitive representations of reality are based on previous learning experiences (e.g., Strupp, 1978; Strong, 1978). Similarly, many clinicians have maintained that a useful understanding of the relationship of these events to disturbed behavioral patterns must take place at a molar rather than a molecular level (e.g., Sollod and Wachtel, 1980; Wolf, 1980; Alexander, 1963). In other words, man forms abstractions of reality and these abstractions serve to organize future perceptions and to guide behavior. Various authors have referred to these abstractions using different terms: e.g., Sullivan's concept of personification (1953), Piaget's use of the term *schemata* (1948), the concept of abstract and referential modeling in social learning theory (Rosenthal and Bandura, 1978), George A. Kelly's notion of personal construct systems (1955), the concept of introjection in object-relations theory (Kernberg, 1976), and even the concept of transference in classical psychoanalysis (Alexander, 1963).

The point I am attempting to establish is that to understand human behavior in interpersonal contexts, one must consider how man organizes his experience. In interpersonal relationships, there is considerable reason to assume that man forms general representational models of significant others. It matters little if one prefers to label these models internal objects, personifications, or schemata. These models, or templates for organizing interpersonal stimuli, are the mechanism by which the past influences current reality. This mechanism was clearly described by Wolf in 1966: "An individual's characteristic patterns of behavior to other people, as much as to objects, are learned principally during the formative years of childhood in the course of interactions with significant members of the nuclear family. The interpersonal patterns thus acquired are, with greater or lesser modifications, transferred by way of social generalization into relationships with comparable, equivalent, or derivative human figures" (Wolf, 1966, p. 7). It is of note that analysts such as Alexander (1963) and Rado (1962) have advanced similar notions. As previously reviewed in this text, social psychologists have hypothesized analogous mechanisms.

Numerous theoreticians and therapists concerned with the relationship of organismic variables to psychopathology have focused on events within the organism. Thus, Meichenbaum (1977) has stressed the importance of internal speech and self-control. Mahoney (1974; Mahoney and Arnkoff, 1978) emphasizes the importance of thought control. Ellis (1962) and Beck (1976) point out the importance of self-statements in the genesis of unpleasant emotions. Even Bandura (1969) stresses the importance of concepts such as internal reinforcement and expectations of personal effectiveness. In many ways, such a concern over the interrelationships of events within the organism is analogous to the concern of dynamic therapists with personality organization (Strupp, 1978).

What I am suggesting is that it may be more profitable to focus attention on the relationship between a patient's molar conceptualizations of significant others and his environmental adaptation. I suggest this for both clinical and empirical reasons. The whole area of feelings toward the self is an extremely difficult one both conceptually and methodologically. In fact, metapsychological theory about the self was one of the forces that originally contributed to the formation of a school of behaviorism, in reaction to the mentalism of psychoanalysis. It is ironic that many members of this original rebellion are now leading the counterswing. It would appear far wiser to begin our search for links between mental events and observable behavior in the interpersonal environment. Within this context, one can specify hypothesized links between inner mental events and observable behavior. If one's theory is properly constructed, false linkages can be disproven and abandoned or replaced. Such a methodological rigor is virtually impossible to achieve in self-statements and conceptualizations about the self.

Similarly, it is unclear to what extent clinical theory need concern itself with feelings about the self or with aspects of personality organization. Whereas such concerns may prove necessary in certain patient populations, currently described as borderline or narcissistic, in the majority of patients seen in psychotherapy such issues may not be paramount: "The most common conflicts begin when the child has already a distinct feeling of being a person (ego awareness) and relates to his human environments, to his parents and siblings as individual persons" (Alexander, 1980, p. 7). It would appear that most neurotic, marital, and character pathology can be understood as disturbances in interpersonal relationship. If one conceptualizes self-concept as predominantly the result of reflected appraisal from others, it is possible that poor self-concept is the result rather than the cause of disturbed interpersonal behavior. If a patient has a history of chronic interpersonal disturbance, he may well have produced an interpersonal environment in which the predominant reflected appraisal is neglect.

Ultimately, one will need an empirically based clinical theory that addresses the issues of the reciprocal interrelationship of self and other representational systems and between reflected appraisal and representational systems for significant others. What I am proposing is that such an integration is premature at this time. I am suggesting that we begin with a simpler model and test its limitations. Such a model should focus on the interrelationship between molar representations of significant others and one's adaptational behavior.

## Psychotherapy as Social Influence

After a period during which the efficacy of psychotherapy was seriously doubted, considerable evidence now exists that psychotherapy is beneficial for the majority of patients (Bergin and Lambert, 1978). However, the effective mechanisms of therapy and the relative contributions of nonspecific and specific factors remain unclear (Strupp, 1978). It is unclear to what extent factors unique to the therapeutic context facilitate patient change in ways different from other helpful human relationships. Studies comparing the relative effectiveness of one form of therapy versus others have by and large yielded inconsistent results (Meltzoff and Kornreich, 1970), leading some investigators to conclude that all therapies may be effective because of similar mechanisms (Frank, 1973). For this and other reasons, some theorists have tended to view the therapeutic process as a form of social influence (Johnson and Matross, 1977). This unquestioned assumption by social psychologists is, of course, objectionable to many therapists who conceptualize their activities as promoting insight or personal growth. Psychoanalysts undergo personal analysis on the assumption that this therapy will ameliorate some of their unconscious tendencies to influence patients in counterproductive ways.

It appears reasonable to assume that all interpersonal interaction involves influence to an extent and that psychotherapy is a special form of social influence. Psychotherapy is concerned with behavior and personality change. This change can be effected only if the therapist brings to bear some influence on the patient. From this perspective, the psychotherapies can be differentiated to the extent that the nature of the intended influence is made explicit. On the one extreme, the behavioral therapies are quite explicit in that they intend to change targeted behavioral abnormalities. The cognitive therapies are reasonably explicit in that they specify certain belief systems and cognitive processes as targets of change. The dynamic therapies are unusual in that the targeted changes often appear more elusive and unspecified. However, certain notable exceptions are available in the psychoanalytic literature. In particular, the recent interest in brief dynamic psychotherapy has produced an analytic literature that is more specific as to the intended impact of therapy. Authors such as Malan (1976), Sifneos (1972), and others (Balint et al., 1972; Mann, 1973) emphasize the need for the therapist to focus his interventions on targeted focal and nuclear conflicts. These therapists model their approaches on pioneering work by Franz Alexander. Alexander was one of the first analytically oriented therapists to attempt to specify the necessary influence on the patient and the ways to augment this influence.

It would appear that many discussions of analytic technique—e.g., timing of interpretations, the triangle of insight, the need for a therapeutic alliance, the necessity of interpreting the defense and anxiety before the impulse—are highly sophisticated discussions of the optimal conditions under which the therapist can influence the patient. For a patient to achieve insight as to the nature of his character structure or transference reactions, that patient has to undergo a change in his personal belief system. The analyst influences this change in the patient's belief system or it doesn't occur. The nature of this influence may range from the fairly obvious to more elusive forms. For example, the therapist can provide an interpretation that brings together various elements in the patient's experience in a coherent, helpful manner, or he can, by his subtle and perhaps unconscious choice of interventions, implicitly reinforce the patient in certain forms of internal problem solving that lead to appropriate "insights." In other cases, the patient may infer the therapist's approach to internal problem solving and apply this to his own difficulties.

It is important to note that the concept of social influence in the psychotherapeutic context is not used in a derogatory sense. It is assumed that both dynamic and humanistically oriented therapists influence patients in beneficial ways, and the "insights" derived from therapy are useful and perhaps correct. It is, however, ironic that dynamic therapists are some of the most skilled diagnosticians of the nature of social influence needed in patients but do not use the full force of their skill because of their reluctance to acknowledge the process involved.

Strong (1978), in an attempt to apply social psychological theory to psychotherapy, concludes that psychotherapeutic change occurs by inducing discrepancy: "Change in psychotherapy results from the application of therapist power to gain acceptance of new information that is inconsistent with some existing client behavior (thoughts, feelings, or actions), and thus leads to change as the client reasserts congruity. For psychotherapy to have any effect on clients, therapists must introduce ideas discrepant from existing client ideas . . . therapists introduce two kinds of information to clients. First, therapists bring to the client's awareness existing incongruencies among client behaviors and consequences of behavior. The facts brought to the client's awareness may be aspects of events the client had not previously noticed, aspects he has distorted, denied, or repressed, or aspects he has attributed to external circumstances and thus not personally owned. The second kind of information the therapist presents that creates incongruency in the client is different standards for evaluating perceived events and different relationships and causal connections among event elements. This information can lead to changes in the client's processing of information, including different conceptions of his or her definition as a 'person' " (Strong, 1978, p. 112). Strong then outlines four main mechanisms of inducing discrepancy: (1) different attribution, (2) different perspective, (3) interpretation, reflection, and instruction, and (4) counterattitudinal-forced compliance.

The fourth mechanism, counterattitudinal-forced compliance, is probably closest to one that occurs in marital or family therapy. Strong uses this mechanism to refer to therapeutic contexts in which the patient is induced to act in ways discrepant from his belief system. In marital or family therapy, a slightly different mechanism is presumably involved. Through specific forms of therapeutic influence, the therapist induces a change in the interactional system, which then produces information discrepant with the spouses' usual beliefs about one another. If one spouse can be induced to act differently, this spouse is presenting different eliciting interpersonal stimuli to the second spouse. The second spouse's behavior will thus be different.

## Choice of Therapeutic Intervention

All too often, therapists tend to artifically separate themselves into various camps, according to theoretical orientation (e.g., psychoanalytic, behavioral) or by treatment modality (e.g., individual, group, family). Each camp tends to be somewhat isolated and to develop its own mythology (London, 1972). These mythologies, understandably, tend to emphasize the superiority of one approach over the others. Each camp observes psychopathology from a given perspective, and its conclusions about psychopathology are usually correct within the constraints of its observational bias. For example, dynamic individual therapists correctly identify the influence of past and internal psychological events on current environmental adaptation, whereas family therapists tend to emphasize the importance of current environmental events within the family. Behavior therapists are impressed with the power of directly modifying observable maladaptive behavior. The failure of each orientation resides in its restricted range of observation.

In most patients, the same behavioral disturbance occurring in life outside of therapy will manifest itself in therapy. There will be nuances of difference in its manifestation partially related to differences in the interpersonal context and partially related to the observational vantage point of the therapist. In "healthier" patients, this abnormality may be confined to intimate interpersonal situations of some duration, such as marriage, extramarital affairs, and long-term psychotherapy. In individual psychotherapy, the disturbed behavioral pattern gradually evolves in relationship to the therapist as therapy progresses. Analytically oriented therapists refer to this as the emergence of the transference (Offenkrantz and Tobin, 1975). In group therapy, a similar phenomenon occurs but is usually directed to the therapist and other group members. Within this context, it is referred to as a group transference reaction (Meissner and Nicholi, 1978). Within marital therapy, the analogous behavioral abnormality manifests itself immediately and is directed toward the spouses (Sager, 1967). In the previous chapter, cases were described in which individual behavioral interventions elicited analogous phenomena. What I am suggesting is that the same interpersonal abnormality is manifested in varying therapeutic contexts. There is no reason to assume that the abnormality is purer or appears in more pristine form in any interpersonal context.

Similarly, there is no reason to assume that these interpersonal abnormalities are more readily or permanently modifiable in any particular therapeutic or life context. If one assumes that psychopathology within the domain of character disorder consists of interrelated clusters of disturbed interactions with the environment and cognitive-emotional events within the organism, that organismic and environmental events are reciprocally interrelated, and that disturbed behavior primarily occurs in an interpersonal context, it is reasonable to conclude that the goal of therapy is to convince the patient that alternative ways of relating, both subjectively and selectively, are both possible and preferable. This process can occur in individual psychodynamically oriented psychotherapy. The analysis of the transference culminates in the patient's experiencing a different form of relatedness to the therapist. This knowledge is then used by the patient in relationships outside of therapy. Disconfirmatory experiences (experiencing that current reality is different from transference reality) likewise should be able to occur in direct relationships with intimate others. These disconfirmatory experiences should be able to occur in marital, family, or group therapy. Similarly, direct modification of patient behavior that precludes disconfirmatory experience in the natural environment should serve the same purpose. In other words, the choice of the form of therapeutic intervention should be decided on a pragmatic basis. The relationships are illustrated in Figure 1.

## AN INTEGRATIVE MODEL

The proposed integrative model addresses four principal areas: the form of disturbed cognitions in marital discord, the mechanism by which these cognitions relate to interpersonal behavior, the properties of disturbed interpersonal systems that preclude disconfirmatory experiences, and mechanisms of change.

It is important to note that this model is intended to be applicable only to cases of chronic marital discord. This can be arbitrarily defined as discord of more than 1 year's duration. An arbitrary time limit is set to indicate that this model is not applicable to the numerous transitory conflicts that arise in most relationships. Intense interpersonal struggles and considerable individual emotional upset can arise secondary to life stress, misunderstandings, and renegotiation of roles within a relation-

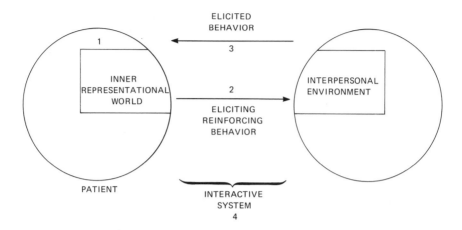

**Figure 1.** Theoretically, psychotherapeutic interventions could be focused at either of the four levels outlined above. In actuality, all interventions probably consist of admixtures. Classical psychoanalysis is an example of a type (1) focus. Fixed role therapy and certain forms of behavior therapy are examples of a type (2) focus. Family therapy, marital therapy, and group therapy are examples of type (4) interventions. Examples of type (3) interventions include classical analysis, where the analyst is truly a non-reactive observer, and certain behavioral interventions, where members of the family are instructed not to reinforce the symptomatic behavior.

ship. Many of these struggles abate or resolve with the passage of time or respond to brief interventions of a different sort. This model is limited to those struggles that are beyond the couple's own resources to solve over time. In these cases, individual character pathology in the spouses appears to play a crucial role and thus intervention requires a different conceptual model. This model is also not applicable to cases where one or both spouses have diagnoses of schizophrenia, paranoia, or affective disorder. This limitation of applicability is imposed as additional factors may be involved.

## Definition

From preceding portions of this text, it is obvious that the author feels that both cognitive and behavioral variables have to be considered in the treatment of marital discord. The proposed model is cognitive and bears a close resemblance to schools of therapy erroneously classified as cognitive-behavioral or as mediational behaviorism. In this regard, a clarification of the term *cognitive* is important. Part of this model focuses on a precise description of the nature of disturbed cognitions in chronic marital discord. For this reason, the terms *cognitive schema* and *cognitive complexity* require definition. Although these concepts were discussed in the previous chapter, they will be briefly redefined.

## Cognition

Cognitions are defined in a general way as referring to the processes involved in the processing of environmental information. It is important to note that cognitions are not restricted to conscious thoughts or self-statements, but "in less technical terms, cognitions are beliefs, thoughts, or items of information which an individual possesses concerning his own internal condition and the nature of the social and physical environment in which he exists. An approach which focuses on cognitive activity, then stresses the role which these sorts of perceptual organizations play as mediations between the stimuli which impinge upon the individual and the responses he makes to them. Cognitions are viewed as an example of what have been called mediating variables in that, though they may not be directly observed, they are held to shape and influence in important ways the relationship between an observable stimulus and a measurable response. Their functioning is presumed to intervene between stimulus and response and to be involved in an important way in determining the meaning which the stimulus has for the individual, and it is in terms of this meaning that a response is initiated" (Stotland and Canon, 1972, pp. 65–66).

## Schema

As outlined in the previous chapter, social psychologists (e.g., Kelly, 1955; Carson, 1969; Stotland and Canon, 1972) have described the encoding of interpersonal information in a different language. The essence of the social psychological framework is the assumption that man forms templates, which he uses to organize environmental information. Thus, man's perception of current reality is codetermined by current reality and by past experiences in similar situations. According to this formulation, past experiences are organized at a molar level. These templates for organizing interpersonal information are frequently referred to as schemas: "Because of the complexity and quantity of interpersonal stimuli and the limited information-processing capacity of the human nervous system, man develops cognitive schemas or templates to organize his interpersonal perceptions. These schemas influence the manner in which new information about people is perceived and assimilated" (Segraves, 1978, p. 452).

Thus, *schema* refers to an internal representational scheme of discrete portions of the universe generated by individuals from their experience of the universe. In other words, schemas are abstractions of events developed by people in order to anticipate events and relate to the universe. Schemas refer to ways of apprehending certain environmental events. It is not assumed that all individuals can verbalize their ways of organizing perceptions or that conscious verbal reports of schemas are in fact correct. Schemas also serve the function of organizing perceptions: "Thus construct systems [schemas] can be considered as a kind of scanning pattern which a person continually projects upon his world. As he sweeps back and forth across his perceptual field he picks up blips of meaning. The more adequate his scanning pattern, the more meaningful his world becomes" (Kelly, 1955, p. 145).

*Cognitive Complexity*

Cognitive complexity refers to the differentiation of object perception. In other words, a cognitively complex person tends to more completely appreciate the complexities of other people and to more fully appreciate subtle differences between individuals. This characteristic is held to be a character trait of individuals. The concept of cognitive complexity overlaps with object relations theorists' descriptions of the structural characteristics of internalized object relations (e.g., Rosenfield and Sprince, 1963; Rinsley, 1977; Kernberg, 1977). The concept of cognitive complexity is assumed to be a continuously distributed trait and is precisely defined.

The basic idea of cognitive complexity is contained in the work of George Kelly and his development of the repertory grid test (Kelly, 1953, 1955). As has been previously described, an individual is given a list of people (role descriptions) presumably important in most people's lives and is then asked to make repeated discriminations on interpersonal dimensions (which he provides) between emotionally significant people in his life. The test is constructed such that the end product is a grid composed of intersections between elements (people) and constructs (ways of perceiving people, schemas). This grid is then capable of being analyzed by mathematical procedures applicable to matrices. The brilliance of this procedure is that it provides a quantitative description of a patient's inner representational world. Thus, one can reasonably define transference as the distance between parent figure and therapist (or spouse) on all relevant constructs for the patient in question. Although minimally appreciated in this country, this procedure has been found to be extremely useful by psychodynamically oriented therapists in the United Kingdom (Fransella and Joyston-Bechal, 1971; Ryle and Lipschitz, 1975; Wijesinghe and Wood, 1976).

Various indices have been derived to measure cognitive complexity. The rationale behind all of these indices is that if two constructs have similar check patterns over different elements, then the constructs are probably measuring the same thing. One method of computing indices is based on the summation of such matches (Bieri, 1965; Olson and Partington, 1977). An individual having numerous such matches would be less cognitively complex in that he uses fewer interpersonal constructs in his perception of people. Another approach to the measurement of cognitive complexity is to calculate the portion of the total variance attributable to the first factor if the matrix is factor-analyzed (Bannister and Mair, 1968).

## Cognitive Factors in Marital Discord

It appears obvious that cognitive factors influence marital adjustment on various levels. Each spouse enters the marriage with certain beliefs concerning the form marriage should take and the role each spouse should take in the marriage. These beliefs appear to be partially determined in the family of origin and partially the result of more widespread cultural influences (Thorp, 1963). Discrepancy in these belief systems is certainly a source of conflict in many marriages. Numerous studies have documented that marital success is related to similarity in personality (Cattell and Nesselroade, 1967; Corsini, 1956; Pickford et al., 1966; Blazer, 1963), religion (Kirkpatrick, 1937; Landis, 1949), ethnic background (Carter and Glick, 1967), socioeconomic background (Hicks and Platt, 1970), and marital role definitions (Thorp, 1963). These studies support the hypothesis that similarity in assumptive worlds between spouses facilitates adjustment.

As noted earlier, differential assessments of the importance of cognitive-emotional events within the organism in the genesis of marital discord has been a source of contention between psychodynamic and behavioral marital therapists. Although behavioral marital therapists have been criticized for ignoring cognitive contributions to marital discord (Gurman and Knudson, 1978), this criticism is not completely warranted. With the growth of "mediational behaviorism," various "behavioral" marital therapists have acknowledged the importance of cognitive factors. For example, in a recent text, Jacobson and Margolin (1979) discuss assessment of relationship dysfunction: "The therapist must be aware that the client's cognitions play a critical role in the problems that they experience. Spouses enter therapy with numerous assumptions about what has caused their relationship problems, with evaluations of themselves and their mates as marital partners and with attitudes about the quality of the relationship. These cognitions play an important role in determining why a couple is seeking marital counseling and how the couple might respond to behavior change activities. For a couple to feel that the therapy experience has been worthwhile, it is important for each partner to change individual cognitions as well as behaviors" (pp. 70–71).

Other behavior therapists have alluded to the importance of modifying both dysfunctional cognitions and behaviors in disturbed marriages (Jacobson and Weiss, 1978; Weiss and Margolin, 1977; Stuart, 1975; Liberman, 1970). When the behavior therapist alludes to modifying cognitions in therapy, he is typically referring to conscious verbalized statements by each spouse. Certain psychodynamic therapists might agree with the behavioral therapists as to the importance of imparting realistic information to the spouses, but they would feel that this intervention overlooks other more important individual organismic variables involved. For example, when Sager and colleagues (1976) conceptualize marital discord as conflict concerning the marriage contract, conscious verbalized expectations make up only one-third of the marriage contract.

Clearly, the behavioral treatment of cognitive factors in marital discord is quite superficial in comparison to other therapeutic approaches. I am proposing that the organismic variables influencing marital discord are far more complex than this and are organized at a molar level. Central to my proposed model is that a crucial factor in marital discord resides in the object representations of spouses. In a review article, Barry (1970) succinctly summarized a comparable position by stating that "in any interpersonal situation, behavior is at least partly determined by the internal reference system (of each of the actors) of self to others and others to self, which is the product of each one's experience with significant others up to that point in time" (p. 41).

Numerous skilled therapists have observed that spouses in disturbed marriages demonstrate a consistent misattribution of characteristics and motives to the other spouse, which outside observers would find less than totally representative of the mate's character. This defect in central information processing has been noted mainly by analytically oriented therapists and has been described in a different language form. These therapists note that transference, "the transfer of relations exhibited toward objects in infancy onto contemporary objects" (Greene and Solomon, 1963, p. 444), presents as a perceptual distortion regarding a significant other (Sandler *et al.*, 1970) and that in marital discord this distorted perception is in regard to the mate's character (Sager, 1967; Litz, 1976). Grotjahn (1960) makes this point quite clearly: "Psychoanalysis invites the transfer of infantile ways into a therapeutic situation; marriage makes it possible for us to transfer our unconscious childhood images of family life—its happiness, disturbances, or fears and anxieties—into the realistic present. A good marriage thus has, in this respect, a potential similarity to a good psychoanalysis" (p. 92). He continues, "Trouble begins with the marriage neurosis, which may be defined as the transfer and projection of unresolved, unconscious conflicts from the pasts of both partners into the present; that is, from childhood families into the marriage situation. . . . The woman may unconsciously see an image of her father or brother in her husband" (pp. 92–93). Working from a different theoretical framework, object relations theorists have noted the character of selective misperception in marital discord. For example, Zinner (1976) discusses the role of projected identification in marital discord: "Highly fluid role attributions occur in which a husband, for example, may parentify his spouse, or on the other hand, infantilize her by experiencing the wife as the child he once was" (p. 297). Dicks (1967) likewise notes that character disorder and marital discord are often characterized by a certain rigidity of personality, which forces patients to be blind to certain aspects of themselves and others. Greenspan and Mannino (1974) discuss the same process in a manner illustrating the perceptual nature of the disorder: "Even though the object of the misperception may not acknowledge the other's perception or misperception, his or her behavior is interpreted as validating the misperception, since aspects of reality that do not fit the perceptual distortion go unnoticed. When the process is operative in both partners, each misperceives the other, each acts in response to only selected misperceived or partially valid but exaggerated aspects of the other, and both become locked into a discordant relationship pattern perpetuated through misperceptions and actions that endure solidly over long periods of time" (p. 1103). Certain behavioral marital therapists have fleetingly acknowledged the role of misperceptions of the spouse. For example, Liberman (1970) described his treatment of a couple in which the husband was intolerant of his wife's "helplessness": "I actively redirected his attention from his wife 'the unhappy, depressed woman' to his wife the coping woman" (p. 338). Jacobson and Margolin (1979) discuss the importance of misattribution of motives in marital discord: "From the absence of expressive behavior, the wife inferred that her husband neither trusted her nor loved her. While her request for expressions of positive feelings from her husband (particularly toward her) is perfectly legitimate and understandable, her inferences were unwarranted. The husband's lack of expressiveness in this case was more accurately construed as a skill deficit which in turn was partially due to his being punished by his mother for such feeling expressions in the past" (p. 143).

The point I am calling to your attention is that, at a clinical observational level, therapists of different disciplines have noted that perceptual distortions of the mate's character are important in the genesis of chronic marital discord. This phenomenon has been emphasized mainly by psychodynamically oriented therapists. This is not surprising in that dynamically oriented therapists receive considerably more training in understanding the nuances of interpersonal behavior than do therapists of other theoretical persuasions. Psychoanalytically oriented therapists have been justifiably criticized for confusing observation with inference in their clinical writings (Eysenck and Beech, 1971). Partially for this reason, many behavioral therapists have totally dismissed all contributions by psychodynamic therapists. I feel that this is unfortunate. Whatever one may think of psychoanalytic theory, psychoanalytic therapists are extremely skilled observers of interpersonal behavior. I am suggesting that some of these observations can be recast in a data-based language system that will be acceptable to a larger group of social scientists and also subject to empirical validation.

If one restricts one's retranslation of analytic contributions to the understanding of marital discord to those phenomena occurring in the interpersonal sphere and to descriptions that are close to the level of clinical observation, a consistent theme emerges in the analytic literature. All of these therapists emphasize the pivotal role of misperceptions of the spouse's character and motivations in the genesis and maintenance of marital discord (Segraves, 1978). This concept clearly overlaps with the use of the terms *transference* and *projective identification* without becoming entangled in metapsychological theory about events within the organism. Thus, analytic theorists posit that marital discord is related to a misperception of the spouse and that the direction of this misperception is such that figures in current reality are erroneously misperceived as similar to people in the patient's past life. Theorists of the object-relations school would also emphasize that these internal object representations are usually negative and poorly differentiated in chronically disturbed couples.

This retranslation of psychoanalytic concepts such as transference into the language system of cognitive social psychology is more than simple transliteration. If one can capture part of the clinical observations of analytically oriented therapists in a data-based language, one of the principal reasons that behavioral therapists dismiss the contributions of analytic therapists can be challenged. An advantage of the term *schema* is that it describes part of the analytic perspective without becoming entangled in associated assumptions of that theoretical model. A considerable social psychological literature exists on the conditions facilitating modification of interpersonal schemas. Schemas are modifiable by direct behavioral disconfirmation as well as by the method of verbal persuasion. Thus, this shift into terminology of a different conceptual model facilitates the integration of behavioral and psychodynamic approaches to therapy. This point will be returned to in subsequent sections of this chapter.

## The Clinical Context

In this section I will attempt to define the perceptual/cognitive disturbances noted in marital discord in an empirically testable manner. Four specific hypotheses, their supporting evidence, and empirical predictions will be presented. Prior to the presentation of these hypotheses, it is important to anchor the hypotheses in the clinical context. For this purpose, I will briefly describe a case seen by the author several years ago.

A rather introverted radiologist and his vivacious wife, a former nurse, consulted me ostensibly for an opinion as to whether their marriage could survive. The radiologist complained that his wife was stubborn and became explosively angry when she didn't get her way. On those occasions, he had no alternative but to give in. Shaking his head, he said, "It's a hopeless situation. That's just the way she is. I can't do a thing with her." What the therapist observed was slightly different. When the radiologist voiced a position contrary to what his wife wanted, she, being more vocal, tended to interrupt. The radiologist would then become silent and withdrawn. He was never observed to object to her interruptions or to talk over her interruption. The radiologist tended to control his wife by passive manipulation. Whenever his wife insisted on a social function that he really wanted to avoid, he would halfheartedly voice his opposition and then agree to go. Somehow, convenient last-minute medical emergencies necessitated his late arrival to these functions. Due to obscure forces influencing patient flow, he rarely had to be late to functions that he wanted to attend. Whenever the radiologist was upset with his wife, he tended to silently withdraw, change the subject, or indirectly criticize her. For example, if his wife looked upset, he usually would tell her how much he loved her. In the next breath, he might begin discussing how a friend's wife really understood the demands made on physicians and how she was a real ally to her husband. If the therapist inquired if he was saying that his own wife was deficient in this manner, the radiologist replied that he meant nothing of the kind. The radiologist tended to passively manipulate his wife until she became explosively angry and would threaten divorce in a fit of anger. At these times, the radiologist would become anxious and try to reassure his wife. He might, for example, begin to talk of buying her a fur coat. It seemed reasonable to infer that he saw his wife as an angry, powerful woman whom he had to placate but could never overtly influence.

Although his wife outwardly appeared competent and self-assured, especially in comparison to her more socially awkward husband, it was clear that she required considerable reassurance. What the radiologist did not *observe* was the effect of silent withdrawal upon his wife. During these times, she would become visibly anxious and then use her vivaciousness to draw out her husband. That vivaciousness had a frantic quality to it until she was able to get her husband to smile. She had a "little girl" quality, continually looking for reassurance of her lovability. She was an exceptionally attractive and flirtatious blonde, but few men would have found her seductive.

One subject of contention concerned the living arrangements for his aging mother. The radiologist's father had recently died, and the mother, whom the radiologist described as domineering and controlling, expected to come live with her son. The radiologist felt that his mother had dominated his father and perhaps contributed to his father's heart attack by the stress she put on the poor man. In spite of this, he felt that he should provide for his mother. His wife was quite upset about the prospect of her mother-in-law living in their home. As the wife expressed the extent of her opposition to the proposed living arrangements, her husband became increasingly sullen. At this point, the wife became increasingly nervous and turned to the therapist. "You have to help. I haven't been able to sleep all week. When he gets upset like this, I can't stand it. I've started getting migraine headaches for the first time in my life." She continued, "If I have to, I'll put up with her to save my marriage. I think that it would be a horrible mistake."

The therapist turned to the husband and asked what he had just heard his wife say. The husband acknowledged everything except the influence of his behavior on her. At this point, the therapist repeated verbatim what the wife had said about the effect of his behavior on her and her willingness to compromise. He asked the radiologist if this was what his wife had said. The radiologist concurred, but with nonverbal cues suggesting that he dismissed this as not having any significance.

The therapist then inquired as to whether he felt that his wife was lying. The radiologist became visibly anxious and reconsidered. One could almost feel his struggle against trying to assimilate this information along with the contradictory image he had maintained of his wife for 10 years of marriage. As the session progressed, the husband reluctantly accepted the idea that his wife might be frightened of his disapproval but clearly did not know how to integrate this information with his image of her as an autonomous, powerful being. This omission from his awareness of a part of her character was a crucial element in their interaction. For example, he would not consistently challenge his wife on any decisions regarding their children but would passively manipulate situations to get his way. For example, his wife insisted that their children go to sleep by 9:00 p.m. on school nights. The radiologist felt that this was too early and would somehow always manage to keep the children up later. He might take the older son with him to the hospital at night and have to return late because of some unforeseen problem.

In most instances the wife did not strongly insist that her husband recognize her need for reassurance. Her parents had separated when she was young, and her mother had been devastated by this. She appeared to become frightened when openly acknowledging the degree of her dependence upon her husband.

For purposes of explication, let us focus on the nature of the radiologist's defect in processing information about his wife. From the available data, we can reasonably infer certain characteristics of this central information-processing defect. He consistently misperceives the character and motivations of his wife. This misperception or partial perception is based on the perception of environmental stimuli fitting a conceptual scheme. Information not fitting this scheme is omitted. The image he has of his wife is similar to his image of his mother. Both of these images are negative and relatively undifferentiated. He describes both his wife and his mother in blanket categorical terms denying the multidimensional complexity of human personality. The nature of these misperceptions can be stated in four hypotheses.

## Hypothesis One

It is hypothesized that in cases of chronic marital discord one or both spouses have schemas for the perception of the mate that are markedly discrepant with the mate's personality. Clinicians of multiple theoretical persuasions will observe certain behavioral abnormalities in marital discord. Erroneous and maladaptive cognitions about the forms of possible relationships with the mate and about the mate's personality will be found to coexist with these behavioral abnormalities. If one observes how mates in disturbed marriages process information about the other, one will observe certain repetitive and characteristic cognitive distortions of this information. Information about the mate will be consistently and cognitively distorted and assimilated into a preexisting schema. Clinically, one will observe one or both spouses having a fixated way of misperceiving the other's character and motivations. In the clinical context, schema is roughly equivalent to the psychoanalytic concept "transference reaction." It refers to a consistent cognitive and perceptual distortion of emotional information.

This hypothesis leads to the prediction that individuals in happy marriages will tend to more accurately perceive their spouses' characters than will individuals in poorly adjusted marriages. A small body of research supports this hypothesis. R. Dymond (1954), reported recruiting 15 couples and requesting each individual to complete the Minnesota Multiphasic Personality Test twice, once for self and once as he or she predicted the spouse would complete the questionnaire. Couples judged by the author to be more happily married were more accurate in their prediction of spouse answers. Kotlar (1965) reported similar findings. Fifty couples in marriage counseling and 50 volunteer couples having high scores on the Wallace Marital Adjustment Inventory were asked to complete the Leary Interpersonal Check List for self and spouse. Adjusted couples demonstrated less discrepancy between self-perception and mate's perception of that self. Murstein and Beck (1972) reported similar findings in 60 volunteer couples completing the Locke-Wallace Marital Adjustment Scale and adjective checklists for self and spouse description. More recently, Christensen and Wallace (1976) studied perceptual accuracy in groups of happily married volunteer couples, couples in marital therapy, and couples seeking divorce. The happily married couples tended to be more accurate than the unhappily married in their prediction of spouse answers. Frank and Kupfer (1976) reported similar findings in another recent study. In other studies (Luckey, 1960; Taylor, 1967; Stuckert, 1963) marital adjustment has been found to be related to the wife's accurate perception of her husband, but not to the husband's perceptual accuracy. To my knowledge, only one study has reported the absence of a relationship between perceptual accuracy and marital adjustment (Corsini, 1956). This study employed only 20 subjects. Indirect evidence supporting this hypothesis was recently reported by Gottman and his associates (1976) at the University of Illinois. In two studies, distressed and nondistressed couples did not differ in the way they intended messages to be received by the spouses, although they consistently differed in their perceptions of messages. Distressed couples consistently perceived messages from spouses to be more negative, regardless of the sender's intent.

This research can perhaps be adequately summarized by the statement that individuals in happy marriages tend to be more accurate than individuals in unhappy marriages in their predictions of psychological information about their spouses. This finding may have been stronger for wives than for husbands at the time that most of this research was conducted. In view of recent societal changes in sex roles, this sex difference may be less pronounced today.

Various explanations could be offered as to why couples in happy marriages demonstrate greater perceptiveness about their spouses' personalities. These explanations might include (1) greater interpersonal sensitivity as a character trait among the happily married, (2) a history of greater self-disclosure among the happily married, (3) a by-product of greater personality similarity among the happily married. The relevance of this discussion is to establish that the research on perceptual accuracy among spouses is supportive of the first hypothesis, but not definitive. If faulty schemas are postulated to contribute to the genesis of marital discord, this phenomenon needs greater precision in definition and measurement to be specifically examined. Additional postulates will aid in the provision of greater specificity.

## Hypothesis Two

It is hypothesized that these schemas or tendencies toward misperceptions were learned from previous intimate relationships with the opposite sex. This is an attempt to restate the concept of transference in social learning theory. It differs from the concept of transference in several important ways. Although these schemas are presumed to be learned mainly in the family of origin, this hypothesis allows for the effects of later learning. In older individuals, traumatic experiences with a previous spouse may be as significant as experiences with a parent figure. In other words, this model emphasizes the continual growth and change in the human in his interaction with the environment and does not assume the absolute primacy of early childhood events in the determination of adult personality.

As this redefinition is a change from the assumptive world of many dynamic therapists, it is worth a brief diversion to discuss the effects of early childhood events. Considerable evidence suggests that the effects of early childhood experiences can be reversible with adequate experiences later in life (Davis, 1976; Koluchoua, 1976; Clarke, 1968; Kagan, 1976; Rutter, 1976). In other words, it is the total life experience that counts. In a review of the empirical evidence concerning the impact of early childhood events on adult personality, Clarke and Clarke (1976) concluded: "Our main general conclusion is that, in man, early learning is mainly important for its foundational character. By itself, and when unrepeated over time, it serves as no more than a link in the developmental chain, shaping proximate behavior less and less powerfully as age increases" (p. 18). This conclusion is deviant from the clinical experience of many dynamic therapists who frequently elicit histories of stressful childhoods in adult patients and conclude that these early experiences are etiologically involved (Bowlby, 1968). No one can refute the clinical observation. One can, however, question the certainty of the conclusion. At least three alternative explanations can be offered for the frequent finding of abnormal childhood experiences in psychiatric patients.

First, the clinician is not in a position to appreciate the frequency of stressful early childhood events in nonpatient populations. Transient separations from parents in early childhood (Douglass *et al.*, 1966) and parental divorce (Bloom *et al.*, 1978) are quite common experiences. Similarly, some evidence exists (Alkon, 1971) that traumatic separations in childhood are not more common in psychiatric patients than in the normal population. A second point emphasized by Clarke and Clarke is that children's family environments are often quite constant. It is highly likely that a child who experiences adverse family influences in early childhood will experience similar influences in middle childhood and adolescence: "That development is correlated with home background is well established. Particularly where adult deviant behavior is involved, clinicians and others will tend, through their pervasive frame of reference, to seek information about the early years. Commonly such data show abnormalities in early rearing and a casual link in thought to be established. As already implied, however, this is a non sequitur, for it ignores the probability that later experiences were also deviant. One could argue, then, that the cumulative effects of deviant rearing are responsible; or that later rearing is prepotent. Without environmental change as an independent variable it is indeed very difficult to determine the nature of this type of relation between early and later development" (Clarke and Clarke, 1976, p. 19). This conclusion is buttressed by findings in Rutter's (1971) study of children on the Isle of Wight. In this study, the rate of childhood antisocial disorder was found to decrease when the home situation changed for the better. A third mechanism for the relationship of early childhood events to later adaptation has been proposed by Clarke and Clarke (1976) and by Wachtel (1977). This mechanism can be referred to as the indirect causality model. In essence, it states that early events may produce certain behavioral predispositions, which interact with the environment, thus prolonging the effects of the early events. In other words, the child may unwittingly and continually elicit adverse responses from the interpersonal environment.

This hypothesis can be tested by comparing a patient's description of his spouse with his description of significant members of the opposite sex in his life. It is specifically predicted that one or both spouses in "bad marriages" will demonstrate such a selective misperception of the mate's character that they will have a tendency to perceive the current partner as erroneously similar to past figures. To my knowledge, minimal published research is relevant to this hypothesis. Ryle and Breen, in an unpublished study, compared seven maladjusted and seven volunteer adjusted couples on a modification of the Kelly repertory grid. This study reported that clinic couples are more likely than control couples to see their partners in a parental role. Because of procedural modifications and small sample size, this study can only be suggestive. This hypothesis can also be tested by using standard adjective checklists (e.g., LaForge and Suczek, 1955). If the adjective checklist method is employed, couples in unhappy marriages would be expected to demonstrate greater similarity in the pattern of adjectives checked to describe spouse and opposite-sex parent (or previous spouse).

## Hypothesis Three

The first two hypotheses specify that in cases of chronic marital discord one or both spouses have cognitions about the form of possible relationships with the mate that are erroneous and similar to memories of previous relationships. These two hypotheses are essential retranslations of the role that "transference" plays in marital discord. From this perspective, the persistence of chronic marital discord is partially related to the failure of spouses to adequately discriminate between the external reality of the current spouse and internal schemas for the perception of the opposite sex. Thus, chronic marital discord is related to a failure of discrimination learning.

The third hypothesis concerns a possible explanation for the failed discrimination learning. It is assumed that part of the failure of spouses in disturbed marriages to appropriately perceive the character of their mates is an individual characteristic or trait. One or both spouses will be observed to have a relative paucity of conceptual dimensions relevant to perception of intimate members of the opposite sex. This habitual cognitive structural characteristic of the spouses is known as low cognitive complexity.

In the clinical context, one will observe spouses assimilating information about their mates into simplistic and relatively undifferentiated forms. To varying degrees, subtleties of complex interactions will be overlooked and the complexity of the spouse's personality and motivational set often will not be perceived. For example, the spouse's personality will be perceived in shallow images or described in global terms such as *insensitive, selfish, stubborn, rigid, helpless*. These perceptions overlook obvious ambivalences and contradictory information about the spouse's personality. The character of perceptions is analogous to clinical descriptions of the perceptions of patients diagnosed as borderline personality disorders (Kernberg, 1972). However, this perceptual characteristic exists on a continuum. One or more spouses in cases of chronic marital discord will display this perceptual characteristic more than spouses in happy marriages. This characteristic is inferred from the spouses' habitual manner of relating to one another. One will often hear one refer to the other as if he or she were a fixed, undifferentiated being. The perceptions do not allow for ambiguity, uncertainty, and inconsistency.

This hypothesis specifies that the unhappily married will be characterized by their tendency to have less differentiated perceptions of their spouses and of the opposite sex.

This hypothesis can be tested by comparing the similarity of descriptions of all significant members of the opposite sex. In the unhappily married, there will be less differentiation of these descriptions. If the Kelly repertory grid method is used, the chronically unhappily married, as compared with the happily married, will demonstrate less cognitive complexity in the perception of the opposite sex. This can be documented by any of the standard ways of computing cognitive complexity using this instrument. The advantage of the Kelly repertory grid technique is that it is an instrument that provides a reliable map of an individual's private universe. One can use this procedure to estimate the distance between people in a patient's private universe as well as to estimate the degree of differentiation in this universe.

Although this instrument was available in the 1950s and has recently been utilized by dynamically oriented marital therapists (e.g., Ryle and Lunghi, 1970; Wijesinghe and Wood, 1976), the author is not aware of any study that has compared the cognitive complexity of happily and unhappily married couples. Crouse *et al.* (1968) compared happily and unhappily married couples on a far less sophisticated instrument. Unhappily married couples were found to have lower levels of integrative complexity, indicating intolerance of ambiguity and uncertainty. Indirect evidence supports the hypothesis that measures of cognitive complexity should be related to marital adjustment. For example, studies have indicated that measures of cognitive complexity are related to social behavior in other contexts. Olson and Partington (1977) reported that cognitively complex students were better able to view interpersonal situations from the perspective of other participants. Similarly, Bieri (1965) reported that cognitive complexity was related to the accurate perception of interpersonal intimates. Some work also demonstrates a relationship between cognitive complexity and interpersonal behavior. Czapinski (1976) found that prosocial behavior is positively related to the degree of one's cognitive differentiation of that person, and Hayden and associates (1977) reported that cognitive complexity is related to perceptual accuracy and the degree of social adjustment in emotionally disturbed boys. Several investigators have examined the relationship of cognitive complexity, personal perceptiveness, and assimilative projection (Bieri, 1965; Adams-Webber *et al.*, 1972). Assimilative projection refers to the tendency to see others as similar to oneself. As might be expected, individuals who see others as similar to themselves are less accurate in perceiving the viewpoint of others.

## Hypothesis Four

It is hypothesized that these relatively undifferentiated images of the opposite sex will be more negative in the unhappily married. Couples in disturbed marriages will tend to view the spouse and the opposite sex in general as more negative. That the unhappily married view their spouses more negatively than the happily married is almost a truism and is confirmed in the literature (Kelly, 1941; Udry, 1967). The author, however, is unaware of any empirical documentation of the unhappily married's perception of the opposite-sex parent or previous partner as compared to the happily married. This hypothesis can be examined by simply comparing the number of unfavorable adjectives checked for spouse description and opposite-sex parent description on a standard instrument such as the Adjective Check List (Gough and Heilbrun, 1965).

Clinically, these negative perceptions will often be manifest at an overt level (i.e., men are ungiving, men are only interested in sex, etc.). In other couples, this negativity may be restricted to interpersonal situations of individual emotional significance (i.e., it is dangerous to admit or express vulnerability to someone you love, etc.). In the latter instance, documentation of the distorted image may require greater methodological sophistication. In other words, I am referring to an element of risk (dangerousness) in one's apprehension of emotionally significant members of the opposite sex. These nuances of feeling and thought may be present only in established relationships and may not be verbalizable at a conscious level. They refer to one's apprehension of the opposite sex.

Clinically, one immediately thinks of two seeming exceptions to this hypothesis. This hypothesis would appear to have difficulty accounting for the situation in which one spouse denigrates his partner in relation to some romanticized ideal (i.e., my ex-husband never treated me that way). I am positing that in such situations, a sophisticated examination will reveal disappointment in all relationships with the opposite sex, although this may not be obvious on casual examination. On closer examination, evidence will appear that the romantic figures are dangerous as well. In certain couples, one or both spouses may have distorted, idealized perceptions of the other. These idealized perceptions restrict the possible behaviors of the other spouse. However, severe discord usually erupts when the idealization is broken. Thus, this situation does not appear to be an exception to the hypothesis.

## Relationship of Cognitions to Interpersonal Behavior

An integrated model of marital therapy needs to relate events within the organism to events in the environment. This step is necessary to bridge the contributions from both dynamic and behavioral therapies. Clearly, both organismic and environmental factors are important. In this section two hypotheses are offered to explain the influence of intrapsychic events on the environmental field. One of these hypotheses relates to the tendency of humans to induce and reinforce behavior in others that is congruent with the inner object world. The other hypothesis relates to the reactivity of humans in prolonged relationships.

In the case example of the radiologist and his wife, one can observe that the husband provokes his wife into angry outbursts by his passive-aggressive behavior toward her. Her expressions of weakness or need for reassurance are ignored by him and thus unreinforced. His behavior toward her is such that he never elicits behavior from her that challenges his way of construing her personality. He clearly influences his wife to act as if she is autonomous and powerful. The influence of his behavior on her over the years is deducible from her description of previous relationships. In a previous affair with a more assertive cardiologist, she had been concerned over her incredible passivity. She had felt protected by his assertiveness and was much less lively socially.

## Hypothesis Five

One mechanism by which schemas persist relatively intact in spite of interpersonal relationships with individuals of varying personalities relates to the tendency of individuals to reliably elicit behavior from others that is confirmatory to one's inner representational world. People tend to act toward significant others in such a way as to invite behavior that is confirmatory to the inner representational model for the opposite sex. Most individuals tend to avoid interactions for which they do not have conceptual maps. This standard assumption of contemporary social psychology permits a linkage between behavioral and psychodynamic models of marital therapy. It implies a primary role for perceptual distortions (transference reactions), predicts that they should precede observable signs of discord, and also predicts that there should be demonstrable relationships between perceptual distortions and observable interactional patterns.

Clinically, one observes spouses restricting the range of each other's behavior by the contingencies they provide for that behavior. This observation has been made by behavior therapists (Goldiamond, 1965), family therapists (Jackson, 1965), and dynamically oriented marital therapists (Sager, 1967). In the clinical context, one observes this control of spouse behavior occurring by a variety of mechanisms. This restriction of spouse behavior will range from blatant outrage when the spouse deviates from a prescribed range of behavior to much more subtle delivery of reinforcement and aversive stimuli. For example, if one spouse breaks an interactional "rule" (engages in proscribed behavior), the other spouse may be noted to begin criticizing that spouse about a seemingly unrelated behavior. If the criticized spouse shifts his initial behavior, the criticism will cease. The total interactional sequence may well be out of conscious control. Observations such as this lead some family therapists to speak of family interaction as a rule-governed system. It appears as if the interaction is controlled by a series of unspoken rules. In other cases, one may hear one spouse complain that the other is insensitive and emotionless. If one observes the complaining spouse carefully, one will often note that he does not provide reinforcement for the other spouse's expression of affect. By selective inattention to the mate's emotional state, the first spouse essentially extinguishes the supposedly desired behavior. Another frequent example is the spouse who complains that the mate is never tender. Whenever the mate is seemingly about to be intimate, the other spouse can be observed to consistently provoke anger in the mate. Most family therapists can provide numerous other examples of how spouses shape their mate's behavior.

In the marital context, I am positing that one spouse's actions based upon erroneous beliefs about the other spouse will channel social interaction in ways that cause the other spouse's behavior to confirm these beliefs. In other words, spouses both elicit and reinforce in the mate behavior that is congruent with the inner representational model. This process can be observed in marital therapy and has been documented in analogue studies (Snyder and Swann, 1978). Investigational documentation of this process in ongoing relationships is obviously difficult. One is postulating that elicited confirmatory behavior from the spouse will be related to the first spouse's image of the other through the mechanism of eliciting stimuli and reinforcement provided by the first spouse.

However, reliable coding schemas for interpersonal behavior have been developed by the Marital Studies Center at the University of Oregon (Vincent *et al.*, 1975) and by John Gottman's lab at the University of Illinois (Gottman *et al.*, 1976). Evidence is accumulating that certain forms of interactional behavior (Fineberg and Lounan, 1975; Birchler *et al.*, 1975) and communication styles (Gottman *et al.*, 1976; Thomas *et al.*, 1974) differentiate distressed from nondistressed couples. Indirect measures of cognitive schemas can be obtained from the Kelly repertory grid and adjective checklists. If this hypothesis is correct, cognitive measures, such as low cognitive complexity and negative perception of the spouse, should be related to maladaptive behavior toward the spouse and to elicited behavior from the other spouse. If one assumes that these cognitive states are relatively constant, the demonstration of linkages between measures of perceptual disturbance and coded interactional behavior should not be that difficult. If such a linkage can be demonstrated, an important bridge between clinical observation and behavioral research can be established.

### Hypothesis Six

In disturbed marriages, one often observes peculiar contrasting personality types (Sager, 1977; Sarwer-Foner, 1961; Jacobs, 1974). This observation has been the subject of much speculation. Most dynamically oriented therapists assure that the personality contrasts are the result of unconscious assortive mating. Neurotics are posited to unconsciously select partners who will help to perpetuate their neuroses (Lassheimer, 1967; Ostow and Cholst, 1970). For example, a man who is unconsciously afraid of his own sexual feelings might be attracted to a woman who is essentially devoid of sexual interest. Other theorists have speculated that complementary needs partially determine mate selection (Winsch, 1958). For example, a person with a need to be dependent would be expected to marry a mate who needs to be in control and take care of others. This novel hypothesis has received minimal support from empirical studies of mate selection (Thorp, 1963; DeYoung and Fleischer, 1976).

The author's model assumes that the peculiar contrasting personality styles often observed in chronic marital conflict are partially the result of the interactional history of the couple and are not necessarily reflective of enduring personality traits in the individual spouses. This hypothesis is clearly an extension of hypothesis five, which states that each spouse's behavior in the marriage is partially the result of contingencies offered by the other spouse. In other words, spouses train each other how to behave. In many couples, one will observe a remarkable congruence of the actual behavior of the spouse with the mate's representational model for the opposite sex. This hypothesis emphasizes the relative reactivity of social behavior and personality style in intimate relationships.

Some evidence exists as to the power of interactional forces in marriages. For example, it has been repeatedly found that the concordance of mental illness in married couples exceeds the expected frequency calculated from the prevalence rates for such disorders (e.g., Slater and Woodside, 1951; Gregory, 1959; Penrose, 1944; Kreitman, 1968; Crago, 1972). Two primary explanations have been offered to explain this concordance: assortive mating and interactional hypotheses. The assortive mating hypothesis assumes that the concordance of mental illness in marital pairs is primarily the result of the mentally unfit tending to marry one another. By contrast, interactional hypotheses tend to emphasize the impact of interactional processes on the spouses.

Kreitman and his associates (Kreitman, 1968; Nelson *et al.*, 1970; Kreitman *et al.*, 1970) have studied this phenomenon in considerable detail. From their work, it appears that the assortive mating hypothesis may explain the concordance of psychotic illness but does not explain the concordance of neurotic disturbance in spouses. This concordance has been found to increase with the duration of marriage and to be related to the quantity of shared activities. The finding that psychological improvement in one spouse is occasionally associated with psychiatric decompensation in the well spouse also offers support for the interaction hypothesis (Kaplan and Kohl, 1972; Kohl, 1962). A longitudinal study by Uhr (1957) also attests to the power of interactional forces in the unhappily married. In this study, the unhappily married were found to be more alike in personality at the time of marriage but to be more different than the happily married after 18 years of marriage.

This particular hypothesis has therapeutic implications. Clearly, if one assumes that marital discord is the result of clashes between relatively fixed personality entities, a degree of therapeutic pessimism and a restricted range of interventions are mandated. From this viewpoint, a therapist would logically concentrate his efforts on modifying personality structure, where possible. However, if one assumes that the observed "personalities" are largely the result of the interactional history between the spouses (each spouse's training the other how to behave), a more optimistic approach to therapy is possible. From this perspective, one would assume that the spouses could be trained to offer different contingencies for each other's behavior.

## Properties of Interactional Systems

Hypotheses one through four related to perceptual disturbances posited to be present in cases of chronic marital discord, and hypotheses five and six concerned mechanisms whereby these organismic variables contribute to interactional disturbances. The next two hypotheses are offered to try to account for the maintenance of disturbed interaction over years of marriage. In other words, if inner representational events and observed interaction are assumed to be reciprocally interrelated, why don't chance events lead to spontaneous remission over time? It appears that in many disturbed marriages, certain properties of the interactional system lead to stability and maintenance of the discord. General systems theorists, of course, have noted these features of disturbed marriages and have described marriages as a rule-governed system. As noted earlier, this is a metaphoric explanation and does not address the possible mechanism of action. Behavioral therapists also have not really addressed this issue. If marital discord is simply disturbed interactive behavior, a random change in the behavior of one spouse should modify the system. If one returns to the case example, what factors led to this man's misperceiving his wife's character for over 10 years of marriage? Somehow, their interaction was such that this misperception was never called into question.

## Hypothesis Seven

The observable recurring maladaptive behavior patterns observed in disturbed couples are hypothesized to be the result of an equilibrium reached between the spouses' attempts to provoke behavior confirmatory to inner representational models of the opposite sex. In other words, the interaction remains stable as each spouse resists efforts by the other spouse to act consistently in a manner discrepant with the schema for intimate members of the opposite sex. If one spouse deviates too radically from the prescribed range of behavior, the other spouse will work to restrict that range of behavior. Each spouse resists the anxiety of recognizing events that do not fit his or her cognitive scheme of things. In other words, the actual observable interaction pattern between the spouses is confirmatory to each spouse's inner representational world.

If we return to the case example, we observe a repetitive pattern of the husband passively manipulating his wife until she becomes explosively angry. Her outbursts reinforce his image of her as an angry tyrant. The wife sees her husband as a man that she has to please in order to be loved. She gives in to his passive manipulations in order to receive that reassurance of love until she becomes furious. At these times, she loses his love and reassurance. This confirms her perception of him. Her angry outbursts, of course, reinforce his image of her. In other words, the influence of both their inner representational worlds is such that the system remains in equilibrium. I don't believe that the construct of unconscious collusion is necessary to explain the interactional sequences.

A hypothesis such as this can be tested only in the clinical context. If it is true, however, certain indirect tests are possible. First, a consistent change in the interactional sequence should lead to a change in the inner representational worlds. Second, couples in chronic discord should demonstrate a relationship between their restricted images of one another and the restricted range of their behavior.

## Hypothesis Eight

The persistence of certain interpersonal patterns in disturbed couples is related to a process of stimulus–response chaining in interpersonal systems. An interpersonal stimulus from one spouse elicits a response from the other spouse, which serves as a stimulus to the first spouse. If the spouses have a limited response repertoire (presumably related to limited understanding of one another), a chaining or circular effect will be observed. This concept is similar to the general systems concept of circular causality or Don Jackson's notion of family rules (Jackson, 1965). It is also similar to the behavioral concept of environment trap. In the behavioral literature, this concept is used to explain how a given behavior becomes self-sustaining—although the therapist no longer provides reinforcement. It is assumed that the behavior in question elicits reinforcement from the natural environment. In marriage, I am proposing that each spouse can serve as an environmental trap for the other. These "traps" can maintain either adaptive or maladaptive behavioral patterns.

This hypothesis is necessary to explain the common recurring behavioral abnormalities in disturbed marriages. In many couples, the cycles of maladaptive behavior appear remarkably similar and nonspecific. As a therapist, one is often amazed how unimaginative and repetitive the ways are in which couples can disagree. A repetitive theme of attack–counterattack reappears. This theme appears in the clinical literature of behaviorists (e.g., Stuart, 1969), analysts (e.g., Brody, 1961), and general system theorists (e.g., Haley, 1963). If each spouse serves as the predominant environmental contingency for the other and each spouse has a limited response capability to perceived threat, the system can evolve a life of its own.

Behavioral marital therapists tend to refer to these interactions as coercive cycles (e.g., Patterson and Reid, 1970) and aversive reciprocity (Stuart, 1969). In coercive cycles, one spouse attempts to gain positive reinforcement from the other by using negative reinforcement as an interpersonal strategy, i.e., spouse desires a reward at minimal personal cost or risk. For example, "a husband might wish his wife to express greater affection; following the failure of his amorous advances, he might become abusive, accusing his wife of anything from indifference to frigidity, abating his criticism when he received the desired affection" (Stuart, 1969, p. 176). According to this formulation, the strategy elicits abusiveness from the wife, which can then lead to a standoff. Neither spouse will give the other what she wants until he gets what he wants first. Most therapists have observed such a process in disturbed couples but would find the behavioral formulation too simplistic. The question is, why do some couples repetitively become locked into such interactions whereas others don't? It does not appear to be a simple lack of skills, as most couples are more cooperative with opposite-sex strangers than with their spouses (Birchler *et al.*, 1975), suggesting that they have the requisite interpersonal skills. Indeed, disturbed couples appear more reactive than nondistressed couples to displeasing behavior from the spouse (Gottman, 1980), suggesting that the problem may be partially an individual variable. In the preceding example, the cycle could easily have been aborted if the wife had replied to her husband's abusive behavior in a different way. For example, she could have exclaimed, "I never knew that you wanted me so badly. Gosh, that's really exciting."

What I am suggesting is that at a certain level of intimacy, failures of accurate perception of the spouse allow the cycles to become self-perpetuating. If each spouse perceives the other in a relatively undifferentiated manner as threatening and attacking, the only possible response is counterattack. Although the cycles may be a nonspecific effect of marital discord, couples getting repetitively caught in such cycles should be differentiable from couples who don't.

Basically, this hypothesis maintains that reciprocity of behavioral exchanges will be observed in couples and that the ranges of exchanged behaviors will be more restricted in disturbed couples. A demonstrable relationship should exist between limited conceptual complexity and limited response plasticity within the individuals and the interactional system.

## Mechanism of Change

Theoretically, marital discord should be modifiable through a variety of therapeutic interventions and treatment modalities, ranging from psychoanalytically oriented individual psychotherapy to behavioral marital therapy. Disconfirmatory experiences can occur in various modalities. Because of the action–reaction nature of events and the subtle nuances of meaning in interpersonal systems evolved over time, it is difficult to identify what is eliciting and what is elicited behavior. For this reason, most conjoint therapy approaches will initially have to be focused at the interactional level. The goal of disrupting these intereactional sequences is to provoke behavior that is discrepant with the inner representational systems of each of the spouses. Similarly, modifying dysfluent forms of verbal communication in disturbed couples should facilitate change by increasing information exchange. In other words, the behavioral interventions such as reciprocity counseling and communication training are construed to work by disrupting old sequences and providing new information that is incongruent with inner representational worlds.

If we return to the case example, the husband sees his wife as an angry woman who is unresponsive to his wishes. By his behavior, he never tests this assumption about her. If this couple had consulted a behavior therapist who emphasized contingency contracting, one can envision the probable intervention. To disrupt the coercive cycle, each spouse would have been coached in expressing his or her wishes and working out an equitable exchange of goods. If this couple remained in therapy and complied with the behavioral program, eventually the husband would have expressed what he wanted from his wife and a compromise would have been reached whereby he would have obtained these goods. The very structure of the behavioral intervention disrupts the old pattern and provides a literal disproof of the victim–tyrant model. This diconfirmation, if sustained, must influence the inner representational model.

In the case example, the author utilized a technique similar to procedures employed by behavior therapists who emphasize communication training. The therapist forced the husband to acknowledge discongruent information about his wife. If this couple had enrolled in a behavioral marital therapy program containing a communication training module, each spouse would have been instructed and coached in using clear and direct expression of feelings and desires. Each spouse would have been coached in listening skills and paraphrasing the statements of the other. Again, the husband would have been forced to acknowledge and incorporate information about his wife that was discrepant with his inner representational image of her.

These two processes can be captured in empirical predictions.

## Hypothesis Nine

If the perception of the spouse at any given moment is partially a function of the actual behavior of the spouse and partially a function of the representational model evoked, the degree of influence of the representational model should be a function of the ambiguity and salience of the perceived situation. Unless persistent, unambiguous, and unusual information about the spouse is available and attended to, erroneous cognitions about the spouse will remain unmodified. This implies that the use of clear and explicit communication patterns (verbal and nonverbal) between spouses should minimize the amount of distortion possible. Repeated unambiguous verbal feedback discrepant with the inner representational model for the spouse should modify that model.

Two predictions follow logically from this hypothesis. First, couples with chronic discord should be observable to have communication styles promoting obfuscation. Second, and more important, disruption of these communication patterns should decrease the influence of the cognitive misrepresentation. Some evidence supports the first prediction. To my knowledge, the second prediction has not been adequately tested to date. Numerous clinicians have observed the presence of dysfluent communication in disturbed couples. Satir (1967) in particular observed that disturbed couples often employ language that poorly differentiates self from other, and imprecise language that augments the amount of distortion and projection. Thomas and associates (1974) have reported extensive research developing a 49-category coding scheme for verbal behavior in marital dyads. They have reported provisional data suggesting certain dysfluent communication categories as being more common in disturbed couples. The categories rated in Thomas's group are similar to the ones suggested by Satir. Gottman and associates (Gottman *et al.*, 1977) investigated 28 distressed and nondistressed couples in terms of their verbal and nonverbal communication styles. Couples were asked to resolve a current marital problem while their interaction was videotaped. These videotapes were then independently rated by separate coders for both verbal style and nonverbal affect expression. Certain combinations of verbal and nonverbal codes were found to reliably distinguish distressed from nondistressed couples. It is of note that disturbed couples were more often observed to display channel inconsistency, agreeing verbally while concurrently displaying an inconsistent nonverbal message. Kahn (1970) reported somewhat similar findings. Forty-two couples were asked to communicate messages nonverbally to their spouses. Adjusted couples were distinguished from poorly adjusted couples by the greater effectiveness of their nonverbal communication, suggesting the presence of a communication deficit in disturbed couples.

As previously reviewed, the University of Oregon group has similarly reported communication problems in disturbed couples using the Marital Interaction Coding System.

The second prediction provides a more exact test of this hypothesis. If the hypothesis is correct, treatment approaches that modify dysfluent communication patterns should also modify the cognitive representation of the spouse. For example, if a couple in discord can be reliably identified as having specific communication deficits, is behaviorally treated such that the deficit is removed (brought to a reasonable criterion level), and a reasonable follow-up demonstrates persistence of the new communication patterns, the perception of the spouse should be demonstrably changed. If this does not occur, the hypothesis is false.

### Hypothesis Ten

Repetitive observation of spouse behavior discrepant with the internal representational model for that spouse will result in a change in the representational model. Schemas can be disproved or modified if the individual can be induced to remain in disconfirmatory life experiences. In the terminology of Ezriel, if a marital interaction pattern can be modified such that each spouse experiences the avoided interpersonal relationship, significant intrapsychic change will occur in one or both spouses. This may be a change in cognitive complexity (the new description for the spouse will be dissimilar to descriptions of other significant members of the opposite sex) or simply a change in the unitary representational model for the opposite sex from a negative to a more positive valence. In other words, I am postulating that transference distortions can be modified by a consistent external reality discrepant with the perceptual distortion. Within the marital context, disproof of the transference reactions requires a modification of the interaction system.

Several well-developed behavioral treatment interventions exist for the modification of maladaptive marital interaction patterns (Jacobson and Martin, 1976; Azrin *et al.*, 1973; Stuart, 1969). This hypothesis predicts that if couples are brought to a reasonable behavioral criterion in such programs, their perceptions of their spouses will shift. The technology for assessing this prediction is available.

## CONCLUSIONS

This chapter was written in the form of specific hypotheses. In this section, I will attempt to summarize my theoretical framework in less precise language, in a form perhaps more usual to clinicians.

The crux of this theoretical model is the assumption that fixated misperceptions of the opposite-sex partner play a primary role in the genesis and maintenance of chronic marital discord. These schemas, derived from learning in earlier life situations, appear more readily elicited by interpersonal situations of emotional significance and duration. Typical eliciting events might be marriage or intensive psychotherapy. The primary difference between the two settings is the primary target of misperception, the misperception being of the spouse in marital situations. As illustrated in Chapter Three, this hypothesis is similar to ones posited by psychodynamic therapists who have indicated the importance of transference distortions in marital contexts. This model differs from dynamic models in that transference is retranslated into the terminology of social psychology. This retranslation allows a more precise definition of the posited cognitive-perceptual process in a testable form.

A second major feature of this theoretical model is the specification of relationships between inner representational events and external reality. I am postulating that certain individuals become trapped by their inner representational systems because they influence their interpersonal environments in such a way as to obtain confirmatory data. This hypothesis has been entertained as well by dynamically oriented therapists under the rubric of self-fulfilling prophesies. I differ from many dynamic therapists in my insistence on a reciprocal interaction between inner representational events and environmental confirmation. I am postulating that repetitive environmental disconfirmation will be perceived by patients and that these disconfirmatory events can lead to intrapsychic change. In different language, I am postulating that transference distortions can be disproved as well as modified by interpretation. This seemingly radical change from traditional psychodynamic theory is actually implicit in much of analytic writing. Certainly, most of us as therapists have been disappointed when a patient making significant progress precipitously breaks off an outside relationship that would be a healthier experience for that patient. Implicit in our disappointment is the assumption that a different form of life experience would have been beneficial for that patient.

I am positing that inner representational systems often remain intact because of the patient's skill in eliciting confirmatory data from significant others and because of the extreme complexity of attributing correct motivation in interpersonal systems. For example, a couple can easily become locked in a mutual misperception. A husband may be afraid that his wife will leave him if she becomes more independent, and his wife may fear that men will dominate and destroy her autonomy if she is emotionally dependent on them. On one level, such a conflict appears irreconcilable as a power struggle. On another level, the true concerns of each spouse are not in conflict. The subtlety of the disconfirmatory experiences contributes to this couple's persistent difficulty.

This model differs primarily from existing models of therapy because of its explicit recognition of person–environment interaction. This feature of the theory leads the therapist to a different consideration of therapeutic interventions. In other words, equivalent psychological change might be produced by internal organismic change or environmental restructuring. With this focus on the person–environment interaction, the therapist can use behavioral or psychodynamic interventions under a unified conceptual framework.

Another feature of this model is the assumption that behavioral abnormalities observed in marriage and in therapeutic contexts are similar. In other words, the development of schools of therapy around different forms of interventions is unnecessary. There are indeed peculiarities to marital therapy requiring different classes of intervention. However, these peculiarities do not require differing theoretical frameworks, as the same phenomena are involved.

## REFERENCES

Ackerman, N. W. *Treating the troubled family.* New York: Basic Books, 1966.

Adams-Webber, J. R., Schinenker, B., and Barbeau, D. Personal constructs and the perception of individual differences. *Canadian Journal of Behavioral Science,* 1972, 4, 218–244.

Alexander, F. The dynamics of psychotherapy in light of learning theory. *American Journal of Psychiatry,* 1963, 120, 440–448.

Alexander, F. The dynamics of psychotherapy in light of learning. In J. Marmor, and S. M. Woods (Eds.), *The interface between the psychodynamic and behavioral therapies.* New York: Plenum, 1980.

Alkon, D. I. Parental deprivation. *Acta Psychiatrica Scandinavica, Supplementum,* 1971, *233,* 7–8.

Azrin, N. H., Naster, B. J., and Jones, R. Reciprocity counseling: A rapid-based procedure for marital counseling. *Behavior Research and Therapy,* 1973, *11,* 365–382.

Balint, M., Ornstein, P., and Balint, E. *Focal psychotherapy.* London: Tavistock, 1972.

Bandura, A. *Principles of behavior modification.* New York: Holt, Rinehart & Winston, 1969.

Bandura, A. *Social learning theory.* Englewood Cliffs, N.J.: Prentice-Hall, 1977.

Bandura, A., and Barab, P. G. Conditions governing non-reinforced imitation. *Developmental Psychology,* 1971, *5,* 244–255.

Bannister, D. The rationale and clinical relevance of repertory grid technique. *British Journal of Psychiatry,* 1965, *111,* 977–982.

Bannister, D., and Mair, J. M. M. *The evaluation of personal constructs.* London: Academic Press, 1968.

Barry, W. A. Marriage research and conflict: an integrative review. *Psychology Bulletin,* 1970, *73,* 41–54.

Bateson, G. *Naven.* Stanford: Stanford University Press, 1958.

Beck, A. T. *Cognitive therapy and the emotional disorders.* New York: International Universities Press, 1976.

Beck, A. T., Rush, A. J., Shaw, B. F., and Emery G. *Cognitive therapy of depression.* New York: Guilford Press, 1979.

Bergin, A. E., and Lambert, M. J. The evaluation of therapeutic outcomes. In S. L. Garfield and A. E. Bergin (Eds.), *Handbook of psychotherapy and behavior change: An empirical analysis.* New York: Wiley, 1978.

Bieri, J. Cognitive complexity-simplicity and predictive behavior. *Journal of Abnormal and Social Psychology,* 1965, *51,* 263–268.

Bieri, J., Atkins, A. L. Briar, S., Leaman, R. L., Muller, H., and Tripodi, T. *Clinical and social judgment.* New York: Wiley, 1966.

Birchler, G. R., Weiss, R. L., and Vincent, J. P. A multi-method analysis of social reinforcement exchange between maritally distressed and non-distressed spouse and stranger dyads. *Journal of Personal and Social Psychology,* 1975, *31,* 349–360.

Birk, L., and Brinkley-Birk, A. W. Psychoanalysis and behavior therapy. In J. Marmor and S. M. Woods (Eds.), *The interface between the psychodynamic and behavioral therapies.* New York: Plenum, 1980.

Blazer, J. A. Complementary needs and marital happiness. *Marriage and Family Living,* 1975, *25,* 89–95.

Bloom, B. L., Asher, S. J., and White, S. W. Marital disruption as a stressor: A review and analysis. *Psychological Bulletin,* 1978, *85,* 867–894.

Bowen, M. Family therapy after twenty years. In D. X. Freedman, and J. E. Dyrud (Eds.), *American handbook of psychiatry,* Vol. 5. New York: Basic Books, 1975.

Bowlby, J. Effects on behavior of disruption of an affectional bond. In J. M. Thoday and A. S. Parker (Eds.), *Genetic and environmental influences on behavior.* Edinburgh: Oliver and Boyd, 1968.

Bowlby, J. The making and breaking of affectional bonds. *British Journal of Psychiatry,* 1977, *130,* 201–210.

Brody, S. Simultaneous psychotherapy of married couples. In J. Masserman (Ed.), *Current psychiatric therapies.* New York: Grune and Stratton, 1961.

Carson, R. C. *Interaction concepts of personality.* Chicago: Aldine, 1969.

Carter, R. D., and Thomas, E. J. Modification of problematic marital communications using corrective feedback and instruction. *Behavior Therapy,* 1973, *4,* 100–109.

Carter, H., Glick, P. C. *Marriage and divorce: a social and economic study.* Cambridge: Harvard University Press, 1976.

Cattell, R. B., Nesselroade, J. R. Likeness and completeness theories examined by 16 personality factor measures on stably and unstably married couples. *Journal of Personal and Social Psychology*, 1967, 7, 351–361.

Christensen, L., and Wallace, L. Perceptual accuracy as a variable in marital adjustment. *Journal of Sex and Marital Therapy*, 1976, 2, 130–136.

Clarke, A. D. B. Learning and human development. The 42nd Maudsley Lecture. *British Journal of Psychiatry*, 1968, 114, 161–177.

Clarke, A. M., and Clarke, A. D. B. The formative years? In A. M. Clarke and A. D. B. Clarke (Eds.), *Early experience: Myth and evidence.* New York: Free Press, 1976.

Corsini, R. J. Understanding and similarity in marriage. *Journal of Abnormal and Social Psychology*, 1956, 52, 237–332.

Crago, M. A. Psychopathology in married couples. *Psychological Bulletin*, 1972, 77, 114–128.

Crockett, W. H. Cognitive complexity and impression formation. In B. A. Maher (Ed.), *Progress in experimental personality research*, Vol. 2. New York: Academic Press, 1955.

Crouse, B., Karlins, M., and Schroder, H. Conceptual complexity and marital happiness. *Journal of Marriage and the Family*, 1968, 30, 643–646.

Czapinski, J. Prosocial behavior as affected by the structure of the cognitive representations of psychotherapy. *Polish Psychological Bulletin*, 1976, 7, 155–162.

Davis, K. Final note on a case of extreme isolation. In A. M. Clarke and A. D. B. Clarke (Eds.), *Early experience: Myth and evidence.* New York: Free Press, 1976.

DeYoung, G. E., and Fleischer, B. Motivational and personality trait relationships in mate selection. *Behavior Genetics*, 1976, 6, 1–6.

Dicks, H. V. *Marital tensions.* New York: Basic Books, 1967.

Douglas, J. W. B. Broken families and child behavior. *Journal of the Royal College of Physicians of London*, 1970, 4, 203–210.

Douglass, J. W. B., Ross, J. M., Hammond, W. A. and Mulligan, D. C. Deliquency and social class. *British Journal of Criminology*, 1966, 6, 294–302.

Dulany, D. E. Awareness, rules, and propositional control: A confrontation with S-R behavior therapy. In T. R. Dixon and D. L. Horton (Eds.), *Verbal behavior and general behavior theory.* Englewood Cliffs, N.J.: Prentice-Hall, 1968.

Dymond, R. Interpersonal perception and marital happiness. *Canadian Journal of Psychology*, 1954, 8, 161–171.

Ellis, A. *Reason and emotion in psychotherapy.* New York: Stuart, 1962.

Eysenck, H. J. The place of theory in psychology. In H. J. Eysenck (Ed.), *Experiments in personality*, Vol 2. London: Routledge and Kegan Paul, 1960.

Eysenck, H. J., and Beech, R. Counter conditioning and related methods. In A. E. Bergin and S. L. Garfield (Eds.), *Handbook of psychotherapy and behavior change.* New York: Wiley, 1971.

Fineberg, J. and Lounan, A. Affect and status dimensions of marital adjustment. *Journal of Marriage and the Family*, 1975, 37, 155–160.

Frank, J. D. *Persuasion and healing.* Baltimore: Johns Hopkins University Press, 1973.

Frank, E., and Kupfer, D. J. In every marriage there are two marriages. *Journal of Sex and Marital Therapy*, 1976, 2, 137–143.

Fransella, F., and Joyston-Bechal, M. P. An investigation of conceptual progress and pattern change in a psychotherapy group. *British Journal of Psychiatry*, 1971, 119, 199–206.

Goldiamond, I. Self-control procedures in personal behavior problems. *Psychological Reports* 1965, 17, 851–868.

Gottman, J. M. Consistency of nonverbal affect and affect reciprocity in marital interaction. *Journal of Consulting and Clinical Psychology*, 1980, 48, 711–717.

Gottman, J., Notarius, C., Markman, H., Banks, S., Yoppi, B., and Rubin, M. E. Behavioral exchange theory and marital decision making. *Journal of Personality and Social Psychology*, 1976, *34*, 14–23.

Gottman, J., Markman, H., and Notarius, C. The topography of marital conflict: A sequential analysis of verbal and non-verbal behavior. *J. Marriage and the Family*, 1977, *39*, 461–477.

Gough, H. G., and Heilbrun, A. B. *The adjective checklist manual*. Palo Alto, California: Consulting Psychologist Press, 1965.

Greene, B. L., and Solomon, A. P. Marital disharmony: concurrent psychoanalytic therapy of husband and wife by the same psychiatrist. *American Journal of Psychotherapy*, 1963, *17*, 443–457.

Greenspan, S. I., and Mannino, F. V. A model for brief interventions with couples based on projective identification. *American Journal of Psychiatry*, 1974, *131*, 1103–1106.

Gregory, I. Husbands and wives admitted to mental hospitals. *Journal of Mental Science*, 1959, *105*, 457–462.

Grotjahn, M. *Psychoanalysis and the family neurosis*. New York: Norton, 1960.

Gurman, A. S., and Knudson, R. M. Behavioral marriage therapy. A psychodynamic systems analysis and critique. *Family Process*, 1978, *17*, 121–138.

Haley, J. Marriage therapy. *Archives of General Psychiatry*, 1963, *8*, 213–234.

Hayden, B., Nasby, W., and Davis A. Interpersonal conceptual structures, predictive accuracy, and social adjustment of emotionally disturbed boys. *Journal of Abnormal Psychology*, 1977, *86*, 315–320.

Hicks, M. W., and Platt, M. P. Marital happiness and stability: a review of the research in the sixties. *Journal of Marriage and the Family*, 1970, *32*, 553–574.

Jackson, D. D. Family rules. *Archives of General Psychiatry*, 1965, *12*, 589–594.

Jacobs, L. I. Sexual problems and personalities in four types of marriage. *Medical Aspects of Human Sexuality*, 1974, March, 160–178.

Jacobson, N. J., and Margolin, G. Marital therapy. New York: Brunner/Mazel, 1979.

Jacobson, N. S., and Martin, B. Behavioral marriage therapy, current status. *Psychological Bulletin*, 1976, *83*, 540–556.

Jacobson, N. S., and Weiss, R. L. Behavioral marriage therapy III. Critique. The contents of Gurman et al. may be hazardous to your health. *Family Process*, 1978, *17*, 149–164.

Jackson, D. D. Family rules—marital quid pro quo. *Archives of General Psychiatry*, 1965, *12*, 589–594.

Johnson, D. W., and Matross, R. P. Interpersonal influence in psychotherapy: A social psychological view. In A. S. Gurman and A. M. Razin (Eds.), *Effective psychotherapy, a handbook of research*. Oxford, England: Pergamon, 1977.

Kagan, J. Resilience and continuity in psychological development. In A. M. Clarke and A. D. B. Clarke (Eds.), *Early experience: Myth and evidence*. New York: Free Press, 1976.

Kahn, M. Non-verbal communication and marital satisfaction. *Family Process*, 1970, *9*, 449–456.

Kaplan, H. S., and Kohl, R. N. Adverse reactions to the rapid treatment of sexual problems. *Psychosomatics*, 1972, *13*, 185–190.

Kaufman, A., Baron, A., and Kopp, R. E. Some effects of instructions of human operant behavior. *Psychonomic Monograph Supplement*, 1966, *1*, 243–250.

Kelly, G. A. *A theory of personality*. New York: W. W. Norton, 1953.

Kelly, G. A. *The psychology of personal constructs*, (Vol. 1), *A theory of personality*. New York: W. W. Norton, 1955.

Kelly, E. L. Marital compatibility as related to personality traits of husbands and wives as rated by self and spouse. *Journal of Social Psychology*, 1941, *13*, 193–198.

Kernberg, O. F. The structural diagnosis of borderline personality organization. In P. Hartocollis (Ed.), *Borderline personality disorder*. New York: International Press, 1972.

Kernberg, O. F. *Objects-relations theory and clinical psychoanalysis*. New York: Jason Aronson, 1976.

Kernberg, O. F. The structural diagnosis of borderline personality organization. In P. Hartocollis (Ed.), *Borderline personality disorders*. New York: International Universities Press, 1977.

Kirkpatrick, C. Factors in marital adjustment. *American Journal of Sociology*, 1937, *XLIII*, pp. 270–283.

Klerman, G. L., and Neu C. Manual for short-term interpersonal psychotherapy for depression. Boston-New Haven. Collaborative Depression Project, Version #5. Unpublished, February 1977.

Kohl, R. N. Pathological reactions of marital partners to improvement of patients. *American Journal of Psychiatry*, 1962, *118*, 1036–1041.

Koluchoua, J. Severe deprivation in twins: A case study. In A. M. Clarke and A. D. B. Clarke (Eds.), *Early experience: Myth and evidence*. New York: Free Press, 1976.

Kotlar, S. L. Middle-class marital role perceptions and marital adjustments. *Sociological and Social Research*, 1965, *49*, 283–293.

Kreitman, N. Married couples admitted to mental hospitals. *British Journal of Psychiatry*, 1968, *114*, 699–718.

Kreitman, N., Collins, J., Nelson, B., and Troop, J. Neurosis and marital interaction. *British Journal of Psychiatry*, 1970, *117*, 33–46.

Kuhn, T. S. *The structuce of scientific revolutions*. Chicago: University of Chicago Press, 1970.

LaForge, R., and Suczek, R. F. The interpersonal dimension of personality: III An interpersonal check list. *Journal of Personality*, 1955, *24*, 94–112.

Landis, J. T. Marriage of mixed and non-mixed religious faith. *American Sociological Review*, 1949, *14*, 401–407.

Lassheimer, P. The diagnosis of marital conflict. *American Journal of Psychoanalysis*, 1967, *27*, 127–131.

Leary, T. *Interpersonal diagnosis of personality*. New York: Ronald, 1957.

Liberman, R. P. Behavioral approaches to family and couple therapy. *American Journal of Orthopsychiatry*, 1970, *40*, 106–108.

Litz, T. *The person*. New York: Basic Books, 1976.

London, P. The end of ideology in behavior modification. *American Psychologist*, 1972, *27*, 913–920.

Luckey, E. B. Marital satisfaction and congruent self-spouse concepts. *Social Forces*, 1960, *39*, 153–157.

Mahoney, M. J. *Cognition and behavior modification*. Cambridge, Mass: Ballinger, 1974.

Mahoney, M. J., and Arnkoff, D. Cognitive and self-control therapies. In S. L. Garfield and A. E. Bergin (Eds.), *Handbook of psychotherapy and behavior change: An empirical analysis*. New York: Wiley, 1978.

Malan, D. H. *The frontier of brief psychotherapy*. New York: Plenum, 1976.

Mann, J. *Time-limited psychotherapy*. Cambridge, Mass.: Harvard University Press, 1973.

Marmor, J. Psychoanalytic therapy and theories of learning. In J. Marmor and S. M. Woods (Eds.), *The interface between the psychodynamic and behavioral therapies*. New York: Plenum, 1980.

Meichenbaum, D. *Cognitive-behavior modification*. New York: Plenum, 1977.

Meissner, W. W., and Nicholi, A. M. The psychotherapies: Individual, family and group. In A. M. Nicholi (Ed.), *The Harvard guide to modern psychiatry*. Cambridge, Mass.: Harvard University Press, 1978.

Meltzoff, J., and Kornreich M. *Research in psychotherapy.* New York: Atherton Press, 1970.

Menninger, K. *Theory of psychoanalytic technique.* New York: Basic Books, 1958.

Minuchin, S. Families and Family Therapy. Cambridge: Harvard University Press, 1974.

Mischel, W. *Personality and assessment.* New York: Wiley, 1968.

Money-Kryle, R. E. The Kleinian school. In S. Arieti (Ed.), *American handbook of psychiatry,* Vol. 1. New York: Basic Books, 1974.

Murstein, B. I., and Beck, G. D. Person perception, marriage adjustment and social desirability. *Journal of Consulting and Clinical Psychology,* 1972, *39,* 396–403.

Nelson, B., Collins, N., Kreitman, N., and Troop, J. Neurosis and marital interaction. *British Journal of Psychiatry,* 1970, *117,* 47–58.

Offenkrantz, W., Tobin, A. Psychoanalytic Psychotherapy. In D. X. Freedman and J. E. Dyrud (Eds.), *American handbook of psychiatry,* Vol. 5. New York: Basic Books, 1975.

Olson, D. H. A critical overview. In A. S. Gurman and D. G. Rice (Eds.), *Couples in conflict.* New York: Jason Aronson, 1975.

Olson, J. M., and Partington, J. T. An integrative analysis of two cognitive models of interpersonal effectivness. *British Journal of Social and Clinical Psychology,* 1977, *16,* 13–14.

Ostow, M., and Cholst, B. Marital discord. *New York State Journal of Medicine,* 1970, *70,* 257–266.

Patterson, G. R., and Hops, H. Coersion, a game for two: Intervention techniques for marital conflict. In R. E. Ulrich and P. J. Mountjoy (Eds.), *The experimental analysis of social behavior.* New York: Appleton-Century-Crofts, 1972.

Patterson, G. R., Reid, J. B. Reciprocity and coercion. Two facets of social systems. In C. Neuringer and J. Michael (Eds.), *Behavior modification in clinical psychology.* New York: Appleton-Century-Crofts, 1970.

Penrose, L. S. Mental illness in husband and wife. *Psychiatric Quarterly, Supplement,* 1944, *18,*161–166.

Piaget, J. *The moral judgment of the child.* Glencoe, Ill.: Free Press, 1948.

Pickford, J. H., Signord, E. I., and Rempel, H. Similar or related personality traits as a factor in marital happiness. *Marriage and Family Living,* 1966, *28,* 190–192.

Rado, S. *Psychoanalysis of behavior: Collected papers,* Vol. 2. New York: Grune and Stratton, 1962.

Rinsley, D. B. An objects-relations view of borderline personality. In P. Hartocollis (Ed.), *Borderline personality disorders.* New York: International Universities Press, 1977.

Rosenfeld, S. K., and Sprince, M. P. An attempt to formulate the meaning of the concept of borderline. *Psychological Study of the Child,* 1963, *18,* 603–635.

Rosenthal, T., and Bandura, A. Psychological modeling: Theory and practice. In S. L. Garfield and A. E. Bergin (Eds.), *Handbook of psychotherapy and behavior change: An empirical analysis.* New York: Wiley, 1978.

Rutter, M. Parent–child separation: Psychological effects on children. *Journal of Child Psychology and Psychiatry,* 1971, *12,* 233–260.

Rutter, M. Parent–child separation: Psychological effects on the children. In A. M. Clarke and A. D. B. Clarke (Eds.), *Early experience: Myth or evidence.* New York: Free Press, 1976.

Ryle, A., and Lipschitz, S. Recording change in marital therapy with the reconstruction grid. *British Journal of Medical Psychology,* 1975, *48,* 39–48.

Ryle, A., and Lunghi, M. A. The measurement of relevant change after psychotherapy: Use of repertory grid testing. *British Journal of Psychiatry,* 1969, *115,* 1297–1304.

Sager, C. J. Transference in conjoint treatment of married couples. *Archives of General Psychiatry,* 1967, *16,* 185–193.

Sager, C. J. Marriage contracts and couple therapy. New York: Brunner/Mazel, 1976.

Sager, C. J. A typology in intimate relationships. *Journal of Sex and Marital Therapy*, 1977, *3*, 83–112.

Sandler, J., Dare, C., and Holder, A. Basic psychoanalytic concepts: III. Transference. *British Journal of Psychiatry*, 1970, *116*, 667–672.

Sarwer-Foner, G. J. Patterns of marital relationships. *American Journal of Psychotherapy*, 1962, *23*, 31–44.

Satir, V. *Conjoint family therapy*. Palo Alto: Science and Behavior Books, 1967.

Schroeder, H. M., Driver, M. J., and Steufert, S. *Human information processing*. New York: Holt, Rinehart & Winston, 1967.

Segraves, R. T. Conjoint marital therapy: a cognitive behavioral model. *Archives of General Psychiatry*, 1978, *35*, 450–455.

Sifneos, P. E. *Short-term psychotherapy and emotional crisis*. Cambridge, Mass: Harvard University Press, 1972.

Slater, E., and Woodside, M. *Patterns in marriage*. London: Cossell, 1951.

Slater, P. The use of the repertory grid technique in the individual case. *British Journal of Psychiatry*, 1965, *111*, 956–975.

Slater, P. Theory and technique of the repertory grid. *British Journal of Psychiatry*, 1969, *115*, 1287–1296.

Sollod, R. N., and Wachtel, P. L. A structural and transactional approach to cognition in clinical problems. In M. Mahoney (Ed.), *Psychotherapy process, current issues and future directions*. New York: Plenum, 1980.

Stotland, E., and Canon, L. C. *Social psychology, A cognitive approach*. Philadelphia: W. B. Saunders, 1972.

Strong, S. R. Social psychological approach to psychotherapy research. In S. L. Garfield and A. E. Bergin (Eds.), *Handbook of psychotherapy and behavior change: an empirical analysis*. New York: Wiley, 1978.

Strupp, H. H. Some comments on the future of research in psychotherapy. *Behavioral Science*, 1960, *5*, 60–71.

Strupp, H. H. Psychotherapy research and practice: an overview. In S. L. Garfield and A. E. Bergin (Eds.), *Handbook of psychotherapy and behavior change: an empirical analysis*. New York: Wiley, 1978.

Stuart, R. B. Operant-interpersonal treatment for marital discord. *Journal of Consulting and Clinical Psychology*, 1969, *33*, 675–682.

Stuart, R. B. Behavioral remedies for marital ills. In A. S. Gurmann and D. G. Rice (Eds.), *Couples in conflict*. New York: Jason Aronson, 1975.

Stuckert, R. P. Role perception and marital satisfaction—A configurational approach. *Marriage Family Living*, 1963, *25*, 415–419.

Sullivan, H. S. *The interpersonal theory of psychiatry*. New York: W. W. Norton, 1953.

Taylor, A. B. Role perception, empathy, and marriage adjustment. *Sociological and Social Research*, 1967, *52*, 22–34.

Thomas, E. J. *Marital communication and decision making*. New York: Free Press, 1977.

Thomas, E. J., Walker, C. L., and O'Flaherty, K. A verbal problem checklist for use in assessing family verbal behavior. *Behavior Therapy*, 1974, *5*, 235–246.

Thorp, R. G. Psychological patterning in marriage. *Psychological Bulletin*, 1963, *60*, 97–117.

Udry, J. R. Personality match and interpersonal perception as predictors of marriage. *Journal of Marriage and the Family*, 1967, *29*, 722–725.

Uhr, L. Personality changes during marriage. Unpublished dissertation. University of Michigan, 1957.

Vincent, J. P., Weiss, R. L., and Birchler, G. A. A behavioral analysis of problem solving in distressed married and strange dyads. *Behavior Therapy*, 1975, *6*, 83–94.

Wachtel, P. L. *Psychoanalysis and behavior therapy*. New York: Basic Books, 1977.

Watson, J. P. A repertory grid method of studying groups. *British Journal of Psychiatry*, 1970, *117*, 309–318.

Watzlawick, P., Beavin, J. H., and Jackson, D. D. *Pragmatics of human communication.* New York: W. W. Norton, 1967.

Weiss, R. L., Margolin, G. Marital conflict and accord. In A. R. Ciminero, K. S. Calhoun and H. E. Adams (Eds.), *Handbook of behavioral assessment.* New York: Wiley, 1977.

Weissman, M. M. The psychological treatment of depression. *Archives of General Psychiatry*, 1979, *36*, 1242–1249.

Wijesinghe, O. B. A., and Wood, R. R. A repertory grid study of interpersonal perception within a married couples psychotherapy group. *British Journal of Medical Psychology*, 1976, *49*, 287–294.

Wilson, G. T. Cognitive behavior therapy. In J. P. Foreyt and D. P. Rathjen (Eds.), *Cognitive behavior therapy.* New York: Plenum, 1978.

Winsch, R. F. *Mate selection.* New York: Harper & Row, 1958.

Wolf L. Learning theory and psychoanalysis. *British Journal of Medical Psychology*, 1966, *39*, 1–10.

Wolf E. Learning theory and psychoanalysis. In J. Marmor and S. M. Woods (Eds.), *The interface between the psychodynamic and behavioral therapies.* New York: Plenum, 1980.

Zinner, J. The implications of projective identification for marital interaction. In H. Gruenbaum and J. Christ (Eds.), *Contemporary marriage: structure, dynamics and therapy.* Boston: Little Brown, 1976.

# Clinical Application

This chapter concerns the clinical application of the author's model. The chapter will begin with a conceptional overview concerning the psychotherapy of marital discord. This section will be followed by brief discussions of technical considerations, the goal and length of marital therapy, and the indications for marital therapy. Then the typical stages of marital therapy will be discussed. The chapter will end with a brief discussion of the differing needs of practicing clinicians and clinical researchers.

## CONCEPTUAL OVERVIEW

As outlined in the previous chapter, analogous phenomena are assumed to operate in individual psychotherapy and in conjoint marital therapy. Disturbed interpersonal relationships are assumed to be related to individual psychopathology through the mechanism of fixated and distorted interpersonal perceptions. These distorted perceptions are posited to be self-sustaining through the mechanism of individuals inadvertently provoking confirmatory behavior from significant others. Although this perceptual abnormality has origins in the patient's past experiences in analogous situations, current environmental information is crucial for its maintenance. The perceptual abnormality is assumed to have both past and present determinants.

Although similar processes are assumed to be involved in individual psychotherapy and marital therapy, differences in interpersonal context require modifications of technique. In individual psychotherapy, the potency of past determinants of behavior is clear-cut and impressive. The therapist notes that the patient seemingly is attempting to provoke him into feeling and acting certain ways, notes the analogy of this to events in the patient's family of origin, interprets this to the patient, and unravels a complex history of emotions and fantasies in other interpersonal relationships. Through the interpretation and working through of the transference neurosis, the patient learns to discriminate between his own feelings and inner representational systems for perceiving the person of the therapist and the reality of the therapist. By contrast, in marital therapy the potency of current determinants of symptomatic behavior are more evident. The transference reactions are directed from spouse to spouse, and neither spouse is a passive observer of the other's pathology. The couple has a long history of training each other how to behave in accordance with inner representational reality. Similarly, a characteristic of most interpersonal systems is the ability of certain defensive behavior to elicit behavior of a similar kind from the other participant. These evolving cycles serve to obfuscate the resolution of issues, as they are open to multiple interpretations. When the couple is in the midst of an ongoing argument, it is difficult for the therapist to ascertain the relative influence of each spouse's pathology. Thus, where the individual therapist might be able to rely mainly on interpretation and insight for psychological change, the marital therapist does not have the same luxury. He finds himself suddenly in the midst of an ongoing interactional system. This system has a reality far greater than the therapist's influence. For example, an interpretation by the therapist that the husband has a need to see his wife as weak and demanding is not particularly useful when her actual behavior (partially and unknowingly provoked by the husband) can be legitimately described as weak and demanding. Clearly, the marital therapist has to be ready to modify interactional systems in a systematic way. Another difference between marital and individual therapy concerns modification of transference distortions. The marital therapist is concerned with transference only to the extent that it interferes with current relationships with the spouse. Detailed insight as to the past origins of the perceptual problem may be interesting but are not germane to the treatment objectives. In fact, insight as to the nature of the transference distortion is not necessary as long as the spouse is perceived in a manner more congruent with reality.

The overall goal of marital therapy is analogous to the goal of individual therapy. The therapist seeks to modify maladaptive behavioral patterns and related internal cognitive-emotional events. Because the marital therapist is working with an interactive social system, he has to employ procedures that the typical individual therapist would consider unconventional. It is only at the latter stages that events in marital therapy bear a resemblance to events within individual psychotherapy. The end stages of marital therapy are analogous to interpretation of the transference in individual therapy. However, the marital therapist has to make many interventions before this stage is reached.

Figure 2, which is a slight modification of Figure 1, illustrates the possible avenues of intervention in a schematic manner. If one assumes that the observable interaction is codetermined by each spouse's inner representational system, one has at least four different types of possible psychotherapeutic interventions into marital discord. One could attempt to interpret the transference in one or both spouses, modify eliciting behavior in one or both spouses, modify confirming behavior in one or both spouses, or attempt first to modify the interactional system.

In actual practice, a certain sequence of events will usually prove more fruitful. In the initial stages of therapy, the therapist encounters a confusing morass of innuendos, reference to past events, list of past injustices, and quickly escalating battles. In these cases, it is virtually impossible to ascribe primary responsibility for any action to either spouse. One is observing an interactional system out of control. This system has to be brought back into control before any other types of interventions

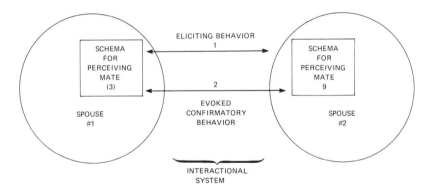

**Figure 2.** Each spouse has a representational system for the perception of the other spouse. This schema is related to behavior toward that spouse, and serves to elicit that stimuli for the behavior of the second spouse. If the evoked behavior from the second spouse is interpreted by spouse #1 as congruent with the schema for the opposite sex, the couple becomes locked into an interactional system.

The therapist has three possible levels of intervention: 1. modifying eliciting behavior, 2. modifying confirmatory behavior, or 3. attempting direct change of the schema (interpretation, cognitive relabelling, discrimination training). As all components are integrally related, an intervention on one level will influence the other two.

will be useful. At this point, the therapist's interventions will probably resemble those of behavioral marital therapists and general system therapists. He will be concerned with modifying the interactional system, and his interventions will be nonspecific attempts to accomplish this. By nonspecific, I mean that similar types of procedures will be employed in different couples. Later, the therapist will be able to focus on interventions specific to the couple. At this point he may work specifically to disrupt sequences that elicit confirmatory behavior. His interventions at this point bear a resemblance to the type of interventions frequently employed by individual behavior therapists. In the end phases of therapy, after the disturbed behavior patterns are disrupted, the actions of the therapist will begin to resemble those of the individual psychodynamically oriented therapist. During this stage, he will emphasize the discrepancy between perceived reality and past reality. His interventions will differ from individual psychotherapy in that the target of misperception will be the spouse rather than the therapist. Table 1 outlines the sequence of interventions, associated procedures, and their rationale.

As the reader is probably thoroughly confused at this point, I will go through each of the stages in a little more detail. In the initial interviews, the therapist will note certain repetitious maladaptive interac-

Table 1.   Level of Intervention

| Level | Procedures | Rationale |
|---|---|---|
| Interactional | Reciprocity Training Communication Training Cognitive Relabelling Prevention of Escalation | Non-specific modification of interaction on assumption that current interaction confirmatory to both representational worlds |
| Eliciting behavior | Label; identify probable influence on spouse; teach alternative way to achieve stated goal | Modify behavior that elicits confirmatory behavior |
| Evoked behavior | Label; identify probable influence on spouse; teach alternative ways of responding | Modify spouse behavior confirmatory to inner representational world |
| Inner representational system | Discrimination training; repetitive emphasis of discrepancy between mate's behavior and interpretation of that behavior | Direct verbal challenge of validity of inner representational world |

tional sequences. These sequences will be remarkably similar across couples. Regardless of the driving forces in marital discord, its manifestation is often remarkably similar in all cases. Arguments escalate, issues are not resolved, behavior is variously interpreted, and speech is tangential or obscure. Each spouse experiences a range of emotions from utter despair and hopelessness to unmitigated desire to destroy the partner. If one assumes that the observable interaction is confirmatory to each spouse's inner representational world (hypotheses 7 and 8), the initial thrust of the therapist will be to modify the interactional system. As the disturbed behavior is partially confirmatory to each spouse's inner representational world, a modification of the interactional pattern is an initial move toward a bilateral disproof of the transference distortions.

Various procedures described by nondynamic therapists are ideally suited to the task of modifying interactional systems. Reciprocity counseling was reviewed in a previous chapter. This can be a potent technique for a start at interrupting behavioral sequences marked by anger and disappointment. The therapist can begin the actual process of behavior change without the couple's having to acknowledge the underlying issues. It offers the additional advantage of possibly provoking a small but tangible disproof of the assumption that cooperation with the spouse at any level is dangerous or impossible. Similarly, as each spouse decides on the goods or services desired from the other, a successful barter or exchange of desired services contradicts the image of the other as always ungiving, selfish, or bad. Although the spouses are aware only of negotiating around a series of seemingly minor issues, the therapist has made a movement toward disrupting the system.

The therapist may also begin disrupting the system in a nonspecific way by focusing on modifying faulty communication patterns. In disturbed couples, information exchange is full of innuendos, incongruence between verbal and nonverbal messages, topic switching, and poor referent specification. In the heat and confusion of the interaction, multiple interpretations of the spouse's intent are possible and issues are seldom brought to resolution. Because of the lack of clarity, each spouse is spared the difficulty of accommodating clear but disconfirmatory information from the mate. Similarly, the confusion and lack of resolution generate a sense of hopelessness and unfocused anger. The vagueness of the interchange does not challenge usual assumptions. Again the therapist's actions serve the purpose of beginning to set the system into disequilibrium. This disequilibrium is necessary so that the observable interaction begins to be discrepant with inner representational events.

The therapist will want to begin gradual cognitive relabeling of events early in therapy. This relabeling also serves to set the system into disequilibrium. The spouses will observe that the therapist does not agree with their usual ways of construing events. Clearly, this procedure has to be used judiciously if the therapist is to maintain credibility. In many couples, the actual interaction will have to be slightly modified in a concrete manner before the spouses will entertain alternative ways of construing events.

Once nonspecific interventions such as those outlined above have been successful in modifying the interactional system, a different level of intervention is possible. After the chaos has been reduced by assisted bargaining and modified communication patterns, the system returns to a sense of order. At this point, the therapist can begin to discern the actions of each individual spouse and the influence of those actions on the other spouse. By now, the therapist also has a provisional formulation about each spouse's distorted image of the other and how the other spouse's behavior confirms this image.

If reciprocity counseling and communication training have been successful, the couple are able at this stage to discuss reasonably most issues without major fights escalating. Similarly, many of the minor issues providing the fuel for the frequent arguments have been settled by negotiated compromise (reciprocity counseling). Once this state of relative tranquility has been reached, one will observe seeming atttempts by one or both spouses to provoke the other into more usual ways of behaving. These attempts, often extremely subtle in sophisticated patients, need to be interrupted quickly before the couple manages to return the system to its prior state. Prompt labeling of the behavior and its probable effect on the spouse, inquiry as to the response desired from the spouse, and firm coaching of alternative ways of achieving the stated goal will usually suffice if one intervenes prior to a counterattack by the second spouse. A case example may help to illustrate how the therapist intervenes to circumvent eliciting behavior. A couple seen by the author has entered therapy with constant arguments about everything from politics to in-laws. After approximately 6 weeks of therapy focused on negotiation and communication skills, the couple has begun almost to enjoy being together, and their sex life has noticeably improved. Suddenly, the husband begins to complain that his wife is not responsive sexually. He then proceeds to say how this illustrates his knowing all along that, underneath it all, his wife is self-centered and cold. Before the wife can react, the therapist quickly inquires as to what happened sexually this past week. With a bit of inquiry, he discovers that the husband unsuccessfully made sexual advances while his wife was cooking, pouted after dinner when she was in the mood, and then attempted another initiation in an irritated voice tone when she was watching her favorite television show. In this instance, the therapist points out how his choice of times was hardly likely to be successful, how he was unlikely to have a willing partner after he pouted while she was in the mood, and that his voice tone tended to elicit anger. The therapist points out how one instance doesn't prove his case and how the evidence is biased. He emphasizes that the husband knows his wife's probable reponse, given these circumstances, and that the husband, not the wife, is responsible for her nonresponding. The therapist also uses this example to illustrate to the wife how her behavior unwittingly plays into her husband's view of her. He emphasizes her behavioral alternatives. For example, she could have said that she was in the mood but preferred to wait until after dinner when she could devote her full attention to the activity. When her husband was pouting, she could have asked if she had inadvertently hurt his feelings. The therapist wryly comments that she could have turned off the television, saying that she found her husband so desirable that she was unable to concentrate on the show. By his voice tone, the therapist suggests that her husband would have been frightened by this turn of events. In other words, the therapist is attempting to play on the element of sadism in most relationships to get the wife to purposely act in defiance of her husband's inner representational system.

In a different case, the wife suddenly began attaching her husband for being rigid and incapable of letting go. The more the wife criticized her husband, the more rigid and ungiving her husband became. The impact of her behavior on her husband was pointed out. She was asked what she wanted from her husband. In a circuitous reply, she finally mentioned that she wanted for them to go dancing with another couple, and her husband had refused. A little more inquiry revealed that the night chosen was before an important business day for the husband. The wife was known to be difficult to get home at a reasonable hour after she had been drinking. The therapist points out that the wife could agree in advance to leave at a specified hour, regardless, or that she could ask the other couple to reschedule to a night more convenient to her husband's schedule. The therapist points out how the wife is partially responsible for her husband's "rigidity" in this case. The therapist inquires as to why the husband passively allowed his wife to characterize him that way. He points out that the husband could have suggested alternative dates. He wryly suggests that the husband should dance her into the ground.

In the initial stages of therapy, the therapist made nonspecific interventions to disrupt the interactional system and to restore a sense of cooperation and hopefulness. In the sequences just described, the therapist specifically intervened to disrupt interactions specific to the couple. If his interventions are successful and the couple doesn't outwit the therapist, one enters a peculiar stage in therapy. The actual behavior of the spouse has been modified and each one of the couple is rendered powerless by the therapist in his or her attempts to provoke customary behavior from the other. In many couples one can almost sense an uneasy tension. Certain therapists might refer to this uneasiness as a fear of intimacy. I would agree if by fear of intimacy they mean of experiencing the spouse as he or she really is. This stage appears to be characterized by a fear of the unknown. Both spouses' usual tactics have been rendered powerless, and they are in a situation of encountering information about the spouse that does not fit their habitual ways of perceiving the spouse. A change is being forced. Thus, they are forced either to leave the field of new experience (find a new way to outwit the therapist and escalate a fight out of control, seek another partner, terminate therapy) or to form new ways of perceiving the spouse.

At this point in therapy, the therapist has modified the behavioral interaction such that the actual behavior of the spouses is no longer totally confirmatory to inner representational worlds. The therapist begins to note a clear-cut discrepancy between the spouses' descriptions of one another and their actual observable behavior. It is now that the therapist uses verbal redirection of attention to augment the perception of the discrepancy between actual behavior and inner representational worlds. The therapist's actions are somewhat similar to those of the individual therapist when he interprets the transference. However, rather than interpret the transference, the therapist facilitates discrimination between current and past reality. In other words, he pinpoints discrepancies between the inner image of the spouse and current reality. The therapist's comments will emphasize contradictory information about the spouse. He will emphasize unseen portions of the spouse's character, especially those aspects that are positive, more differentiated, and complex, and those parts that are dissimilar to past objects in the first spouse's life.

A few case vignettes may help to illustrate the process. A husband who remembered his mother as weak and depressed began describing his wife as dependent and helpless. From the husband's voice tone, the therapist had an image of a leech sucking its host dry. In actual fact, the wife was a reasonably autonomous person, but she was stuck at home with several children. She desired her husband's companionship for obvious reasons. Due to the strain in their relationship, she was concerned whether the marriage would survive. For this reason, she frequently solicited her husband's opinion on things. Her husband interpreted this as a sign of weakness on her part. In this case, the therapist emphasizes aspects of the wife's personality that don't fit the husband's image of her. For example, the husband had stayed late at an office party the previous evening. While he was gone, the electrical system in their house had malfunctioned. In a home repair book, by flashlight, his wife calmly read how to replace fuses and remedied the problem. This was particularly important in that the husband was deathly afraid of electricity. The therapist emphasizes this fact and asks the husband how this fits with his image of his wife. The therapist suggests that there are parts of his wife's personality that he tends to dismiss. At a later point in therapy, the couple disagrees over vacation plans. The husband wants to go gambling in Reno. The wife would much prefer a camping trip in the Smoky Mountains but is tentative in expressing her wishes. The therapist knows that she is violently opposed to a trip to Reno, as her husband has a tendency to gamble too much. The therapist purposely forces the issue, getting the wife to clearly express her wishes and "bottom line." It quickly becomes apparent that she will not go to Reno with her husband. If he insists on Reno, she plans to take the children on a camping trip by herself. The therapist asks if the husband believes her. He asks how the husband can reconcile this with his image of her. The therapist emphasizes the wife's contradictory feelings. She wants the marriage to work, wants the husband's love and approval, and is willing to compromise only up to a point. The therapist points out how the husband has the wife in a "Catch-22." She is either helpless or unconcerned about his feelings.

In another case, the wife was on the verge of tears complaining of how controlling and unloving her husband is. In actuality, the husband is a man who has considerable ambivalence about giving up control. He both wants to be taken care of and fears loss of control. In this case, the therapist points out how the husband had recently agreed to let his wife manage their household budget, although saying that this frightened him, as he had seen his mother destroy his father by driving the family into debt. The therapist also emphasizes that the husband had recently been able to respond when his wife was more sexually aggressive. Understandably, he had erectile problems at first, but this no longer seemed to be a problem. The therapist points out that the wife's image of her husband is too simple. She is seeing only a part of him. Her husband is in the process of trying to give up control and is finding it a difficult struggle. If the wife continues to complain and push, she will make him more frightened and thus confirm her fears about him. If, instead, she rewards his gains and discusses his fears with him, she will obtain what she says she wants from him.

A disproof in action usually carries far more weight than simply a verbal redirection of attention by the therapist. For example, a clinical psychologist in her 50s was complaining that her husband was weak and dependent and that she needed a strong man to be happy in life. In actuality, her husband was somewhat unsure of himself sexually. Previous behavioral sex therapy had reversed a lifelong problem with premature ejaculation and he was still in the process of recovering his sense of self-confidence. Evidence that this was occurring consisted of his reporting that women at work were beginning to flirt with him. Interpersonally, he appeared to appease others and to be ready to compromise. However, this man had managed to establish a multimillion-dollar business in his lifetime. This suggested that he got his way when it was important. Also, he didn't appear in reality to be that dependent on his wife. When she was gone on professional trips, he managed quite well and actually seemed a bit happier with her gone. When she was in town, he had numerous activities that did not involve his wife. Efforts by the therapist to point this out to the wife had been unconvincing. She steadfastly interpreted her husband's difficulty as a character defect related to early childhood experiences. The minor exceptions emphasized by the therapist were thus insignificant. The therapist judged that the husband had regained considerable self-confidence now that his sexual difficulty was over. In the past, he had been afraid to displease his wife because of his fear that no other woman would want a sexually disabled partner. The therapist also noted that the husband, although silent, had seemed quite angry during his wife's monologue. Therefore, the therapist began questioning the husband about how he felt about what his wife had just said. During this inquiry, the therapist purposely sought out the husband's anger. Eventually, the husband began to speak of how angry he was that his wife was impossible to please and how other women were not that way. He eventually stated emphatically that if she did not change, he would seek another partner. The therapist made certain that the wife heard clearly what her husband's position was. The therapist commented that the wife was perceiving only part of her husband. Along with his desire to please her and make the marriage work was considerable anger. The therapist wondered out loud if the husband's facade of appeasement was a defense against his anger.

In other cases, the therapist is seeking a more subtle discrimination. What one spouse is attributing to the other is correct, but it is only part of the story. An assistant professor in the humanities at a local college was anxiously awaiting a tenure decision, with no likely alternative job prospects. He continually characterized his wife as self-centered and not caring about him. When he was discussing his concerns, his wife looked quite upset. Of course, the husband was looking away at that moment. So the therapist comments that he missed seeing how concerned his wife is. The professor observes that his wife is only concerned about the impact of a loss of income on their lives. She doesn't care about his feelings. At this point, the therapist asks the wife to discuss her feelings honestly. She discusses how she is concerned about the pressure her husband is experiencing. She is concerned that her husband has all sorts of psychosomatic complaints and is having trouble sleeping. She wonders if maybe things would be better if he got a different sort of job. She would miss the university life, but her husband might be happier. Then she wonders if their income might be better in a different type of job. The husband focuses on her last statement as indicating her concern about money. The therapist then asks the husband to repeat all of what his wife said. The therapist insists until the husband complies. At this point, the therapist points out how the husband only listens to the part of what his wife says that fits his image of her. He points out that most spouses would have both concerns. He also points out how the husband is depriving himself of emotional support at a time when he clearly needs it.

In most of these vignettes, the therapist's intervention was predominantly unilateral. In other words, he focused primarily on one spouse's misperception. This raises the question of whether the therapist should attempt a bilateral disproof of transference distortions. The answer to this question concerns a relative focus of effort. In most cases, some disproof of both spouses' perceptual distortion will occur. It appears that if the interaction has been changed and the spouses have the skills to maintain the new interaction, a concentrated disproof of one spouse's contribution may be sufficient. This degree of intervention should be enough to permanently shift the interactional pattern. The other spouse's inner representational world should shift as the result of further interaction. The choice of spouse for primary focus rests upon the therapist's decision as to the spouse most amenable to change.

During the forced discrimination training, it is not unusual for a spouse to spontaneously recall events in the family of origin. For example, a wife who begins to realize that her husband does care for her but has difficulty expressing feelings may begin crying, talking about how her father was never available. At this point, the therapist comments that this may have been true in her relationship with her father, but it is not true in her relationship with her husband. In actuality, her memory of her father is probably also distorted. A diversion into this would extend the objectives and time frame of the current treatment. In other cases, the wife may begin to describe her husband differently and wonder if perhaps she misunderstood her father while growing up. In these instances, the therapist agrees that this is possible and suggests that she might want to check this out when therapy is over. He suggests that for the time being, her relationship with her husband is more important. After all, they are different people.

To recapitulate briefly, the thrust of the proposed therapy is a combined behavioral and cognitive program with the express purpose of systematically disproving transference distortions in one or both spouses. As the transference distortions are assumed to be partially maintained by current environmental feedback, the first goal of the therapist is to restructure the marital interaction system. The purpose of this is to gradually shape a new interactional pattern that is incongruent with inner representational worlds. His first interventions are relatively nonspecific and are techniques borrowed from behavioral marital therapists. Thus, he assists the spouse in negotiating compromises around issues of current concern. This intervention begins to shift the nature of the interaction and to disconfirm the undifferentiated image of the spouse as ungiving and bad. Techniques are also borrowed from communication training programs on the assumption that clear verbal feedback discrepant with inner representational models will likewise contribute to an internal cognitive change. These interventions are supplemented by interventions specific to the couple. In the more specific interventions, the therapist purposely interrupts behavior that helps to maintain the cognitive distortion. After a new interactional system has evolved, the therapist then has an environment in which discriminations between inner and external reality are possible.

For a therapy such as this to be successful, the therapist has to attend flexibly to observable behavior and to the inferred inner representational systems connected with that behavior. As one is attempting a disproof of both spouses' habitual ways of perceiving one another and structuring their intimate interpersonal lives, the timing of interventions is crucial. If one proceeds too rapidly, the magnitude of the shift in internal reality may be too overwhelming. Similarly, a premature attempt at discrimination training will not be effective and may increase anxiety to unacceptable levels. The advantage of the combined behavioral and cognitive approach is that the therapist can first engineer considerable behavioral change without either spouse having to acknowledge the meaning of that change. Once the change has been established, the therapist uses the altered interpersonal environment for cognitive restructuring. The difference between this approach and other approaches is that the therapist uses the incredible power of behavior therapy to change maladaptive behavior and then follows this intervention with a systematic effort at cognitive restructuring.

## INDICATIONS

There is little empirical evidence documenting when one form of therapeutic activity is indicated over another, with the possible exception of certain behavioral interventions for specified symptoms (Segraves and Smith, 1976). All too often, the choice of intervention reflects the therapist's theoretical bias rather than the patient's needs. Clinical opinion as to the indications for marital therapy varies considerably. Certain analytic therapists (e.g., Lussheimer, 1966; Giovacchini, 1965) feel that individual therapy is always the preferred intervention, whereas other analytic therapists (Mittlemann, 1944; Malan, 1976) feel that marital therapy is indicated only when current life relationships trap a patient in a neurotic form of relating. Marital therapists, of course, tend to feel that the indications for marital therapy are much broader (Fitzgerald, 1973; Martin, 1975).

From the author's viewpoint, the choice of therapeutic modality is a pragmatic decision. Clearly, disturbed behavioral patterns can be interrupted in individual therapy, marital therapy, or nontherapeutic life experiences of some lasting impact. The ultimate decision as to the form of intervention rests upon the therapist's judgment of the patient's primary area of failed adaptation, the context in which this will become manifest, and the therapeutic format that is most likely to have a lasting impact. Of course, the therapist's assessment and recommendations need to be acceptable to the patients. In cases of chronic marital discord, the choice of modality is seldom an issue, as both spouses define the problem as marital and the therapist agrees. Given the evidence suggesting the importance of marital relationships to individual functioning, a marital intervention may be a more effective use of the therapist's time than an individual intervention. Seeing the patient in relationship to a spouse may help the therapist gain a greater understanding of the nuances of interpersonal behavior that sustain the patient's difficulty. Often these nuances of behavior surface only after lengthy individual therapy. Even then, the behavior directed toward a same-sex therapist may be quite unlike the behavior directed toward an opposite-sex spouse. The primary advantage of the marital context is that the therapist can observe the disturbed behavior in its natural habitat. This can be a crucial advantage in patients who tend to describe their life difficulties in abstract intellectualized ways. The emotional intensity of marital therapy militates against this interpersonal strategy.

If both therapist and patients agree that the problem is marital, there would appear to be minimal justification for preferring an individual therapy context. In certain cases, the interaction may appear so intense and out of control that the therapist doubts that the couple can withstand the intensity of marital therapy. He may feel that the anxiety level is too high for anything to be accomplished. In my experience, this is a relatively rare occurrence if the therapist is willing to be quite active and to exert considerable control over the interactions. If the therapist is more passive and purely interpretive in his interventions, these couples may well prove untreatable. This conclusion may reflect the therapist's style as much as the couple's ability to profit from therapy. In other instances, the therapist may encounter situations where one spouse appears "too sick" for therapy to progress. In such cases, one often notes that the "healthier" spouse subtly and persistently provokes the irrational, destructive outbursts by the other spouse. The therapist needs to intervene quickly to interrupt these destructive cycles. Clearly, the therapist can modulate the patient's anxiety levels by the degree of support and structure he provides. One way of modulating anxiety is for the therapist to be purposely concrete and simplistic in all of his interactions with the couple. Although the intensity of the emotional struggle between the spouses clearly indicates that the struggle has a symbolic meaning, the therapist can defuse the struggle by stubbornly refusing to accept the behavior at that level. He can simply define the issue as failure to learn how to compromise and provide movement toward resolution of the struggle without acknowledging its symbolic meaning. Use of the interplay between behavior and its internal meaning can give the therapist great latitude in modulating anxiety levels.

## LENGTH OF THERAPY

The goal of this therapeutic model is to provide the clinician with guidelines from which to conduct brief, time-limited, and structured interventions into marital systems. This model was developed with the goal of keeping the length of therapy to fewer than 20 sessions. In most cases seen by the author, couples were seen for 15 sessions or less. Different therapists will vary the degree of structure and time limitation depending on their style and goals.

Brevity of intervention was an important consideration in the development of this model. Clearly, interventions have to be brief if large populations are to be served. Given the frequent absence of insurance coverage for marital therapy, brevity of intervention has a direct financial consequence for most patients. Several other considerations mandated the development of a brief intervention model. Within the field of individual psychotherapy, considerable evidence suggests that most psychological interventions are brief (Butcher and Koss, 1978). Patients tend to leave therapy when their goals are reached or once they feel that minimal progress is being made toward those goals. Many patients will be reached only by time-limited interventions. The goal of this model is modest in comparison to the goal of individual dynamically oriented psychotherapy. The expected outcome is for the couple to have the knowledge and skills to avoid future conflict and thus serve as supports for one another. A healthy relationship with the spouse is assumed to be more beneficial than a long-term relationship with the therapist. Similarly, there is minimal evidence that lengthy interventions are more effective than briefer interventions (Bergin and Lambert, 1978).

Several factors suggest that brief psychotherapy can be effective. Within the field of individual psychotherapy, numerous therapists maintain that much of the work in long-term therapy can be accomplished in briefer time periods if the therapist actively structures his interventions toward clearly formulated goals (e.g., Malan, 1976; Mann, 1973). The same rationale applies to marital therapy. Certain characteristics of marital therapy contribute to the probable effectiveness of brief contact. In individual therapy, transference reactions usually take time to become fully manifest. In fact, one major rationale for increasing the frequency of sessions is to mobilize transference reactions (Offenkrantz and Tobin, 1975). In marital therapy, this time consideration is seldom operative, as numerous clinicians have noted that the couple presents for treatment with already full-blown transference reactions to one another (Meissner, 1978; Sager, 1967). In marital therapy, the clinician's task is to quickly decipher the nature of these distortions rather than wait for their development. Once they are deciphered, he can then proceed with a systematic disproof of these distortions. Another advantage of marital therapy is that therapy doesn't end with the termination of sessions. If a change in interaction is successfully introduced, there is a chance of its being sustained if at least one member of the couple works to maintain the change. Similarly, there are at least two witnesses to therapeutic interventions. The spouse who conveniently forgets any of the therapist's comments that he doesn't like will most likely have his memory jogged by the less forgetful spouse (Haley, 1935).

## TECHNICAL CONSIDERATIONS

The therapeutic model has been outlined in broad conceptual terms. As such, it should be transposable to a variety of clinical settings. However, the clinical reader is probably interested in the actual application of this model by the author. Questions of frequency of sessions, presence or absence of cotherapy teams, and the relative use of individual versus conjoint sessions are crucial concerns to most clinicians. Thus, I will attempt to outline my practice according to these variables. Obviously, the model can be employed with modifications of these basic technical variables.

The model was developed in a brief, time-limited format, with couples being seen once weekly in most instances. The time limitation is usually established in the first or second session. At this point, the therapist says that they should plan to meet approxmately 10–15 sessions on a once-a-week basis. In most cases, the therapist and the couple know if the model will be effective by about 8–10 sessions. In infrequent cases, the number of sessions may be extended beyond this. By and large, extended therapy presents considerations beyond the scope of this model. In other words, one is led into detailed considerations of individual personality difficulties. Session length is usually 1 full hour. Typically, I have found 45 minutes to be too brief for a full replay of the interactional difficulty, still allowing time for an intervention to be effective. For certain couples, it is necessary to extend therapy sessions to 1½ hours. This is particularly necessary for couples who constantly battle with great ferocity. It is difficult for a couple to maintain a full-fledged war for extended periods of time. By extending the contact time, the therapist increases the probability of a lull during which an intervention will be heard.

Sessions are typically set at a once-a-week frequency. This timing allows for the couple to have a week to employ new learning and for the therapist to have a chance to monitor the impact of the therapy in the natural environment. In rare instances, the model has been used in extended blocks of time when life circumstances (impending move to another city) precluded extended therapy. The author has had limited experience with the outcome from the more massive focused application of the model. One would suspect that the long-term effectiveness of a briefer intervention would be less. Too many stimuli would be operative to restore the system to its original state.

The use of individual sessions, as opposed to conjoint sessions, remains a concern to therapist trainees, especially those with extensive exposure to individual psychotherapy. I personally have found individual sessions to be of limited usefulness. In particular, the initial use of formal individual diagnostic sessions appears to be a waste of time. As this viewpoint is counter to the position of others in the field, I will briefly explain. Individual diagnostic sessions can be useful in eliciting data related to early social learning experiences and inferring the probable nature of the distorted perception. However, the past is of concern only to the extent that it is operative in the present. From this perspective, the important past information can be gathered in conjoint sessions as the therapy evolves. The elicitation of this information in the presence of both spouses is useful in evoking a greater understanding of one another as complex beings.

The model proposed has typically been done using a solo therapist, although on occasion a dual therapy team has been utilized. The advantages and disadvantages of a solo therapist versus a cotherapy team relate to the role of the therapist. As the final resolution of the difficulty comes from the couple, the therapist's role is to be outside of the system unless making a planned intervention. This element of the therapist's role is more easily accomplished by a solo therapist. With two therapists, a different social system evolves. This system, by its nature, tends to change the couple's interaction and involve the therapists in a different manner.

## GOAL OF THERAPY

The therapeutic goal of this model is to reduce marital discord on the assumption that a well-functioning marital system can serve to prevent individual distress. If one assumes a reciprocal connection between individual distress and interpersonal interactions with intimate others, the reduction of interpersonal distress is a logical goal of therapy. An individual's sense of personal worth is partially the result of reflected appraisal from intimate others. If one's interactions with others is peaceful, this reflected appraisal will be more positive. Similarly, it appears that most individuals require well-functioning interpersonal relationships with significant others as a buffer against the impact of life stress (Brown et al., 1975). Individuals without such social support systems appear to weather adversity with less resilience (Burke and Weir, 1977).

The primary goal of this therapeutic modality is to reduce interpersonal discord and those factors that prevent satisfactory pairing. As the individual past lives of the participants contribute to the functioning of the system, these variables have to be considered. However, the goal of therapy is not insight as to the past contributors to present discord. These variables are considered only to the extent that is necessary for the completion of the therapeutic task. In other words, the focal point of intervention is the marital unit and the variables that are crucial to this understanding.

The peculiarities of marital therapy require the use of a variety of procedures alien to the usual psychodynamically oriented individual psychotherapist. The use of such procedures does not require the adoption of two sets of conceptual frameworks—one for individual therapy and one for marital therapy. The same framework is applicable to both, but the peculiar circumstances of marital therapy require a framework encompassing both past and present determinants of distress and the interplay of intrapsychic and interpersonal realities. The author's framework attempts to allow the clinician to utilize procedures derived from differing theoretical models without drifting into unstructured clinical eclecticism.

## STAGES OF THERAPY

Earlier, a conceptual overview of the author's theoretical model was presented. Skilled therapists, of course, realize that events in therapy don't always follow clearly from a conceptual model. The therapist has to put in a considerable amount of work to engage and maintain patients in therapy. In this section, I will attempt to discuss events occurring in a typical therapy sequence. Although the actual sequence of events will vary from couple to couple, certain regularities of events can be described across couples. For purposes of discussion, these regularities of events will be arbitrarily grouped into early, middle, and late phases of therapy.

### Early Phase (Entrance into Therapy)

The therapist has three primary goals in the early stages of therapy: (1) to establish a working alliance with the couple; (2) to observe the interactional difficulty, detail its history, and form provisional hypotheses about its maintaining variables; and (3) to formulate provisional hypotheses about the most effective and least threatening ways to begin to set the interactional system into disequilibrium.

Clearly, the primary goal of the therapist in the first several sessions is to engage the couple in an amiable working relationship. If this isn't satisfactorily accomplished, further work may be extremely difficult. The therapist has three principal objectives in this regard: (1) to make sure that each member of the couple feels that his or her position has been heard and is respected, (2) to lower defensiveness as much as possible, and (3) to restore some hope of change.

Most individual psychotherapists are skilled at establishing working relationships with patients of varying personality styles. This is usually accomplished by statements from the therapist indicating that he understands the subjective world of the patient. The skilled therapist makes these statements in a language form familiar to the patient and with a degree of intimacy tolerable to the patient. The same factors are involved in marital therapy. The process is more complicated in that the therapist needs also to maintain his neutrality in the marital dispute and to avoid unnecessary escalation of the dispute. Several basic ground rules are useful in couple therapy: (1) The therapist must make certain that each spouse expresses his or her views and should attempt to have each spouse speak for roughly comparable periods of time; (2) the therapist should attempt to give each spouse a reasonably uninterrupted period in which to express his or her viewpoint; (3) the therapist should paraphrase what he has heard from each spouse; (4) in this paraphrasing it should be emphasized that the opinion is one spouse's viewpoint only, but to be respected as such; and (5) in the paraphrasing an attempt must be made to modulate inflammatory comments. In couples with a long history of heated discord, the therapist should be prepared to be quite active and to assume control of the situation.

Many couples will come to the first session, wait for the therapist to indicate that they should speak, hesitate a moment, and then begin speaking simultaneously. A familiar variation is for one spouse to begin speaking while the other is silent except for frequent signs of disagreement. In such situations, the therapist should politely interrupt, indicating that he needs to hear the viewpoint of each and that it is difficult to obtain a coherent history of the problem if both speak at once. At this point, the therapist might turn to one of the spouses and ask him (or her) to explain his (or her) reasons for coming into marital therapy. Frequently, the therapist might turn initially to the partner who had previously been silent except for voicing disagreement. This maneuver disarms the usual interpersonal strategy of that partner and disrupts the typical interaction pattern of the couple. The therapist might request that the other spouse attempt not to interrupt for the time being, with the assurance that his turn will come shortly. During the time that the first spouse is speaking, the therapist looks at this spouse, while carefully monitoring the emotional state of the silent spouse. If the silent spouse appears about to interrupt, the therapist politely but firmly gestures for that spouse to remain silent. If the spouse resists that request, the therapist may need to say something on the order of "It's crucial that I understand each of your viewpoints. To do that, I need to listen to each of you one at a time. In a few minutes, I want to hear your version." Once the second spouse appears reasonably quiet (perhaps now sulking in his chair), the therapist turns back to the first spouse. The therapist at this point is seeking a brief focused discussion of one spouse's viewpoint. The therapist may need to interrupt for clarification and focus, particularly with long and diversionary discourses. If the first spouse continually switches the subject and seems out of control, the therapist may request that the spouse attempt to focus on the main difficulty. During his requests for clarification, the therapist attempts as much as possible to get the spouse to describe his feelings and his desires relevant to the mate rather than simply cast aspersions on the mate's character. In most cases of marital discord, the attribution of deplorable characteristics to the mate obfuscates what the first spouse desires from that mate. This dysfluent style of communication becomes part of the interactional systems maintaining the discord. At this point, the therapist is beginning to see how much this spouse is capable of speaking about his own feelings. At the end of the discourse, the therapist interrupts and says, "Let me see if I understand clearly what you are saying." Then, the therapist paraphrases what he thinks the first spouse is saying. This paraphrasing, if possible, should emphasize the first spouse's pain and noble efforts at solution, without casting aspersions on the second spouse. To maintain his neutrality, and in an attempt to clearly separate each spouse's subjective experience, the therapist may begin his paraphrasing with the phrase "From your viewpoint." If the second spouse expresses violent disapproval, the therapist may need to reassure that spouse again that he is simply trying to understand things from each person's point of view and that he wants to hear that spouse's viewpoint in a few minutes. Whenever possible, in the paraphrasing, accusations against the other should be shifted to statements about self. For example, if a wife yells that her husband is never interested in her feelings about things, the therapist may emphasize her desire to communicate with her husband and her frustration when she feels misunderstood. This paraphrasing leaves interpretation of blame nebulous. Each spouse is able to feel that his own position is understood without the other spouse feeling blamed. As Haley and others (e.g., Haley, 1963) have emphasized, each spouse would like the therapist to agree that the other is at fault. Thus, it is important that the therapist be extremely careful that no comment of his will be misconstrued in that manner.

In the beginning of therapy, it is especially important that the therapist maintain his neutrality and disrupt the pattern of attributing blame rather than specifying problems to be resolved. Thus, it is usually advisable, because of each spouse's desire to attribute blame to the other spouse, to avoid interpretation or clarification of one spouse's role in the genesis of discord in initial sessions and thus avoid confronting the real difficulties. The therapist is attempting to disrupt this interactional pattern. Later in therapy, when this pattern is disrupted and an element of interpersonal trust has been reestablished, the therapist can clarify individual contributions to the interactional problem. If clarification of one spouse's maladaptive behavior is attempted, I recommend the use of paired clarification such that blame is equally distributed. For example, if one spouse continually digresses into extraneous subjects while talking, so that the therapist has difficulty understanding what that spouse is saying, the therapist may need to point this out while asking for clarification. If the other spouse seems to gloat over this, the therapist may casually mention that he also notes that the other spouse has the same difficulty. Because of the need to continually counterbalance clarifications and the difficulty of doing this effectively early in therapy when anxiety levels are high, it is usually preferable to avoid such maneuvers early in therapy. On rare occasions, individual interpretations may lead to a shortening of the therapeutic work. All too often, it will not work.

Once the interaction with the first spouse reaches a logical conclusion, the therapist then repeats the process with the second spouse. At the conclusion of the interaction with the second spouse, the therapist may then seek further clarification of discrepancies from both spouses. During this interaction, the therapist modulates the amount of interaction between spouses. He wishes to observe their interaction and at the same time prevent a full return to their nonproductive arguing. This modulation of the interaction is similar to the individual therapist's modulation of the patient's anxiety level. If the individual patient's anxiety becomes intolerable, the individual therapist subtly shifts the focus of discussion until the patient's anxiety level is manageable. With couples, the therapist can modulate emotion by topic shifting and by the degree of his participation. Throughout this process, the therapist is gathering information as to each spouse's perception of the other spouse and of the marital difficulty. He is also gaining information as to how their current behavior sustains the problem. At the same time that the therapist is gaining information and establishing rapport with each of the spouses, he is beginning to establish the ground rules of therapy. He has already communicated that he wishes for them to speak one at a time, that he feels attribution of blame to be counterproductive, and that an understanding and respect of each spouse's subjective experience is important. These ground rules are, of course, quite different from the usual interaction in disturbed marriages and are a beginning effort to disrupt the typical interaction.

In order to engage the couple in therapy, it is necessary that the therapist attempt to lower defensiveness in the spouses. In spite of the seeming ease with which couples attack one another with devastating impact on occasion, it is reasonable to assume that each spouse feels a sense of shame in openly displaying his gross inadequacy in working out an interpersonal relationship. In individual psychotherapy, many patients feel shame as they describe their interpersonal failures to the therapist. To control their degree of embarrassment, many patients only gradually reveal the full story to the therapist. In marital therapy, this degree of personal protection is absent, and the shame is compounded because the spouses are openly demonstrating their inadequacy to a stranger. There are few secrets available to the patient. What the therapist can't decipher, the spouse knows. The couple may also feel embarrassment that they had to seek professional help to solve problems that they think should be solved by healthy people on their own. In many couples, the intensity of the attack–counterattack cycles appears directly proportional to the degree of personal shame and hopelessness experienced. Attacking the spouse seems less painful then experiencing one's own feelings. In interpersonal systems, unfortunately, attacks usually generate counterattacks.

To lower defensiveness, the therapist needs to convey his nonjudgmental acceptance of the couple's difficulty, emphasize positive attributes whenever credible, and help prevent the couple from embarrassing themselves further. Undoubtedly, the therapist's major impact is not a therapeutic maneuver but an attitude conveyed in nonverbal gesture and tone as he seriously listens to complaints and attempts to understand each spouse. The attitude of the therapist is usually transparent to most couples. This impact of the therapist may be augmented by general statements as to the universal difficulty of working out close interpersonal relationships and the shared pain and disappointment of almost all couples.

If possible, the therapist should emphasize positive aspects of the relationship. In some couples, this is exceedingly difficult. However, the therapist can comment on their attempt and efforts to solve problems and the pain they've endured as a couple. In other couples, he may discover that the relationship was satisfactory until some event. In these cases, he can emphasize the hidden strengths of the relationship. In most couples, there will be some valued attribute in the spouse at some time in the present or past. An expression of a possible feeling about the spouse, however miniscule, can help to lower defensiveness. These efforts by the therapist to discover and emphasize positives in the relationship need not be considered as manipulations. If indeed the couple has stayed together all of this time in spite of their disappointments, positive features to the relationship undoubtedly exist. From this perspective, the therapist is simply working to have the couple verbalize and experience things as they really are. The added advantage is the power of the expression of positive feelings on the other spouse. The second spouse will usually reciprocate either by a similar expression of positives or by being less intractable over some minor issue. Eventually, the therapist hopes to facilitate cycles of cooperation and expression of positives and to decrease cycles of attack–counterattack.

Much of the defensiveness in couples appears to result from what Haley (1963) described as runaways and behavioral marital therapists (e.g., Patterson and Hops, 1972) describe as coercive cycles. One spouse purposely or inadvertently makes a comment that arouses the ire of the mate, who responds in kind. This soon escalates into a situation that both spouses feel powerless to control. These escalations are seldom productive and generate considerable defensiveness and anger. From an individual level, behavioral marital therapists refer to this as a negative reinforcement behavioral change strategy, i.e., I'll stop complaining, arguing, etc., when you do what I want. Interpersonal therapists might describe this as bargaining from a position of relative safety, i.e., you have to change first. However one conceptualizes these events, the therapist has to assume control early and prevent or reduce the number of unnecessary escalations. These escalations have clearly not been helpful in the past. For therapy to succeed, something has to change. If an escalating battle begins, the therapist should intervene quickly to interrupt the sequence. Rephrasing, changing the subject, and numerous other tactics can be used. In certain extremely combative couples, it may be necessary for the therapist to make some unusual movement to gain attention. He needs to divert the combatants' attention long enough for them to hear an invervention. For example, the therapist might abruptly stand up without saying anything. Eventually, during pauses for breath, the spouses notice his standing, wonder why, and momentarily stop arguing. Then the therapist intervenes. Usually, such unconventional gestures aren't necessary. It is mentioned to underline the absolute necessity of the therapist's gaining control when events escalate. For the theoretical perspective offered by the author's model, these destructive, self-perpetuating cycles are epiphenomena in the interpersonal sequence and serve to confuse deciphering of the underlying issues. The couple understandably view these problems as central. They are central in that nothing can be accomplished by the therapist until these cycles are brought under control. Later in the therapy, the therapist will work more definitively to alter linguistic habits that contribute to escalations. In this regard, he will attempt to get each spouse to describe his or her own feelings and desires without attacking the mate. In other words, he will help each spouse to begin to speak for self alone without casting blame on the mate. This relearning of linguistic habits usually takes several weeks of therapy. Thus, early in therapy, the therapist needs to use alternative means to prevent escalations.

Most patients enter individual psychotherapy because they feel demoralized and unable to solve their problems in living (Frank, 1973). Similar motives underlie most couples' entry into therapy. Therefore, it is important, when possible, for the therapist to restore some hope of change. This restoration of hope is partially determined by the couple's perception of the therapist's attitude and competence. If the couple perceives that the therapist understands their difficulty, feels hopeful about a solution, and appears to know what he is doing, this may be a major factor in restoring morale. A statement by the therapist as to his perception of the problem and the tasks to be accomplished can also be helpful in restoring morale. At least, the couple is aware that someone feels there may be a solution and a related plan of action. Clearly, in the initial session, it is difficult to always outline a concise description of the presenting difficulty. However, the therapist can usually summarize his observations at an interaction level and point to the steps to be followed in subsequent sessions. The advantages of the behavioral models is that they give the therapist a positive way of conceptualizing the initial problems and their solutions. For example, if the couple constantly battles over control and argues incessantly over trivial matters, the therapist can state that one source of their problem is that they are both strong-willed and independent and need to learn how to compromise. This characterization is mildly flattering to most individuals and prepares the way for further intervention, such as behavioral techniques to promote negotiation and compromise in the relationship. In the same couple, the therapist could equally truthfully have said that each spouse's sense of autonomy was so fragile that they were afraid to compromise. This intervention would not restore morale and would lead toward a totally dissimilar form of intervention. Similarly, another couple who constantly misattribute motives to each other can be told that they have difficulty with communication, and that this appears to underlie much of their difficulty and should be the focus of future sessions. These comments also serve the purpose of leading into the next stage of intervention. If possible, some minor change of interaction should be attempted in the first session. An actual change in behavior usually carries more weight than the therapist's words. In the first few sesssions, it is important to bring some issues to a resolution. The substance of the resolved issue is less important than the fact of a resolution. The therapist is attempting to demonstrate in action that cooperative action is possible. When this is attempted, it is important to choose a relatively minor issue with minimal emotional charge. For example, the agreement may be on how to choose the time of the next therapy session. If this transaction can occur without a major battle and with the wishes of both spouses being respected, this very act can restore a sense of hope. In other couples, a compromise on a relatively minor issue, such as which movie to go to this weekend, can be a major initial breakthrough. In other cases, the therapist may have to settle for at least getting the couple to agree on a common problem area to discuss in the next session.

Another technique that facilitates the restoration of morale is for the therapist to gradually shift discussion toward the present and future, implying that a detailed review of the past is unnecessary, as the future will be different. This can be a difficult decision. On the one hand, the therapist needs a sense of the development of the difficulty, as this may influence his choice of intervention. For example, if the distress started around a clear-cut precipitant, alternative forms of intervention might be required. In this case, a brief couple therapy based on a modified individual therapy model might be more appropriate. The couple would be helped to explore the event, its meaning to them individually and as a couple. On the other hand, understanding a past event of some significance might help the therapist to comprehend the meaning of a current struggle. However, diversions into past history also present hazards. These discussions can easily escalate into a series of recriminations that do not appear to serve useful purposes. The review of a long chronology of disappointments further augments the sense of hopelessness. If a cycle such as this begins, I find it absolutely essential that the therapist intervene quickly to abort the cycle. One intervention that is often useful is to say, "If your marriage is like most disturbed marriages, each of you is justifiably angered and has been hurt unjustifiably in the past. The point of this therapy is to evolve a different way of interacting. Perhaps, it would be more profitable to focus on current problems." This intervention serves to lead the couple to a new focus while not disagreeing with their perception of events. It also implies that the future may be different.

At the same time that the therapist is beginning to influence the interactional sequences, he is also formulating tentative hypotheses as to the nature of the underlying difficulty. This information can be inferred from various sources. In many couples, one will observe peculiar polarized personalities, such that each spouse in the company of the other appears almost to be a caricature. These peculiar contrasting interactional styles have been noted by numerous therapists. For example, one spouse may always appear to desire greater intimacy and the other spouse usually prefers greater interpersonal distance, or one spouse is always reasonable and the other always irrational. The list is endless. If one assumes that this hyperpolarization of character tendencies is partially the result of the couple's interactional history, one can then begin to speculate as to the reasons for this. One may then notice that certain behaviors of the "reasonable" husband always precede his wife's "irrational" behavior and vice versa. This then gives clues to the partial genesis and maintenance of the personality differences. One can then speculate that the husband plays a role in maintaining his wife as irrational and that such behavior on his part has an explanation. The search for a plausible reason for his behavior will aid the therapist in changing the wife's behavior and deciphering the inner representational events in the husband related to his wife's behavior. On one level, the husband may describe how he wishes his wife to be. But if the therapist observes the husband's behavior, he may observe that the husband subtly discourages movement toward that ideal by his wife. In other words, the husband's behavior reinforces his wife's current behavior. From this observation, one can form provisional hypotheses about the way the wife must be to receive reinforcement from the husband.

Similarly, in verbal disputes, the nature of the character assassinations can provide additional data. In the litany of abuses that each spouse hurls at the other, one can usually observe a consistent theme. This theme usually is close to each spouse's representational model for the other. Another source of information about the inner representational systems comes when the therapist paraphrases each spouse's description of the marital problem. This paraphrasing always involves a certain shift in emphasis. In fact, the therapist is purposely attempting a minor shift in emphasis for therapeutic reasons. Each spouse will overlook many of these minor discrepancies. Certain discrepancies in spouse description will provoke characteristic reactions (anger, disbelief, confusion). These cues, often nonverbal, of a resistance to a minor recharacterization of the mate's personality, can provide additional provisional information about the inner representational system. In other words, one can infer the relatively narrow spectrum of personality characteristics allowable to the mate. Information concerning this is inferred from observation of each mate's reinforcement pattern for the opposite mate and from verbal descriptions of the mate. The thrust of the therapy will be to dislodge these fixed characterizations to allow each spouse a greater freedom of action, a greater sense of being known, and to allow the system greater flexibility. In the early sessions, the therapist is continually monitoring information for its consistency with his provisional hypotheses.

At the end of the beginning stages of therapy, the therapist has formulated a provisional idea of each spouse's distorted perception of the other and how the interactional behavior serves to maintain these distortions, obfuscate the real issues, and prevent change. At this point, the therapist will be seeking information as to the most efficient manner in which the maintaining variables can be weakened. Although the nature of these interventions may focus on different systems of events by necessity, the overriding concern is to achieve a disruption in the interactional system. Only after the interactional system is disrupted will a more careful examination of the inner representational systems be possible. At this point, the therapist is tentatively trying out procedures and gauging the couples reactions to determine his overall strategy.

Although the main goal of the therapist in the early stages of therapy is to engage the couple in therapy, it is clear from this section that the therapist also begins making interventions early in the therapy. For example, the therapist works to take control of the interaction and to modify that interaction. He blocks escalating battles, intervenes to prevent cycles of blame and counterblame, and attempts to shift a pattern of attack and counterattack into a pattern of cooperation.

## Middle Stages

The goals of the early stages of therapy were primarily to engage the couples in therapy and to form provisional hypotheses about the distorted perceptions underlying their difficulty. The goal of the middle stage of therapy is to begin to modify interaction such that it contradicts those underlying assumptions. As the observed behavior and underlying assumptive worlds are posited to be intertwined, the approach is both cognitive and behavioral in focus. The underlying perceptual problem may not become evident until after a behavioral change has occurred. In many couples, one observes a remarkable similarity of behavioral sequences. These sequences have been described by therapists of differing theoretical backgrounds (e.g., Haley, 1963; Patterson and Hops, 1972). These sequences appear in many disturbed relationships and can derive from remarkably dissimilar sources. The interventions in the middle stages of therapy resemble those defined as nonspecific in the preceding section. These interventions are focused on modifying the interactional system.

During the early states of therapy, the therapist purposely intervened to interrupt the couple's usual ways of interacting with one another. In the middle stage, he gradually shifts his focus. At the beginning of the middle stage of therapy, the therapist attempts to reengage the couple in an interactional struggle so that he can observe the difficulty *in vivo*. This assessment stage rapidly blends into an intervention stage. The intervention will consist primarily of the therapist modifying the form of interaction and instructing the couple in ways to sustain these changes. The main interventions utilized by the therapist resemble techniques advocated by behavior therapists under the label of reciprocity training and communication training (Jacobson and Margolin, 1979).

The reengagement in the struggle is accomplished by the therapist purposely redirecting communication between the spouses and removing himself largely from the process. Strategies for accomplishing this have been described by others (e.g., Sluzki, 1978). The point of this intervention is for the therapist to have an opportunity to observe the couple interacting with minimal outside interference. In this manner, one hopes, the behavior in the office is similar to the behavior in the home that preceded the withdrawal. In this stage, the therapist attempts to get the spouses to interact with one another without using the therapist as a conduit. It is common for a couple to attempt to talk directly to the therapist rather than to each other. Presumably, their discussions together have been unfruitful and painful. The tendency to avoid such discussions is understandable, if unhelpful. Eventually, the therapist hopes that the discussion will be largely between the spouses, almost as if he were not in the room. As he watches this interaction, he makes a decision as to the first type of intervention he will make.

With most couples, considerable work is needed to assist in the change of communication patterns. Dysfluent communication helps to maintain the status quo, as new information is not transmitted. Because of this lack of transmission, new information does not reach the participants, forcing a reexamination of their assumptive worlds about one another. Frequently, the communication in disturbed marriages is so vague that it is difficult for either spouse to explain what is being discussed. One spouse may request something from the other in a vague, tangential way. The second spouse isn't aware that something is being requested and changes the subject. Then the first spouse concludes that the mate is insensitive to his or her needs or doesn't care. Feeling justifiably angry, this spouse attacks the character of the other spouse, who replies angrily to an attack. Soon the couple is involved in an escalating battle and neither spouse is certain what the argument is about. Within limits, each spouse is justified in whatever conclusions are drawn about the other's character or motives.

The objective of the therapist in modifying communication patterns is to achieve greater specification of the issues at hand, to eliminate verbal stimuli leading to escalations, to promote the satisfactory completion of communication on any given subject, and to convey the notion of joint responsibility for effective communications.

## Communication Training

The communication training approaches to the treatment of marital discord were reviewed in the previous chapter. These observations, taken both from clinical observation (Satir, 1967) and from clinical investigation (Thomas, 1977), can be utilized flexibly in the approach to couple therapy. The approach I am advocating differs from that of many of the behavioral marital therapists in that the therapist's interventions are superimposed on the couple's interactions rather than presented as a training package. Thus, the form and timing of the interventions will vary from couple to couple. The overall goal is to promote efficient information exchange. In this regard, most of the advocated components will overlap with procedures developed by other clinicians and will serve to eliminate dysfunctions established as prevelant in disturbed couples. The therapist observes a given couple's communication style, notes the principal problems, and pinpoints these for the couple. At first, the therapist models a different way of saying something. Later, he coaches the couple in rehearsing alternative ways of interacting.

Clearly, problems of communication can reside in the sender, the receiver, or the interaction between the participants. Early in the intervention, the therapist will want to establish the notion that communication is a shared responsibility. For example, if one spouse makes an obscure statement, the therapist can turn to the second and ask if he understood what the first spouse meant. If the reply is negative, the therapist may suggest that the second spouse seek clarification. This maneuver serves two purposes: (1) It undermines the tendency of both spouses to avoid clear communication and (2) it gives the second spouse practice in an alternative behavior. Similarly, the therapist at a different time may ask the second spouse to paraphase what he just heard. The first spouse can be asked if the received message corresponds with the intended message. If not, the second spouse can be prompted to ask for clarification. This maneuver reinforces the notion that unclear communication is a joint responsibility. The first spouse needs to strive to convey messages in a form understandable to the second, and the second spouse needs to seek clarification. Occasional interruptions to seek clarification of both the intended and received messages and to facilitate a better exchange of information can illustrate the tragedy of the couple's attempts to communicate as well as a more effective means of achieving that stated goal. If the wife desired her husband to understand her, she needs to attempt to express her feelings in a language form understandable by her husband. Her husband needs to indicate when he doesn't understand.

Problems in the receiver end of communication are usually (1) misunderstanding or (2) failure to validate. Problems in misunderstanding can be minimized by the therapist interrupting and asking a spouse to paraphrase what was just communicated to him. If the paraphrased account differs considerably from the intended message, the therapist points this out and suggests that the spouse attempt to listen more closely. Several repetitions of this sequence can serve to illustrate the communication gap and motivate couples to attempt to communicate more efficiently. The therapist can even instruct one spouse to listen closely to the mate for a few minutes as the therapist requests a paraphrasing. Most spouses will irritatedly comply with such an instruction. Rather than risk therapist disapproval, most spouses will attempt to listen more closely. A series of such exercises will usually eliminate or sharply reduce receiver difficulties. In the receiver difficulty known as failure to validate, one spouse is saying something that the second spouse dislikes. The second spouse interrupts with a rebuttal. The first spouse continues to expound on his position. At this point, the first spouse may desire confirmation that his position is understood as much as he desires agreement or disagreement. In such cases, the therapist may suggest that the second spouse first validate that he has heard what his mate means and only then express his disagreement.

Several common patterns of dysfluent communication in disturbed couples appear to lead to confusion as to the issues being discussed. This confusion leaves each spouse free to draw his or her own conclusions. Examples of communication problems frequently observed in couples include (1) overgeneralization, (2) incomplete messages, (3) vague referents, (4) incongruent verbal and nonverbal communication, (5) impersonal statements in the third person, (6) topic shifting, (7) combining requests with anger, (8) presumptive attribution, (9) use of first person plural, and (10) excessive summarization of positions.

1. *Overgeneralization* refers to the use of statements grossly oversimplifying a situation. For example, an angry husband may complain that his wife never does any housework. This statement usually leads to a denial coupled with a counterattack. The stage is set for an unproductive escalation. The husband in many cases has the intent to critize his wife about some specific omission, for example, not vacuuming his study. In cases like this, the therapist can intervene quickly, saying, "I'm not sure what you mean. Could you be more specific?" He might turn to

the wife and ask her if she understood her husband. Once the husband clarifies his complaint, the therapist might say, "Why don't you ask your wife if she's willing to vacuum your study rather than throwing a global complaint at her? Who knows, a specific nonjudgmental request might work. Why not try it?" In this particular sequence the therapist pinpoints the problem and recommends an alternative strategy.

2. *Incomplete messages* can similarily obscure what is being said. One spouse may begin a sentence, pause in midsentence, and then shift the topic. The other spouse is left confused as to which part of the message to respond to. The first partner feels misunderstood and angry. For example, the husband may say, "My mother felt you should spend more time with the children . . . did you help Johnny with his homework last night?" The second spouse has no way of knowing if the two phrases are interrelated. If so, should she respond to the inferred hidden meaning? In such cases, the therapist can say, "I'm not sure what you're trying to say." Then, turning to the wife, "Did you? No? Why don't you ask him to clarify what he meant?" In this case, the therapist temporarily joins with the wife against the husband. This serves the purpose of reassuring the wife that the statement was ambiguous. If the therapist sides with the wife, the husband is unable to blame the wife for misunderstanding him without also attacking the therapist. Once the husband clarifies his statement, the therapist can underline how this type of statement leads to misunderstanding. He can emphasize how the husband needs to be clear in his messages and how the wife should ask for clarification in uncertain situations.

3. An example of the disruptive effect of *vague referents* is an engineer who was describing how many of his relationships with women had involved insecure women. This discussion had ranged from his mother to previous sexual partners, his first wife, and his current wife. He states, "They all were insecure." The wife concludes that the "they" includes her and becomes defensive. The husband then informs her that he was referring to past relationships, while silently concluding that his current wife may be the same. In such cases, the therapist should point out that the referent was obscure and the reaction understandable. He can also ask the wife why she didn't seek clarification before responding. In this way, the spouses are held equally accountable for the misunderstanding and steered toward alternative forms of communication.

4. Both clinical observation (Satir, 1967) and empirical investigation (Gottman *et al.*, 1976) have emphasized the presence of *incongruence* between levels of communication in disturbed couples. A classic example would be a wife who says, "I agree completely, dear," in a harsh tone with her arms crossed after her husband has just completed a sermon

on how the woman's place is in the home. The therapist can usually disrupt this sequence by turning to the wife and saying with innocent surprise, "Do you really? I didn't realize that you felt that way." Alternatively, he can turn to the husband and ask, "Do you believe that she really means that? Why don't you try to find out your wife's real opinion on this matter?" This sequence may eventually flush out the real disagreement.

5. In many couples, one spouse will repeatedly make *statements in impersonal form*. Most often, these statements will be in the form of general rules of proper conduct. Thinly veiled in such messages is the implied message that the mate should comply with the general rule and is bad if he does not. A typical example would be the wife who says, "All real men initiate sex." Clearly, this woman desires for her husband to initiate sex, but she is not stating this as her own wish. If she states this as her own wish, then she and her husband can have a reasonable conversation about this. In such situations, the therapist may request that the woman express the general rule as her request. He may need to point out that the husband has different general rules, but that such rules are really just disguised personal preferences.

6. A variety of verbal behavior patterns have been observed to lead to interpersonal escalations and to a sense of frustration that nothing can be resolved. A frequent occurrence is for a couple to approach resolution of an issue and then for a sequence of events to gradually erode the progress. For example, a couple may almost reach an agreement about a trivial but recurring conflict when one spouse introduces another issue prematurely. This has been referred to as "off-beaming" (Gottman et al., 1976) and "content shifting" (Thomas, 1977). The shift in focus is often to an emotionally charged issue and elicits a counterresponse. Then the spouses can again assume that resolution is impossible and settle back comfortably into their usual ways of perceiving one another. When one spouse brings up an extraneous subject at precisely the wrong time, the therapist needs to lead the couple back to the problem at hand without alienating either spouse. A useful tactic is to turn to the interrupting spouse and say, "That's an extremely important issue. I'm glad you brought that up. Why don't we focus on that next? But right now, let's resolve this issue." Such an intervention can redirect the flow back to the issue at hand without arousing great animosity. Later in the therapy, the therapist may wish to label the sidetracking behavior as problematic to interrupt a spouse's use of this as an interpersonal tactic.

7. The more experience one has working with couples in conflict, the more one becomes convinced that bitter unresolved disputes are more often the result of stylistic clashes than of disagreement on sub-

stantive issues. Couples become locked into battles over relatively trivial issues with great emotional intensity. Once the confusion has been cleared, the fight may be over how often the couple eats out a week. On further clarification, the real disagreement may be between the wife's desire for three meals in a restaurant per week and the husband's desire for one. On such a trivial issue, one would assume that a compromise of two would have been reached years ago so that the couple could free up this energy to resolve larger problems. The manner in which these negotiations occurs appears to preclude their resolution. Neither spouse states clearly why it is important to him or her, and their requests for change are usually intermingled with thinly veiled disapproval of the other. The spouse being requested to change receives a mixed message, a request for change and disapproval. Few spouses respond positively to such verbal stimuli. Ultimately, the therapist hopes to shape the spouses' behavior such that each will state explicitly what is desired from the other without a value judgment concerning the other spouse. Once this is achieved, the couple is in a position to observe what substantive disagreements really exist. In many couples, these are relatively minor. The therapist can help to shape verbal behavior toward this goal. The desired goal is for each spouse to express his or her wishes without attacking the mate, either overtly or covertly. As the sequence of interaction between spouses progresses, one spouse may request something from the other in a negative voice tone. The therapist can intervene, inquiring about the tone of voice. The spouse will perhaps say, "He'll never agree. He never does anything I want." The therapist can quickly say, "Well, we'll never know this way. How about repeating your request as a genuine request?" Another frequent problem is for one spouse to request something from his mate, and for his mate to reply, "That's a dumb idea." The therapist needs to intervene early to prevent an escalation. A reasonable intervention is "It may or may not be dumb. But that's besides the point. How about responding to the question being asked. He (she) desires this from you."

8. Another source of confusion in clinical couples is deciphering who feels what. Satir (1967) posited that couples in dysfunctional marriages have difficulties with relatedness and differentness. For this reason, their speech often obscures real differences. Other investigations have noted the tendency for disturbed couples to use language that confuses the self–other differentiation. One style of communication that contributes to this has been labeled *presumptive attribution* (Thomas, 1977) or mind reading (Sluzki, 1978). In these instances, one spouse concludes as factual some inference about the other's spouse's inner state. An example would be the husband who replies, "You only said that because

you're angry about last night. There's no possible other reason." The wife may angrily reply that her husband is wrong. This cross-attribution of motives obscures differences between couples in the same manner as the persistent use of first person plural pronouns. Both result in obfuscation of real knowledge about the other partner. In cases of presumptive attribution, the therapist can intervene, saying, "Your conclusion is reasonable, but alternative conclusions are possible. Let's examine the data together." If the husband will go along with therapist, an impartial discussion usually leads to several likely meanings for the event. Then, the therapist can laugh at himself and say, "Hey, why don't we find out the answer by asking your wife?" If successful, this maneuver introduces the concept of faulty attribution of motives and checking reality by asking the spouse. A common pitfall is the mate who links the current misperception to a consistent theme buttressed by a litany of events dating back to an incident prior to their marriage 12 years ago. This occasionally can be disrupted if the therapist agrees that this may have been true in the past but doesn't seem to completely explain the events now. Depending on the emotional tone at the moment, the therapist can casually mention the excitement of discovering new things in a person so different from the self.

9. Many couples avoid open discussion of differences by the excessive *use of first person plural* pronouns. Examples would include "We both think that our sex life is wonderful" and "We don't think about things like that." Presumably, the couple has resorted to this tactic because previous efforts at resolving differences have failed. The denial of differences avoids overt conflict. Eventually, the therapist desires the open expression of differences. If differences aren't acknowledged, resolution is impossible. In cases of the use of the first person plural, the therapist can repeatedly turn to the other spouse and say, "Do you really feel that way?" If the reply is vague and noncommittal, the therapist can pursue greater clarification. If the second spouse appears reluctant to openly acknowledge disagreement, the therapist might say, "Well, maybe you don't agree completely."

10. Another sequence of verbal behavior that interferes with resolution of issues is the "summarizing-self" sequence (Gottman *et al*, 1976). This excessive summarization usually occurs early in an interactional sequence and precludes its progressing further. One spouse summarizes his position. The second spouse does likewise. Then the first spouse restates his or her position again. Such sequences can be repeated ad nauseum. Not only do the sequences prevent a resolution of issues but they essentially stalemate the interactional sequence. The usual technique for interrupting such sequences is to ask one partner and then

the other to summarize what the other has said. Then the therapist can make sure that one spouse's understanding of the other's position matches what the other spouse intended to say. To prevent digression into further summarizing of positions, the therapist can then say, "Well, I think that the two of you now have a better understanding of your differences. How can we now move to resolve this?" This intervention firmly guides the interaction toward a different direction.

Early in the sequence, the therapist will need to interrupt in a timely fashion. These interruptions serve to prevent unnecessary escalations and to provide information about alternative strategies. Similarly, the therapist is modeling alternative ways of dealing with provocative behavior. Once the intervention has been repeated on numerous occasions, the therapist wishes to gradually remove himself from the interaction. For an intervention to be useful, it needs to be self-sustaining. If therapy is only 1½ hours per week, the couple is left with 166½ hours to resort to old patterns. Thus, the therapist hopes for the spouses to eventually perform their own self-modulating functions. In the transition from therapist to couple control, the therapist may need to make occasional prompting statements, such as, "We've been here before. If we keep going like this, another battle will follow. John (Mary), how have you learned to handle this differently? Mary (John), why don't you ask for clarification if your feelings are hurt?"

*Negotiating Differences*

Changing communication patterns and teaching negotiation skills are clearly intertwined. As communication becomes clearer, real differences in preferences become clear. As couples become enmeshed in bitter disputes over seemingly minor compromises, a way of breaking these deadlocks is necessary. Fitzgerald (1973) refers to this as traversing the jungle. One has to eliminate the fog and complexity of transactional difficulties before one can approach core issues. With negotiation problems over trivial issues, it is reasonable to assume that the deadlock is because of some inner meaning of the event to each participant—a "core symbol" (Liberman *et al*, 1980). In the middle stage of therapy, one has at least two alternative strategies. If the level of trust is reasonable, one may help each spouse to decipher the meaning of the core symbol. If the meaning is an emotion known to the other spouse, compromise is more likely. For example, a couple became deadlocked in a dispute over whether to have breakfast at home on Sunday mornings. The husband desired his wife to prepare breakfast at home. His wife had other preferences. The deadlock was broken when the husband spoke of its meaning to him. As a child, it was one time that the whole family was together and thus an emotional symbol of feeling safe and secure. For the wife, eating out with the family was a special time of emotional significance. With this additional information, the real issue became capturing a sense of security and relatedness for both. The place of Sunday breakfast was less significant and easily compromised.

In other couples, elicitation of such information is more problematic, and it may be more expedient to first establish a compromise and later decipher its meaning, if necessary. The advantage of reciprocity training, negotiation training, or bartering exercises is that it breaks deadlocks, shifting the interactional system into new patterns. Once issues of genuine disagreement are clarified, it is usually preferable to choose a relatively minor issue to work on first. The resolution of this issue in and of itself is relatively unimportant. Instead, one is seeking a momentum in changing the interactional system. This momentum builds on gradually accumulating successes. The minor issue might be the wife's wish for her husband to wash dishes. The therapist asks for greater clarification. How often does she wish her husband to wash dishes? Once this is clear, the therapist asks the husband for a small favor he desires from his wife. A list of things from greater sexual responsiveness to greeting him at the door when he comes home from work may be obtained. The therapist can say, "Sex is important, but more complicated. Let's start with the simple things. Later, we'll tackle the big ones." Turning to the wife, the therapist asks, "Is meeting him at the door a reasonable exchange for dishwashing from your perspective?" If so, an explicit agreement is reached. The exact nature of this agreement and possible exceptions are explored. Nonverbal noncompliance is precluded. For example, the therapist may say, "Meeting him at the door with a frown won't work" and "Doing a poor job on the dishes doesn't count." If one spouse, in this case the wife, complains that the other should do this without reciprocity because she already does so many other things, the therapist can preclude this argument by saying, "We're starting at base zero. We've agreed to try to work out a new relationship." In subsequent negotiations, the stakes can be gradually increased until behaviors related to core symbols can be negotiated. The trick in these interchanges is to assure an equality in the trade-offs and an equitable exchange of goods and services. The equity is internally perceived so each spouse is forced to state preferences more explicitly. The use of this procedure can quickly undercut a spouse's interpersonal tactic of passive compliance. As the sequence evolves, that spouse realizes that he or she is being boxed into an undesirable corner with increasingly specificity. The therapist attempts to preclude this by repeatedly seeking reassurance that each spouse feels that the exchange is fair. Exchanges of this sort become problematic when one spouse desires an attitudinal change in the other: "I want him to love me." "I want her to desire me." These problems can be circumvented by pointing out the impossibility of knowing whether this has occurred. The therapist can say, "Those issues are important, but let's stick with things we can see and agree on for the time being."

During these sequences, relatively minor exchanges of behavior are negotiated. Dynamic therapists may question the significance of such exercises. First, the importance of the transactions gradually escalates until spouses are negotiating compromises around issues of important individual symbolic value. Although the symbolism may never be made overt, the fact that something of symbolic value can be obtained from the spouse offers a preconscious (or unconscious) disproof of the spouse as somehow dangerous, evil, or uncaring. If the husband equates a clean house with a loving mother, his wife's housekeeping is a disproof of his perception of her as uncaring. The other importance of focusing on minor problems of communication and interactional problems around negotiation is to achieve a shift in the interactional sequences. The repetitive cycles of deadlocked behavior lock the system into a steady state and limit the range of interpersonal behavior in each of the spouses. By changing the interactional system, each spouse is forced to participate in sequences of behavior and emotions that are unknown and unpredictable. The uncertainty and unknowability contribute to the accommodation of new conceptual systems and schemas.

## Cognitive Relabeling

In the previous sections, we have focused mainly on the therapists's activities to change interpersonal behavior. The activities described so far are analogous to procedures described by behavioral marital therapists. However, if one assumes a reciprocal connection between behavior and cognitions, there is no reason for the therapist to limit his interventions to behavior alone. Therapists identified with general system theory (e.g., Haley, 1963; Lederer and Jackson, 1968) have detailed the manner in which cognitive relabeling of events can put an interactional system into disequilibrium. They have suggested that the therapist actively relabel events as being the polar opposite of how the couple describes them. The implicit assumption is that a cognitive shift will eventuate a behavioral change.

In disturbed couples, one will observe each spouse describing the other as if the other's personality is totally aversive and unchangeable.

Such a description contributes to the other spouse's behavior remaining unchanged. If the other spouse's personality is a fixed entity, the first spouse has no responsibility for the way the mate acts and no reason to expect change. Thus, the system remains in equilibrium and each spouse's belief system remains unchallenged. Over several therapy sessions, the therapist can introduce disequilibrium gradually with a sequence of planned interventions. His comments can gradually challenge the assumptive worlds of both spouses. For example, if a wife continually complains that her husband has no feelings, the therapist can gradually challenge this assumption. Initially, he might reply, "Yes, his family was less emotionally expressive than yours." Subsequently, he might agree that the husband is "a bit gruff." Later, the therapist might say, "Well, your husband has difficulty expressing his feelings." If the wife agrees with the therapist, he can ask, "How do you think that you could help him with that?" At this point, a terminal statement has been converted into an instrumental hypothesis (Hurvitz, 1975). A criticism about the spouse as a fixed entity has been changed into a statement of the husband as an interactional being for whom the wife bears partial responsibility. Similarly, if the husband complains that his wife is too dependent, the therapist can gradually redefine this as her desire for greater emotional intimacy. Eventually, this can lead to a situation where the husband is asked how he might meet his wife's desires. At this point, his wife has been converted from a needy person to someone desiring a healthy intimacy.

Cognitive relabeling occasionally borders on what dynamic therapists would consider interpretation. For example, numerous couples will deadlock in a battle, saying that they're so different that a resolution is impossible. Most often, the situation involves perceived rather than real differences. In such cases the therapist may want to emphasize their similarities. The similarity has to have a basis in fact or his comment will lack credibility and impact. For example, one may see an insecure couple, both of whom could be described as fearing being alone in the world without a partner. The wife may handle this by demanding reassurance of her lovability. The husband may handle the same situation by seeming aloofness. A comment as to their underlying similarity may break the cycle of recriminations.

Similarly, numerous pairs of artifically polarized positions can be broken be relabeling of events. For example, the "strong" husband may repeatedly discuss his desire to leave the marriage. The therapist notes that the husband has stated this desire for 5 years without acting on it. The wife responds by submissively trying to keep her husband interested in her and in the marriage. These sequences play into the definition of the husband as strong and independent and the wife as weak and dependent. Presumably, most humans have greater ambivalences about relationships than are expressed in this sequence. In such sequences, the therapist may begin to pursue one or the other partner for expression of these ambivalences, dislodging the fixated misperceptions. For example, he may question the "helpless dependent" wife about what she would do if her husband left, how long she would passively wait for his uncertain return, etc. Eventually, the wife will express certain conditions that define her stance regarding the situation. The therapist then labels these stances in a way that precludes the wife's later denying her statements. If the couple can be dislodged from this artificial polarization of positions, the real issues confronting the couple can be addressed and perhaps resolved.

## COMMENT

In this section, I have described certain nonspecific interventions for disturbed marriages. Analytically oriented therapists may have difficulty comprehending the significance of such simplistic surface interventions. In these simplistic interventions, the therapist is interrupting general classes of behavior that characterize disturbed interactional sequences. The advantage of these nonspecific interventions is threefold.

First, a focus on behavior alone is often an extremely powerful way to engage defensive couples in therapy. The therapist, after all, is only dealing with behavior. He may purposely avoid any discussion of the symbolic meaning of such behavior. For certain couples, this may be absolutely necessary. At an overt level, the therapy is simply focusing on changing faulty communication patterns and teaching negotiation skills. What couple who overtly say that they want a better relationship can object to such an intervention? Of course, the therapist realizes that he is changing the way the couple structures intimate interactions. In other words, the therapist engages the couple at an ego-syntonic level. By dealing with the conflict-free portion of the ego, he helps the couple change behavior mediated by conflictual portions of the ego.

Second, it is difficult for therapists who have not used these procedures to comprehend the power of these interventions for changing behavior. Couples who enter therapy attacking each other with unrelenting savageness and arguing incessantly over trivia can rapidly be shifted into different forms of interaction. At the beginning of therapy, the interaction is characterized by mutual recriminations. Each spouse feels that the other is responsible for his or her misery in life and that cooperation and compromise are impossible with the spouse because the spouse is insensitive, selfish, rigid, etc. The therapist insists that each spouse's viewpoint is legitimate and that the past is unimportant. He consistently converts attacks into requests for change and then mediates compromises. In the process of doing this, many of the trivial arguments with which disturbed couples fill their time are eliminated. Every conflict is converted into a potential negotiation rather than a chance to ventilate frustration.

Third, a systematic modification of communication patterns can have quite a significant impact. Rather than concluding that communication is impossible, the couple learns that it is possible for them to talk reasonably and to understand one another. The actual impact on changing behavior can be quite profound.

The therapist's insistence that he is only changing behavior is partially tongue in cheek. If one assumes that conflictual interaction is defensive (i.e., the required relationship), the therapist disarms the defense without ever interpreting the defense or anxiety. By removing the defense, he is shifting the couple into a new pattern of interaction (i.e., the avoided relationship.)

A couple of case vignettes may help to illustrate the process. The author saw an Egyptian doctor and his wife in brief marital therapy. This couple argued constantly, with innuendos about the other not filling appropriate sex roles. The wife felt that her husband was supposed to take care of her, and the doctor felt that the wife was supposed to run the family so that the man could pursue activities outside of the home. The actual fights seemed to center around the husband's repeatedly coming home late. When he arrived home, the house was a mess, the children were crying, and his wife appeared overwhelmed. The husband felt that his wife should be on antidepressants so that she could function. The wife wanted me to instruct her husband how to behave. The therapist's initial intervention was to assist the couple in negotiating a series of compromises to tone down the current interactional struggle. Upon inquiry, it was discovered that the husband could probably be home by six o'clock most days without compromising his professional duties. If a rare emergency arose, he or his nurse could notify his wife by telephone. In turn, the wife could make his arrival more pleasant, giving the husband a few minutes to unwind before dinner. During dinner, they both could assist in management of the children. After dinner, the husband could play with the children while the wife cleaned the kitchen. In return, the wife would clean the house before her husband's return. She also agreed not to meet her husband at the door with a litany of her day's struggles. In return, her husband would listen to her after the children were asleep. She also agreed to pay more attention to her physical appearance if her husband would assist with weekend shopping. This series of compromises modified the interactional climate so that collaborative discussion was possible. At this point, a more central issue surfaced. The husband's family disapproved of the marriage and the doctor had not taken a stand with his family. The constant bickering conveniently did not leave time to confront this more substantial issue.

The author saw an Israeli woman who was married to a Hungarian. Their marriage was characterized by continuous fighting. The most recent fight concerned an expected visit by the Hungarian mother-in-law. The Israeli wife was violently opposed to this visit and extremely angry at her husband. She continually spoke of how all Hungarians are mother's boys. Her husband would retaliate, saying Israeli women were cold, heartless bitches with no feelings. To interrupt this interactional impasse, the therapist asks the wife to discuss her feelings about the visit without attacking her husband. He suggests that it might help things if she began her sentence with "I." She begins, "I think he's a mother's boy." The therapist prompts her again to discuss her own feelings without attacking her husband. With a series of prompts, the woman first expresses her extreme anger. Later, the anger is clarified as jealousy. Subsequently, she discusses how she feels left out when the mother-in-law visits. At this point, the therapist asks the wife what she wants from her husband so that she won't feel left out. The husband, no longer being the target of attack, is more willing to compromise. In this way, the couple is able to arrange for the visit in a way at least partially satisfactory to both spouses.

### Specific Interventions

As outlined in the conceptual overview section, nonspecific modifications of interaction are augmented by more specific interventions to disrupt behavioral sequences that partially confirm inner representational reality. In most cases, nonspecific interventions and specific interventions will overlap to a considerable degree. For example, in communication training one modifies the way spouses communicate their wishes to one another. A husband may view his wife as powerful and intractable. The husband accordingly gives his wife commands instead of seeking cooperation. His wife understandably refuses to follow orders. During communication training, the husband would be instructed in alternative ways of expressing his wishes to his wife. These alternative ways of expressing his wishes to her would of course elicit different forms of behavior from her. With the change in his behavior, the self-confirming cycle will be broken. One can further interrupt this cycle by having the wife instruct her husband as to the best approach to elicit her cooperation. Similarly, the therapist can instruct the wife to cue her husband when he resorts to his old way of ordering her. She can be encouraged to remind her husband that by persisting, he won't get what he wants and will provide evidence that she is intractable. The wife could even be asked to go along with her husband whether she wants to or not if he expresses himself differently.

## End Stage

At this point in therapy, the therapist has been successful in modifying communication patterns such that each spouse is receiving information discrepent with each one's sterotyped perceptions of the other. Similarly, each spouse has learned how to compromise so that some desires are satisfied by the mate. The satisfaction of at least some desires means that each spouse is not justified in seeing the mate as completly negative. At this point, the therapy is finally set for a discrimination between inner and external reality. The observed behavior from the spouse if perceived in a broader context, rather than in a restricted, sterotyped manner, and thus the range of the spouse's behavior has accordingly broadened. It is assumed that the misperceptions of the spouse's intentions and personality were one reason why compromise was impossible in the past and obfuscating communication was used.

The major concerns of the therapist in this phase of the therapy are (1) focused discrimination of the differences between inner and external reality, (2) prevention and identification of interpersonal behavior that tends to return the interactional system to its previous maladaptive state and, (3) preparation for termination.

To my knowledge, Greenspan and Mannino (1974) are the only authors who have discussed the technique of forced discrimination training in marital therapy. Working from a Kleinian framework, they suggested that projective identification could be disrupted either by interpreting the hypothetical denied inner feeling or by the therapist repeatedly pointing out how the spouse differed from the projected image. For example, if an overtly healthy spouse repeatedly described the mate as weak and unstable, the therapist would comment on the real hidden strengths of the supposedly weak mate, disrupting the collusion necessary for the system to remain in equilibrium. Working from different theoretical frameworks, therapists identified as general systems therapists (e.g., Haley, 1963) and even behavioral marital therapists (e.g., Liberman, 1975) have suggested similar therapeutic interventions.

Once the interactional difficulties have been sufficiently moderated, the therapist will hear the spouses describe one another in ways that are unlike their current behavior. The descriptions will be the same character descriptions of each other with which the couple entered therapy. At this point, however, the therapist has modified the interaction that confirms these perceptions. He will begin to observe one or both spouses speaking of the other in a manner blatantly discrepant with the other spouse's behavior. At this point in marital therapy, the process is analogous to events in individual psychoanalytically oriented psychotherapy. One observes transference distortions in almost a pure form. The difference, of course, is that the transference is directed toward the mate and may be bilateral.

The goal of the therapist is to begin gently but repetitively to point out the dissimilarities between the mate's actual current behavior and the other spouse's description (schema) of that mate. For example, if a wife continually describes her husband as emotionless, the therapist can comment, "You continually say that your husband has no feelings. Yet you saw tears in his eyes last week when you talked about your sister's death. Your perception can't be completely accurate." Similarly, if a husband describes his wife as dependent and helpless, the therapist can help the husband observe parts of his wife's personality that he has overlooked. The therapist might comment, "You describe your wife as helpless and dependent. But a few minutes ago, she described how she could cope without you. In fact, she's just enrolled in a highly competitive graduate program after being out of school for a long time. You yourself remarked last week what a good job she is doing. Something doesn't quite fit."

The most potent discrimination occurs when one spouse is describing some aspect of the mate with some emotional intensity and can be led into observing current behavior of the spouse that is discrepant with that description. For example, a wife may complain, on the verge of tears, that her husband doesn't care for her. At the same time, the husband may be leaning toward his wife with outstretched arms and a painful facial expression. At this point, the therapist wants the wife to look at her husband and to listen as he describes his feelings for her. The fact of the couple's maintaining eye contact during this interaction is more crucial than any comment by the therapist. The facial expression of the spouse provides the credibility and emotional impact. Without eye contact, it is too easy for the spouse to dismiss the discrepant information as false.

Events like the one described above require a degree of orchestration by the therapist. The therapist clearly has to be accurate in perceiving the emotional state of each marital partner. In the example above, the therapist judged that the wife was emotionally prepared to cope with discrepant information and could assimilate it without extreme anxiety. A premature attempt at a discrimination of this sort might have adverse effects. The wife might have become so anxious that weeks would be required before similar interventions could be reattempted. A premature effort would have made her less receptive to new information. The process is analogous to a premature interpretation of an underlying feeling without first interpreting the anxiety and defense in individual psychotherapy. If the therapist was grossly inaccurate in his perception of the wife's readiness for this perceptual discrimination, the outcome could have been disastrous. The wife could have an affair, begin divorce action, or precipitously withdraw from therapy. The difference between conjoint and individual therapy is that the therapist must also perceive the emotional readiness of the partner. In this example, the therapist correctly perceived the husband to feel warmly toward his spouse in spite of her protestations to the contrary. If the therapist had been mistaken in this regard, and the wife had turned to the husband to receive a bitter attack from him, this would have reinforced her original feeling. In other words, the therapist utilizes his skill to perceive the emotional state of each partner and to gradually shift these states toward a specific time in therapy when such an intervention can be made. Certain dynamic therapists may feel that the therapist is manipulating the couple. In actual fact, the therapist is judging his timing for an intervention in the same way as an individual therapist. In both cases, there is an artistry involved.

During the focused discrimination between the spouse's observable behavior and the habitual way of perceiving that spouse, some patients become increasingly unsettled. Initially they may appear confused and disoriented, as if experiencing information overload. The therapist attempts to lessen anxiety by commenting, "Sometimes, when you're used to seeing someone one way, it's difficult to realize that you've overlooked part of them. It takes some time to refocus." In many cases, the spouse continues to become increasingly anxious as the forced discrimination continues. If the therapist gently encourages the patient to discuss his feelings at that point, a description of rage and/or disappointment at the opposite-sex parent may follow. The similarity between the misperception of the mate and the description of the parent may be striking. The therapist may then honestly discuss the real similarities and dissimilarities between the mate and the remembered parent. He comments that learning about the opposite sex obviously began with the parents. "So thinking that all men are that way was a natural conclusion. After all, your husband is similar in some ways to your father. What you've overlooked are the ways he's different. Many of these ways are qualities you desired but didn't have in your father."

Concurrent with the discrimination training outlines above, another process emerges. As the disturbed interaction has been modified and the discrepancies between the perception of the mate and the mate's behavior are repeatedly pinpointed, the therapist can almost feel the tension in the system rise. Then the therapist will note behavioral sequences that almost seem motivated to return the interaction to its previous dysfunctional state. One spouse will make an unprovoked and unnecessarily provocative statement, almost as if hoping to engage the other in battle. At this point, the therapist has to invervene quickly, labeling the provocative behavior and the probable spouse response. The therapist reminds the provoker that he or she is aware of the probable consequence of a counterattack. He also reminds the attacked spouse of an alternative strategy other than counterattack: "When he attacks you in that way, it's reasonable to assume that he feels threatened in some way. If you argue back, you prevent him from realizing what is going on inside him and go along with the fight. An alternative response might be to inquire what is going on." The explicit labeling of the interpersonal sequence in the presence of both spouses means it is less likely to work in the future. For it to work, both spouses have to collaborate knowingly. The therapist reminds the provoker that he can simply say that he feels tense or angry rather than attacking his spouse.

Clearly, this labeling and defusing of interpersonal sequences has to be repeated numerous times. Once one attempt is defeated, some couples then develop increasingly devious and subtle ways to provoke one another. The therapist remains vigilant and interrupts each sequence. Eventually, the spouses are forced to endure the discomfort of relative tranquility, as all attempts to return to a previous way of relating are blocked. Throughout these sequences, the therapist continually points out how assumptions about the spouse differ from observable reality.

Behavioral therapists might refer to the behavioral sequences described above as final extinction trials for maladaptive behavior. The degree of tension in the partners and the seemingly highly ingenious ways in which couples work to avoid intimacy suggest that a more complex explanation is needed. Psychodynamically oriented therapists would probably explain these sequences as an expression of neurotic needs in both spouses. Although the psychodynamic explanation is plausible, I tend to view this phenomenon as simply a fear of the unknown. The spouses know what to expect in the old way of relating. The new way of relating is unclear. Its dangers are unknown. In people for whom life has been full of dangers and disappointments, the unknown is understandably perceived as dangerous rather than exciting.

When the new equilibrium has been maintained for several weeks, the therapist begins to think of termination. Prior to termination, the therapist helps the couple to summarize what they have learned in therapy. In particular, he is concerned that they are aware of their perceptual biases and how their misinterpretations inadvertently set up confirmatory life experiences. In particular, he reminds the couple of tactics they can employ on their own to prevent or escape from relapses.

Termination differs from individual psychotherapy in that feelings toward the therapist are less central. Most couples, of course, feel gratitude and express fear that they will not be able to maintain their gains. Feelings toward the therapist are less central than in individual therapy, as the primary emotional interaction has been between the spouses.

## COMMENT

My approach in the preceding section differs from what I know of other theoretical approaches. Family therapists are probably aghast that I did not involve the family of origin and try to work out a different relationship with the parents. Dynamic therapists will be upset by this superficial handling of the transference situation. Behavior therapists, if they've continued reading this far, are probably disillusioned, feeling that the model has again returned to the mentalism of psychoanalysis. I will attempt to explain briefly the purpose of my limited intervention. The goal of this therapy is to promote current adaptation in heterosexual pairing. A breakdown in this process appears related to considerable psychological misery. A better relationship with the family of origin may be a useful goal in and of itself, but this therapy is concerned solely with current relationships in the nuclear family. The subtleties of the transference were not pursued. For this therapy, I am only concerned with the past to the extent that it influences the present relationship with the spouse. If the major obstacles of this relationship can be overcome, minor adjustments can occur through the process of living.

## CLINICAL WISDOM

In the preceding sections of this chapter, the implementation of a combined behavioral and cognitive therapy of marital discord was outlined. These sections were concerned with the descriptions of procedures related to the author's theoretical model. In any therapy, factors unrelated to theoretical systems play an important role. The difficulty of documenting the differential impact of differing psychological interventions in individual psychotherapy outcome research partially attests to the importance of these nonspecific factors. In clinical practice, psychotherapists develop a set of reflexes or ways of conceptualizing and handling frequently occurring problems. The therapist's clinical wisdom in this regard is atheoretical and, unfortunately, often unrecorded. In this section, I will attempt to detail as much as possible some of the clinical wisdom involved in marital therapy.

## The Word "Love"

A common theme in many disturbed marriages is the question of whether one spouse is really loved by the other. In many ways, the behavioral techniques to facilitate positive exchanges between spouses is an indirect way of answering this question in the affirmative. If the spouses begin receiving what they want from one another, they are likely to conclude at some level of awareness that each one cares for the other. Later in therapy this topic will probably be discussed explicitly.

When the question of being loved surfaces early in therapy, it can present a difficult therapeutic situation. Part of the difficulty is that *love* is an intensely charged word and has so many idiosyncratic meanings. For some it means: "If you love me, you'll do what I want." In other cases, the question of love appears to be a ploy to interrupt therapy: "I just can't go on with therapy unless I know that he loves me." This comment may be interjected in the middle of a bitter exchange. In these situations, few spouses genuinely feel love at that specific moment. The other spouse might look away in silent anger or say, "I love you," in a voice tone that portrays his real feelings. The first spouse then begins crying, saying, "I knew it. He doesn't love me."

Interactions like this lead rapidly to a stalemate. I tend to try to avoid these situations by substituting the word *care* for *love*. Most spouses, regardless of the intensity of the battle, will acknowledge caring for the other. Sometimes, the minor semantic distinction permits therapy to proceed.

In the previous example, the therapist might intervene, saying, "It's clear that he cares for you. He's struggling as hard as you are to try to change things." In this situation, the therapist substitutes a compromise word in their power struggle. Clearly, the issue isn't resolved. At this point in therapy, it's probably unresolvable. At least, this intervention shifts the therapy away from this topic.

*Chair Placement*

Typically, the therapist is concerned with facilitating the spouses' interaction with one another and discouraging their always talking to the therapist rather than to each other. I attempt to facilitate this by placing chairs in a peculiar lopsided triangular fashion, with the spouses' chairs angled so that their line of vision overlaps and the therapist is slightly out of direct focus.

*Maintaining a Current Focus*

Clearly, this is a rule that has to be judiciously broken. Maintaining a current focus is important, as the main concern of the therapist is to help the couple work out a satisfactory current relationship. The technique can also help to avoid common pitfalls in couple therapy. Couples can use the past as a resistance to working out the current relationship. One common difficulty is for spouses to compete for the title of who has suffered the most injustices at the other's hands. Another common problem is each spouse's searching in the past for further evidence to document his or her diagnosis of the other's personality problem. These diversions into the past are seldom helpful. In particular, it may be advisable to maintain a current focus in the early stages of therapy.

In later stages of therapy, when a sense of trust and cooperativeness has been established, consideration of the past as it relates to current functioning may be appropriate.

*Eye Contact*

On many occasions, one spouse will continually describe the other in a manner grossly discrepant with observable reality. Actual observable data can be far more effective in dislodging these fixated misperceptions than a therapist's comment. For example, one spouse can describe the other as insensitive and unfeeling while looking at the therapist. During this same time interval, the other spouse's face may be contorted with psychological pain. The direct observation of this is of crucial importance. This is one reason for the chair placement and the therapist's continual redirection of conversation between the spouses. I often request or instruct spouses to maintain eye contact while expressing their opinions. On occasion, one spouse may look genuinely puzzled, as the verbal description of the mate is currently discrepant with the actual observation of the mate.

*Breaking out of True Impasses*

Regardless of the therapist's skill, eventually many couples will lapse into silent withdrawl. At this point, the therapist makes a strategic decision. He can either remain silent or intervene. In individual psychotherapy, the therapist's nonintervention during periods of silence often has a beneficial impact. This is seldom true in couple therapy. If the therapist remains silent, the couple's rage and hopelessness may escalate to unmanageable levels. An intervention that is often useful is for the therapist to talk about each spouse's pain and loneliness. He may refer to the joy and expectations in their early marriage, as contrasted with the current situation. If this is continued, eventually one spouse will make a miniscule attempt at reconciliation. The attempt may or may not be noticed by the other spouse and is usually ignored or rebuffed. At this precise moment, the therapist labels and makes explicit the first spouse's attempt at reconciliation, emphasizing the desire for reconciliation. In a few moments, the second spouse will make a miniscule attempt at reconciliation, which is rebuffed by the first spouse this time. Again, the therapist makes the transaction explicit. He may turn to the first spouse and ask why he or she didn't respond. Eventually, a sequence such as this will draw the couple out.

*Physical Metaphors*

On occasion, couples become deadlocked in a power struggle around issues that are clearly symbolic of more than the issue being argued. A common example of this is the husband who desires greater sexual frequency and the wife who refuses. It is seldom possible to negotiate a satisfactory compromise on an issue so emotionally charged. A careful exploration and relabeling of the issue can often help. If the therapist is a male, he may talk of the pain associated with sexual rejection. Later, he may talk of sexual responsiveness in the partner reassuring one of one's attractiveness. Eventually, he may help the husband verbalize that his desire for sex is also partially a desire for physical intimacy. In this sequence, a demand for physical release can be shifted to a desire for emotional closeness. At this point, both partners are verbalizing a similar desire, although achieved by different means. Once the couple approaches this realization, the therapist can shift the couple to trying to work out a way to achieve each of their wishes jointly. In this process, the therapist carefully titrates the balance between the interpersonal desire and its metaphoric expression. The choice of the husband or wife for this attempted retranslation is mainly dependent on the therapist's judgment about who is more likely to shift positions. It is my impression that many husbands are unskilled in speaking in interpersonal terms. For that reason, I tend more often to attempt to convert male metaphors into interpersonal language.

## Indirect Putdowns

This refers to the management of anger in interpersonal systems. Because of the action–reaction nature of intimate relationships, the management of anger can become a crucial variable. Pain directed at a spouse frequently results in equal pain redirected at the self. This point has been aptly described by numerous marital therapists (e.g., Haley, 1963; Patterson and Hops, 1972). A particularly destructive sequence is for one spouse to attack the other indirectly. For example, a husband who knows that his wife is self-conscious about being overweight may begin talking about how slim and attractive a friend's wife is. The wife feels hurt, and knowing that her husband is self-conscious about his masculinity, begins talking about a girl friend whose husband makes love four times a week. In this sequence, the real issues are never addressed directly, thus resolution is precluded. The effect is experienced by the second spouse, who responds in kind, and an escalation occurs.

The therapist can help to prevent these sequences by immediately labeling such events. For example, he might say to the wife, "You sounded irritated by your husband's comment just then. Why don't you tell him how his comment made you feel rather than counterattack?" Alternatively, he might turn to the husband and inquire, "What were you irritated about just then when you talked about your friend's wife? Do you want your wife to diet?"

Once the irritation is expressed, the therapist can coach the couple in alternative ways of expressing anger. Satir (1967) and others (Gottman *et al.*, 1976) have described ways of expressing feelings in a manner more conducive to resolution. The expression of feelings in the form "I feel A in situation B when you do C has certain advantages. The second spouse's total character is not under attack, and he is offered information that may lead to a resolution. The conversational topic is shifted to the problem to be solved rather than involving the character structure of the participants.

## Speaking for Self

This simple device has been advocated by numerous marital therapists (Satir, 1967; Sluzki, 1978) and incorporated into many sex therapy programs (Segraves, 1976). Basically, one requests that each spouse begin sentences with the pronoun "I." This simple device can greatly facilitate resolution of conflict. It aids the therapist in getting the spouses to explore and express their own feelings rather than project these feelings onto the spouse in the form of an attack.

In certain cases, it can render distortions of perception, bordering on what some therapists would label as projective identification, impossible to maintain. For example, in a previously mentioned case, an Israeli woman, married to a Hungarian man, was violently opposed to an impending visit by her Hungarian mother-in-law. She felt that her husband was too dependent on his mother. She began the conversation, "He's a mother's boy. All Hungarians are mother's boys." The husband responded, "You have no feelings. Israeli women are bloodless. . . . " At this point, the therapist has to intervene. He turns to the wife. "Could you describe how you feel about her visit? Try to start the sentence with "I." She responds, "I think all Hungarians are mother's boys." The therapist tries again, "How do you feel? Start the sentence with "I." She responds, "I feel he's a mother's boy." The therapist comments, "That's a little better. Focus on the expression of your feelings.' She responds, "Well, I feel goddamn angry." The therapist replies, "Good. Tell me more about *your* feeling angry." With coaching and prompting and signals to the husband to remain silent momentarily, she eventually speaks of how she feels angry and left out when her husband feels closer to his mother than to her. She describes her lifelong anger at always feeling lonely and left out. At this point, her thinly veiled desire to be dependent and loved is obvious to her husband. He begins to talk of ways to structure his mother's visit so he and his wife will have time to be together.

### Perceived Equality of Power

It would appear that for marriages to work or for discord to abate, there has to be a perceived equality of power. Each spouse needs to feel that his or her wishes have a roughly equal chance of being fulfilled as the other spouse's. This equality can occur in traditional marriages or in contemporary marriages where both spouses work. The equality is not at an objective level. The equality is at a perceived level. It refers mainly to the level of compromise between wishes such that both spouses' subjective worlds are appreciated to an equal extent.

If the therapist assumes that the equality has to occur at an objective level, he will be introducing his value system into the marriage. This may have unfortunate consequences.

*Converting Criticism into Requests for Change*

Numerous therapists have noted the destructive effects of criticism of the spouse. Criticism usually begets criticism. Behavioral marital therapists have spoken of the destructive influence of negative reciprocity in disturbed marriages (Birchler *et al*, 1975), and systems theorists have posited that angry exchanges serve the function of stabilizing the dysfunctional system (Lederer and Jackson, 1978). Psychoanalytically oriented therapists have speculated that criticism of the mate serves to stabilize the other spouse's behavior such that anxiety is not provoked in the first spouse (Brody, 1961). From my perspective, spouse criticism stabilizes the system such that new information about the spouse is not processed.

One way to shift the interactional sequences into a new direction is for the therapist to first rephrase the comment slightly. Later, he can coach the patient in a different form of expression. For example, one spouse may say, "She never listens to me." The therapist can ask, "Are you saying that you would appreciate her listening to you? Maybe this is something the two of you can work out." This converts a negative statement of unchangeable reality into a direct request for change.

*The Strength of the Weak Partner*

In many cases of marital discord, one will observe couples, one of which appears strong and the other weak. One may complain that he or she can't survive without the other, etc. If one watches the actual interaction sequences, most often one will observe the power of the weak partner. The "weak" partner can be observed "using" that weakness to manipulate the other spouse. In many cases, the weak partner will be observed to survive a separation or divorce with much less suffering than the strong partner. Once the therapist realizes the paradoxical nature of "weakness" in marital systems, he can move to redefine the weak partner as strong and to point out the hidden strengths. This serves to change the interactional system, to change that spouse's self-perception, and to change the other spouse's perception of his or her mate.

*The Plasticity of Response Capabilities*

Numerous analytic therapists have noted the peculiar contrasting personalities often observed in marital partners. Individual therapists, who think of personality as more fixed, tend to explain this as the result of mate selection. Family and marital therapists tend to think of this phenomenon differently. All too often, the roles appear to switch. General systems theorists explain this as the system restoring equilibrium. Object-relations theorists refer to this as projective identification. According to this model, as the collusion is broken the couple is forced to recognize previously denied portions of their own personalities.

Whatever explanation is preferred, one observes peculiar polarization of personalities in marital partners. These personality characteristics should not be regarded as enduring and fixed. If the interactional system shifts, the seeming personalities of the spouses often change rather dramatically. This observation frees the clinician to more actively seek behavior change.

### The Unchangeable Agent of Change

In most disturbed couples, each spouse has decided that it is impossible to obtain what he or she wants from the other spouse. This conclusion is usually true as long as each spouse persists in his or her usual manner of attempting to obtain these things. The inflexibility in the system is most often traceable to the rigidity in the spouse desiring change rather than the spouse targeted for change. The husband wants his wife to be more sexually responsive, yet he refuses to consistently do the things that makes his wife more responsive. Because of these failures, the spouses settle into an uneasy truce, marred by occasional indirect attacks on each other. In situations such as this, the therapist might point out to the husband that this is a mock protest. The husband knows how to get his wife to respond sexually, yet he refuses to do so.

### Ambivalence in Intimate Relationships

It is quite common to observe couples in which one spouse seemingly strongly desires one thing and the other spouse seemingly is strongly opposed. If the therapist can move either spouse from his entrenched position, the other spouse will frequently change his position as well. In such cases, the therapist is usually safe in assuming that both spouses are ambivalent about the topic at hand and that the power struggle precludes their realizing that. This orientation can be useful to the therapist.

For example, one spouse seemingly wants an open marriage and the other spouse is violently opposed. The therapist is aware that this argument has gone on for years and that both spouses have been faithful to the marriage vows. The therapist can usually dislodge the seeming impasse by exaggerating the ambivalence. For example, if the husband desires an open marriage, the therapist may question the husband about whom he would have sex with and get him to pursue his fantasies. As the husband's anxiety becomes obvious, the therapist can wonder if the husband ever had sexual problems with other women or whom his wife would go to bed with. He can get the husband to pursue those fantasies. Gradually, the husband may decide against an open marriage, saying that it wouldn't be fair to his wife. At about this time, the wife may reconsider her position, wondering what it would be like to have sex with another man. In some couples, the therapist can watch the roles reverse before his eyes. The variations in themes around which couples can polarize are limitless. With a touch of controlled sadism, the therapist can usually expose the hidden ambivalences. Once the ambivalences are exposed and acknowledged, the couple is free to work to a solution. In the case of the couple above, they were then free to discuss their mutual dissatisfaction with the boredom and monotony of their sex life. An open marriage is, of course, only one of numerous possible solutions to the problem.

## COMMENTS

The more dynamically oriented clinician may be disturbed by some of the clinical procedures described in this text. In particular, he may be unnerved by the degree of control that the therapist assumes and the conscious manipulation of interpersonal sequences. This issue is worth discussing briefly. If one treats severely disturbed marriages, a direct manipulation of interactional sequences is an absolute necessity. The use of interpretations is powerless when the behavioral events contradict what the therapist is saying. In severely disturbed marriages, so much of the interaction is an ephiphenomenon of interaction that it is virtually impossible to decipher the underlying difficulties. It is absolutely necessary to restore order in the system before one can decipher what is distortion, what is provoked behavior, and what is the usual personality.

The predominantly individual psychotherapy is used to observe a seemingly greater consistency in individual personality. Of course, the individual therapist, because of his training, remains predominantly a constant entity. The emotions evoked in the therapist are referred to as countertransference. The therapist uses his emotional reactions as information to better understand the patient. In marriage the spouse responds to the evoked feelings. These powerful forces then evolve into an interactional system. To even decipher the "real" spouses' personalities, it is necessary to restore the system to an equilibrium. The conscious manipulation of the therapist is toward that goal. Once the interaction is under control, the therapist can more clearly observe phenomena resembling those of individual dynamic therapy. Then one can observe "transference" distortions that don't match the spouse's current behavior. In my opinion, many of the same events that occur in individual therapy recur in marital therapy. The peculiarities of marital systems often allow the therapist to have an impact in a much briefer time span.

To recapitulate briefly, the model recommends a combined behavioral-cognitive approach to the treatment of marital discord. The first thrust of therapy is to change the maladaptive behavior sequences. These sequences are often remarkably similar from couple to couple and seem to be a nonspecific sign of disturbed marriages. It is necessary to interrupt these sequences before cognitive relearning can occur. This cognitive relearning is felt to be necessary for the effects of therapy to be permanent.

## DIFFERING NEEDS OF RESEARCHERS AND CLINICIANS

This text is written for the empirically oriented clinician. I have attempted to outline a treatment model that is clinically useful and still anchored to publicly verifiable hypotheses. Although practicing clinicians and clinical researchers have the same overall goal—the provision of maximally effective services to the emotionally distraught—researchers and practitioners unfortunately, often have minimal influence on one another (Strupp, 1978). Each group has different concerns and differing, equally legitimate, standards of evaluation. The clinician is concerned whether the theoretical model is useful in organizing clinical data into a useful plan of action. The clinician relies on data that are subtle, illusive, and difficult to quantify. This is of little concern to the clinician if he is able to organize these data and use them effectively in his clinical practice. The researcher is concerned with the public verifiability of hypotheses and procedures, believing that genuine progress occurs by the slow accumulation of well-established facts. Such an approach compensates for the tendency of the clinician to overgeneralize principles from small numbers of cases or from biased individual perceptions (Rutter, 1971). On the other hand, the practitioner often feels that much of psychotherapy's research is irrelevant to clinical practice (Olson, 1975). For clinical theory to be useful, its basic hypotheses need to be easily relatable to clinical application. Psychoanalytic theory, with its obvious methodological flaws (Eysenck and Rachman, 1965; Maddi, 1976), has survived because practicing clinicians have found some of its tenets to be useful in the clinical context.

The need to operationalize clinical procedures is now apparent to most psychotherapy theoreticians. This need became apparent after Eysenck's (1952) article questioning the evidence supporting the efficacy of psychotherapy. Although his article has subsequently been criticized on methodological grounds (Meltzoff and Kornreich, 1970; Bergin and Lambert, 1978), it served as an impetus for a renewed interest in psychotherapy outcome research. One product of this area of interest was the realization that comparative psychotherapy research requires a specification of procedures. It is impossible to compare the relative usefulness of a given approach to psychotherapy unless one can define the operations constituting that intervention. In more recent literature, the treatment of depression has rekindled an effort to specify psychotherapeutic procedures. The concern with comparing the relative efficacy of psychotherapy and pharmacotherapy has led to the preparation of psychotherapy manuals (Beck *et al.*, 1979; Klerman and Neu, 1977). This approach at first glance appears to be an excellent way to bridge the concerns of the clinician and the researcher.

While recognizing the importance of explicitly formulating psychotherapeutic procedures, it is also important to point out the pitfalls of such approaches. A treatment manual or the description of a treatment module can lead to a false sense of security. Such recipes overlook variables of considerable significance. For example, behavioral therapists are beginning to rediscover the importance of the patient–therapist alliance (Goldstein, 1973; Parloff *et al.*, 1978). A more important flaw in the therapy manual approach is the assumption that a set of procedures is applicable to all patients with a given syndrome. The skilled clinician quickly learns that it is more effective to flexibly modify the treatment module than to attempt to make the patient fit the module (Lobitz and Lobitz, 1978; Kaplan, 1974). Similarly, many psychotherapy researchers realize that technique variables are difficult to separate from the person of the therapist (Strupp, 1978).

What I am trying to say in this section is that at the point of making a given intervention for a particular patient in a given therapist–patient context, the value systems of the researcher and the clinician reach an impasse. Although attempts to bridge this chasm by the preparation of therapy manuals are important thrusts in the right direction, in my opinion they are premature. In this chapter I described a set of therapeutic principles and the interventions associated with those principles. Although the principles will hold across numerous cases of marital discord, their actual implementation will vary from couple to couple, depending on nuances of presentation and timing within the therapeutic context that are currently beyond precise definition. The need for accountability and public verification of the current model is based on the level of central hypotheses rather than on the level of clinical application.

## REFERENCES

Beck, A. J., Rush, A. J., Shaw, B. F., and Emery G. *Cognitive therapy of depression.* New York: Guilford Press, 1979.

Bergin, A. E., and Lambert, M. J. The evaluation of therapeutic outcome. In S. L. Garfield and A. E. Bergin (Eds.), *Handbook of psychotherapy and behavior change: An empirical analysis.* New York: Wiley, 1978.

Birchler, G. R., Weiss, R. L., and Vincent, J. P. A multimethod analysis of social reinforcement exchange between maritally distressed and non-distressed spouse and stranger dyads. *Journal of Personality and Social Psychology,* 1975, *31,*349–360.

Bowlby, J. The making and breaking of affectional bonds. *British Journal of Psychiatry,* 1977, *130,* 201–210.

Brody, S. Simultaneous psychotherapy of married couples: Preliminary observations. *Psychoanalytic Review,* 1961, *48,* 94–107.

Brown, G. W., Bhrolchain, M. N., and Harris, T. Social class and psychiatric disturbance among women in an urban population. *Sociology,* 1975, *9,* 225–233.

Burke, R. J., and Weir, T. Marital helping relationships: The moderators between stress and well-being. *Journal of Psychology,* 1977, *95,* 121–130.

Butcher, J. N., and Koss, M. P. Research on brief and crisis-oriented psychotherapies. In S. L. Garfield and A. E. Bergin (Eds.), *Handbook of psychotherapy and behavior change: An empirical analysis.* New York: Wiley, 1978.

Eysenck, H. J. The effects of psychotherapy: an evaluation. *Journal of Consulting Psychology,* 1952, *16,* 319–324.

Eysenck, H. J. The effects of psychotherapy: An evaluation. *Journal of Consulting and Clinical Psychology,* 1976, *16,* 319–324.

Eysenck, H. J., and Rachman, S. The causes and cures of neurosis. San Diego, California: R. R. Knapp, 1965.

Fitzgerald, R. V. *Conjoint marital therapy.* New York: Jason Aronson, 1973.

Ford, D. H., and Urban, H. B. *Systems of psychotherapy.* New York: Wiley, 1967.

Frank, J. D. *Persuasion and healing: A comparative study of psychotherapy.* Baltimore: Johns Hopkins University Press, 1973.

Giovacchini, P. L. Treatment of marital disharmonies: The classical approach. In B. Greene (Ed.), *The psychotherapies of marital disharmony.* New York: Free Press, 1965.

Goldstein, A. P. *Structured learning therapy.* New York: Pergamon, 1973.

Gottman, J., Notarius, C., Gonso, J., and Markman, H. *A couple's guide to communication.* Champaign, Ill.: Research Press, 1976.

Greenspan, S. I., and Mannino, F. V. A model for brief interventions with couples based on projective identification. *American Journal of Psychiatry,* 1974, *131,* 1103–1106.

Haley, J. Marriage therapy. *Archives of General Psychiatry,* 1963, *8,* 213–234.

Hurvitz, N. Interaction hypotheses in marriage counseling. In A. S. Gurman and D. G. Rice (Eds.), *Couples in conflict.* New York: Jason Aronson, 1975.

Jacobson, N. J., and Margolin, G. *Marital therapy*. New York: Brunner/Mazel, 1979.

Kaplan, H. S. *The new sex therapy*. New York: Brunner/Mazel, 1974.

Klerman, G. L., and Neu, C. Manual for short-term interpersonal psychotherapy for depression. Boston New Haven Collaborative Depression Project. Unpublished, February 1977.

Lederer, W. J., and Jackson, D. D. *The mirages of marriage*. New York: W. W. Norton, 1978.

Liberman, R. Behavioral principles in family and couple therapy. In A. S. Gurman and D. G. Rice (Eds.) *Couples in Conflict*. New York: Jason Aronson, 1975.

Liberman, R. P., Wheeler, E. G., deVisser, L. A. J. M., Kuehnel, J., and Kuehner, T. *Handbook of marital therapy*. New York: Plenum, 1980.

Lobitz, W. C., and Lobitz, G. K. Clinical assessment in the treatment of sexual dysfunction. In J. Lopiccolo and L. Lopiccolo (Eds.), *Handbook of sex therapy*. New York: Plenum, 1978.

Lassheimer, P. The diagnosis of marital conflicts. *American Journal of Psychoanalysis*, 1966, *26*, 127–146.

Maddi, S. R. *Personality theories: A comparative analysis*. Homewood, Ill.: Dorsey Press, 1976.

Malan, D. H. *The frontier of brief psychotherapy*. New York: Plenum, 1976.

Mann, J. *Time-limited psychotherapy*. Cambridge, Mass.: Harvard University Press, 1973.

Martin, P. A. *A marital therapy manual*. New York: Brunner/Mazel, 1975.

Meissner, W. N., and Nicholi, A. M. The Psychotherapies: Individual and Family Group. In A. M. Nicholi (Ed.) *The Harvard Guide to Modern Psychiatry*, Cambridge: Harvard University Press, 1978.

Meltzoff, J., and Kornreich, M. *Research in psychotherapy*. New York: Atherton Press, 1970.

Minuchin, S. *Families and family therapy*. Cambridge, Mass.: Harvard University Press, 1974.

Mittelmann, B. Complementary neurotic reactions in intimate relationships. *Psychoanalytic Quarterly*, 1944, *18*, 479–491.

Offenkrantz, W., and Tobin, A. Psychoanalytic psychotherapy. In D. X. Freedman and J. E. Dyrud (Eds.), *American handbook of psychiatry*, Vol. 5: *Treatment*. New York: Basic Books, 1975.

Olson, D. H. Marital and family therapy: A critical overview. In A. S. Gurman and D. G. Rice (Eds.), *Couples in conflict*. New York: Jason Aronson, 1975.

Parloff, M. B., Waskow, I. E., and Wolfe, B. E. Research on therapist variables in relation to process and outcome. In S. L. Garfield and A. E. Bergin (Eds.) *Handbook of Psychotherapy and Behavior Change: An Empirical Analysis* New York: Wiley, 1978.

Patterson, G. R., and Hops H. Coercion, a game for two: Intervention techniques for marital conflict. In R. E. Ulrich and P. J. Mountjoy (Eds.), *The experimental analysis of social behavior*. New York: Appleton-Century-Crofts, 1972.

Rutter, M. Parent–child separation: Psychological effects on children. *Journal of Child Psychology and Psychiatry*, 1971, *12*, 233–260.

Sager, C. J. Transference in conjoint treatment of married couples. *Archives of General Psychiatry*, 1967, *16*, 185–193.

Satir, V. Conjoint marital therapy. Palo Alto: Science and Behavior Books, 1967.

Segraves, R. T., Primary orgasmic dysfunction: essential treatment components. *Journal of Sex and Marital Therapy*, 1976, *2*, 115–123.

Sluzki, G. E. Marital therapy from a systems theory perspective. In T. J. Paolino and B. S. McCrady (Eds.), *Marriage and marital therapy*. New York: Brunner/Mazel, 1978.

Strupp, H. Psychotherapy research and practice: An overview. In S. L. Garfield and A. E. Bergin (Eds.), *Handbook of psychotherapy and behavior change: An empirical analysis*. New York: Wiley, 1978.

Thomas, E. J. *Marital communication and decision making*. New York: Free Press, 1977.

# Case Illustration

The purpose of this chapter is to illustrate the use of the author's conceptual model in clinical practice. This will be achieved by describing a single case in some detail. Clearly, a single case presentation does not validate the model. The purpose of the case illustration is to demonstrate the technical therapeutic procedures employed by a therapist utilizing the model. This particular case was chosen because of the availability of extensive progress notes and the range of interventions utilized, and because the case is typical of the clinical population treated at the Department of Psychiatry at the University of Chicago.

The couple was seen for 12 1½-hour weekly sessions by the author. The reconstruction of the therapy comes from progress notes. Certain details have been changed to obscure the couple's identity, and the reporting of material has been rearranged for clarity of presentation. For example, since individual diagnostic sessions were not utilized, details about each spouse's background were gradually accumulated during the course of therapy. For the reader's convenience, this information is summarized in one section. In other instances, material has been reorganized to better illustrate certain types of interventions. In all other ways, the case history is an accurate report of the clinical intervention.

## BRIEF HISTORY OF THE RELATIONSHIP

Mr. and Mrs. P were a couple in their early 30s who had been married approximately 5 years. Considerable discord had been present since the first year of their marriage. However, the intensity of their discord appeared to have escalated severely in the last 2 to 3 years. This escalation appeared related to the concurrent appearance of several major life stresses. Approximately 3 years ago, Mrs. P had given birth to their first child. This child had recurrent upper respiratory and inner-ear infections. On two occasions, the child's temperature had spiked, precipitating febrile convulsions. This meant that one or both parents would have to sit up with the child at night to maintain a vigil to prevent dangerously high temperatures. Shortly after birth of the child, Mrs. P developed a severe asthmatic condition. She had several brief hospitalizations for asthma, refractory to outpatient intervention. When she was unusually active, she seemed prone to upper respiratory infections, which complicated her asthmatic problems. For this reason, her personal physician had instructed Mrs. P to severely restrict her activities, to take daily naps, and to have the husband assist with child-rearing activities. Mr. P had begun work in a prestigious, highly competitive law firm, in which few junior partners reached associate status. His position required frequent overnight travel to other cities. The birth, illness, and new job coincided with their move to Chicago from another city. The extended family was now some distance away, and new social relationships were not immediately available. Financial difficulties precluded the hiring of domestic help. Mrs. P's medical condition meant that she could not attend many of the social functions connected with her husband's profession.

Their usual interaction at home apparently consisted of short periods of relative tranquility interrupted by frequent bitter arguments. These arguments centered around Mrs. P's anger that her husband was seldom at home and seldom helped with household tasks and Mr. P's resentment that his wife couldn't manage their home like other wives and thus hampered his career development. These arguments reached bitter extremes with some frequency. Mr. P had spent an average of two nights per week at his office the past year in order to escape domestic turmoil. Neither spouse had outside sexual relationships, and both spouses maintained an uninhibited sexual responsiveness to one another in spite of considerable and frequent discord. Sexual interaction appeared limited to the times after their most bitter interchanges. However, as conflict was so frequent, this association was unclear.

Both Mr. and Mrs. P had dated extensively before meeting one another through a common friend. The courtship had been stormy, with each partner often refusing to compromise on trivial issues. For example, it was not uncommon for them to disagree on movie or theater choice. The ensuing argument would then last beyond show time, and the evening would be spent at home. It was on one of these occasions that they first had premarital intercourse. Mrs. P remembers being attracted to Mr. P because "he was the first man I couldn't run over. The other

men were such pushovers." Mr. P was less clear on why he was originally attracted to Mrs. P. On recollection, he guessed that it was because
"she appeared independent and strong. She would make a good lawyer's wife. She was good socially."

Both families had objected to the marriage, partially on religious
and partially on social grounds. One was Protestant, the other Jewish.
Mrs. P's father was of working-class origins and a fiery labor organizer
with Communist leanings. He wanted his daughter to marry someone
of the honest working class and felt that lawyers were "the crooked
agents of corrupt businessmen." Mr. P's father was a successful busi-
nessman who detested the labor movement. Both of Mr. P's parents felt
that the daughter-in-law was beneath their only child's social position.
Each family was concerned that the children not be brought up in the
religion and ethics of the opposing family. Since the marriage, the opposing in-laws had seldom visited at the same time. They would first
check whether the other in-laws would be there. If so, the trip would
be canceled. Each set of in-laws tolerated the child's spouse and were
civil. Neither spouse felt accepted by the in-laws.

## BRIEF PERSONALITY SKETCH OF MRS. P

Mrs. P was a tall, attractive woman with a rather unkempt appearance. Somehow, her expensive skirts were always wrinkled or a bit too
long. In other ways, she appeared to be the excellent result of a personal
psychotherapy. She was comfortable discussing interpersonal issues and
had an air of personal comfort and direction about herself. A college
graduate from a competitive art history program, she had personally
decided to become a housewife. She stated that she achieved outside
satisfaction from writing children's stories for various publishers and
from exhibiting her art work at local exhibitions. She stated that her life
had changed after completing 4 years of twice-weekly psychoanalytically
oriented psychotherapy in college. She had entered therapy because of
a history of disappointing relationships with men. She felt that this
therapy had resolved her tendency to "feel that men don't give me
enough." She stated that much of her therapy had focused on issues in
her family of origin, in particular her relationship with her father. He
was described as a distant, idealistic man who kept a tight reign on his
feelings, especially anger. For example, she recalled an incident during
her growing up when her mother had been nagging her father. Her
father suddenly left the house during a heavy rain and sat in the rain
under a tree for the next 2 hours. He then returned to the house soaking
wet, and the issue was never discussed again in the family. She remem-

bered always having difficulty feeling close to her father. As a child, the only time she could remember feeling close to him was when she helped him with household chores, such as putting a shelf in the kitchen. On her visits home from college, her father would remain in his workshop. She would seek him out, assist him on some project, and only gradually would he show interest in her college career. Her mother was a medical social worker who had completed a personal analysis. She described her mother as more emotionally available but a "little crazy every so often." Her mother would apparently become overextended at work and then feel that no one appreciated her and that perhaps people were trying to get rid of her. The relationship between her parents had always been strained and the mother had often used Mrs. P, her oldest child, as a confidante. It appeared that the mother had attempted to be a good wife to earn her husband's love and had gone into analysis, when she concluded that this was impossible. After the analysis, the mother was apparently much more comfortable with herself, but the marital tension never abated. Mrs. P stated that in her therapy she had learned that her father did love her but just couldn't express it like other people. Learning this helped her to relate differently to men.

Mrs. P discussed her pain and disappointment in her current marriage and stated that she didn't want to end up like her parents. Her father had recently become ill. During his illness, he had become so disillusioned as to think of voting for Reagan. Her mother was having extreme difficulty coping with her father and life in general. Mrs. P received twice-weekly telephone calls from her mother. Her mother's sense of desperation was frightening to Mrs. P. She wanted more out of life and wanted to work in therapy to change things in the relationship with her husband.

In the initial interaction with Mrs. P, the therapist had the impression of a creative, sensitive, independent woman who had married an impossible husband. For example, Mrs. P would discuss the beauty of hiking in the Vermont woods in the fall enjoying the changing colors. Mr. P would tersely retort that backpacking was for beatniks. At these times, Mrs. P would alternate between episodes of uncontrolled anger and speaking in a whining, little-girl voice. It was almost as if she tried every conceivable interpersonal maneuver to move an immovable object.

## MR. P

Whereas Mrs. P initially appeared to be an artistic, sensitive woman, Mr. P appeared to be a gruff, rigid, insensitive man. He stated that marital therapy was her idea, not his, and that if she would keep the house clean, that there wouldn't be any problem. He stated, "The only problem in our marriage is that I can't trust her not to get sick again. She's supposed to take care of the house so I can work. She's not doing her bit." Illness on her part was characterized by him as her failure to uphold her role responsibility. He continually spoke of not being able to trust her not to make demands on his time. He consistently refused to discuss his feelings and always diverted the conversation back to a discussion of his wife's responsibilities. From the overt discussion, all Mr. P desired from his wife was the fulfillment of certain responsibilities. The other side of Mr. P surfaced when the therapist was paraphrasing Mr. P's position. Mr. P looked amused for a moment and inquired if he really sounded that bad.

A description of Mr. P's family was less revealing. He described his father as "impossible" and his mother as "crazy." From his viewpoint, this was adequate. Further exploration revealed a hardworking, ambitious father who was frequently away from home and a traditional mother who complained about the father's absences. His mother was described as extremely dependent on the father. The father was an independent sort who resisted any effort to restrict his freedom. This central issue appears never to have been resolved between his parents. His parents were able to come together on issues concerning the importance of religious orthodoxy and their only child's well-being.

Mr. P had a highly successful academic career, having graduated from high school early and completing college by age 19. His law school record was equally outstanding. He did not have any history of psychiatric contact prior to his marriage.

The therapist's initial impression of Mr. P was of a rigid, demanding man who conceived of life in impersonal terms. Human interaction consisted of roles and functions. One was concerned with actions instead of feelings. For example, upon learning that a close friend had died in an automobile accident, Mr. P complained that this would require his taking off from work to travel to the funeral. He resisted all efforts by the therapist to discuss his feelings for the friend. Mr. P apparently had a sense of the moral order of the universe and became furious when people did not live up to their roles. Whenever Mrs. P would become childlike and dependent, Mr. P would become increasingly angry.

## ENTRANCE INTO THERAPY

Mr. P originally contacted another psychiatrist because of difficulty sleeping, irritability, and difficulty concentrating at work. He desired information as to whether antidepressant medication might help. This therapist noted that Mr. P had a somewhat rigid, obsessive-compulsive personality, that he appeared out of touch with his feelings, and that he used rationalization and displacement as defense mechanisms. As most of Mr. P's discussion focused on his marriage, this therapist recommended a marital therapist.

They were then seen by a psychoanalytically oriented marital therapist for 6 months. This therapist focused his intervention on the conflictual replay of their parental marriages in the current relationship. In particular, Mr. P was seen as a perfectionistic, demanding man who, like his father, expected his wife to meet his expectations. Mrs. P, like her mother, was seen as a woman trying hopelessly to meet her husband's expectations. This therapy was terminated when the therapist moved to another city. The couple was then referred to the author. This therapist recommended me as a last resort before recommending an individual psychoanalysis for both spouses.

## COURSE OF THERAPY

### First Session

In the first interview, the therapist attempted to obtain further information on the history of their relationship, their previous therapy experience, and each of their views concerning the marital situation. The initial portion of this session was remarkable mainly in that seemingly minor disagreements escalated into major battles before the therapist could discern the issue being argued. It was similarly difficult to discern the point in the interaction when the escalation began. During these arguments, both would speak simultaneously, so that little information other than the affect was exchanged. A litany of complaints and character descriptions passed back and forth. Mr. P expressed his resentment about helping out with household chores after working hard at the office, his anger on the time demands from his wife, his anger that his wife didn't take her asthma medications regularly and thus risked further illness, and his disgust at how messy their house was. Mrs. P complained that her husband never returned home from work on time, that they had little time together, that he didn't understand the difficulty of raising a small child, that they didn't have time for walks in the woods, and that her husband was in general insensitive to her needs. During the arguments, a certain thematic consistency began to appear in their descriptions of one another. Mr. P usually described his wife as helpless, disorganized, dependent, weak, and demanding. Mrs. P usually described her husband as insensitive, rigid, and withholding.

Several characteristics of their interactional behavior were note-worthy.

1. Whenever Mrs. P made direct requests for action from her husband, he diverted the subject away from the original request. For example, Mrs. P would ask her husband to plan a trip in the woods together. Mr. P would complain that the house was messy without acknowledging her request. Arguments usually escalated soon thereafter.

2. Mrs. P's requests were often stated in a manner to induce guilt. "I don't need much to be happy. One weekend away from your work isn't so much to ask, is it?"

3. Many messages between the spouses were confused, consisting of both requests for change and anger that the request probably wouldn't be met. "Most wives know how to vacuum. I don't see why you can't find time to vacuum at least once a week."

4. Mr. P usually stated his requests as categorical imperatives or orders. For example, most of his sentences started with "You should" or "All wives should."

5. Mrs. P usually responded to her husband's orders with passive noncompliance. She would agree verbally to do what he wanted, but her nonverbal behavior would leave little doubt as to her noncompliance with his wishes.

The therapist also noted how their behavior influenced one another. The greater the resistance Mrs. P met from her husband, the more persistent, nagging, and helpless she became. Her voice tone would change from that of an angry adult to one resembling that of a young child. The more persistent she became, the more rigid and unyielding her husband became. Initially, Mr. P would, at least intellectually, concede that being a mother of a young child could be difficult. However, as his wife began to sound more helpless, he became even more rigid and unwilling to consider her emotional state. At these times, his replies would become even more tense and unfeeling.

At this point, the therapist reached certain conclusions regarding his therapeutic strategy and his conceptualization of their difficulty.

1. Their descriptions of one another appeared partially correct. However, it appeared that her helplessness and his rigidity were mainly in response to their interaction together. These personality predispositions appeared to become exaggerated with distressful interaction.

2. For any intervention to take effect, the therapist would initially have to take control of the interaction to prevent escalations.

3. The interactional and communicational morass exhibited by this couple appeared to be the nonspecific result of chronic discord. The therapist could not at this point decipher a thematic uniqueness to this couple's conflict.

4. The first level of intervention should be to restructure the interactional sequences.

The therapist's intervention for the remainder of this session is mainly to give each spouse a sense that his or her position has been heard and to take control of the interaction to prevent future nonproductive escalations. Due to the emotional intensity of the interaction, it appears unlikely that more can be accomplished in this session. During a momentary silence between arguments, the therapist intervenes: "Clearly, the two of you are struggling with great intensity to work out your relationship and clarify your positions. However, when the two of you talk at once, I have trouble figuring out what is going on. For the time being, I want to hear from one of you at a time. That's for my benefit. I can't follow the two conversations at once."

After a short pause, Mrs. P begins. In a disorganized manner, she elaborates a long history of past injustices from her spouse. The theme of her presentation appears to be how hard she has tried in the marriage and how impossible her husband has been. The therapist interrupts frequently to make certain that he understands her correctly. On occasion, he uses these interruptions to retranslate her bemoaning her fate into requests for help. For example, Mrs. P exclaims, "I can't go on any longer. Julie [the child] is so hard to raise. The house is so large. And he is never around." The therapist paraphrases, "It's difficult and lonely to raise a young child. You would appreciate more help from your husband." When she begins to speak, the therapist turns fully to face her, looking out of the corner of his eye to monitor the husband's action. Whenever the husband begins to interrupt, the therapist signals nonverbally for the husband to be quiet. When the husband appears at the boiling point, unable to contain himself, the therapist intervenes, looking momentarily at the husband: "All I'm trying to do is to hear each of your versions of what's going on. In a minute, I'd like to hear your version. But for now, let her continue." The therapist then turns back to face the wife, motioning for her to continue. When her narrative approaches a thematic closure and she is about to begin on another area of past injustices, the therapist intervenes: "Let me see if I understand you clearly. You feel that you've tried to adjust to your husband's wishes but that he doesn't seem willing to reciprocate. The instances you mentioned are examples of this. Now, I'd like to hear your husband's viewpoint." The therapist turns to face the husband.

The husband is explosively angry at this point, having sat still while his wife made allegations against him to a stranger. He begins with a violent rebuttal of her allegations. The therapist listens politely for a while then intervenes while Mr. P is catching his breath. "I'm sure that both of you have experienced considerable pain and rejection in the relationship. Rather than rebutting her version, could you present your version?" At this point, the therapist is attempting to interrupt the sequence of allegations–rebuttals so often present in marital discord. By nonverbal gestures, the therapist continues to shape the husband's behavior away from rebuttal and toward a presentation of his own viewpoint. Again, the therapist interrupts for clarification of the husband's viewpoint and attempts to retranslate some of his statements. For example, when Mr. P states that "women are supposed to take care of the home and help the husband's career," the therapist replies, "You work in a very competitive firm. The pressure must be difficult. I can understand your wish for an ally." In this example, the therapist is attempting to translate the husband's wishes into a form that the wife might understand. When the husband concludes his version, the therapist summarizes what he's heard. "You feel that you've been willing to compromise but that your wife makes unfair demands of you, without holding up her end of the deal. The examples you mentioned typify this for you."

The therapist pauses for a moment, then continues: "When the two of you were dating, things appeared to work out better. However, the two of you have always had trouble working out ways to compromise and meet each other's needs. This became a critical problem when you moved to Chicago and the system became overloaded. Both of you currently need support from one another, but don't know how to get it. We need to focus on the ways you attempt to get needs met by one another and your reactions when that doesn't work. That's the central area. If we can solve that, then maybe we'll understand why you so often come across as a helpless little girl and you appear to be an insensitive bastard every so often. Neither of you likes being that way, but you don't know how to avoid it."

The therapist then suggests that they need to focus on resolving some of the current arguments that keep recurring. He suggests that each begin to think of the small recurring irritations, and to think of what the spouse could do differently that would be pleasing. The therapist recommends that they first think of small changes in behavior that they would desire from the other. In the next session, they will use this information to begin work on negotiation skills.

At this point the therapist is thinking that the current interactional climate is too heated for any educative or interpretive intervention to be effective. Thus, his first decision is to attempt to defuse the interactional sequence of attack–counterattack. His plan is to arrange an equitable compromise on the current disagreements. This, if possible, will shift the interactional sequences into different areas and also challenge their beliefs that nothing can be obtained from the spouse.

The purpose of his intervention was threefold: (1) to indicate that the therapist agreed with how they saw each other but that he didn't feel that the situation was unchangeable (implicit in this statement was the suggestion that each partner played a role in the other's behavior); (2) to give the couple a sense that the therapist knew what was going on and had a coherent plan of action; (3) to focus attention on the solution of problems of current concern (the phrasing of the statement was purposeful in that the therapist is suggesting that these disputes are trivial and should thus be quickly resolved).

The rest of this session then focused on how they attempted to solve problems with each other and their frustration regarding this. This again elicited considerable anger and allegations concerning the other's untrustworthiness.

## Negotiation Training

The main emphasis of the next six or seven sessions is focused on modifying dysfluent communication and helping the couple learn how to compromise. The therapist's initial goal is to get the couple to work out a joint solution to some problem.

The second session opens with the therapist inquiring as to their reaction to the last session, any questions about the therapy, and how things went between them in the previous week. The last question elicits a series of complaints and innuendos about the other spouse. As this interaction may quickly escalate into a major argument, the therapist intervenes: "This week, you were going to come up with a list of minor things that you would like your spouse to do differently. Why don't we work on that now? From the tone of things, it sounds as if that's a good idea."

Before either spouse can agree vociferously, listing the injustices of the previous week, the therapist turns to Mr. P. "Let's start with you. Could you list some things that you would like your wife to do differently? If possible, try to make your requests positive and as concrete as possible. Maybe start with some minor things. They're more easily solvable."

*Comment.* The therapist purposely chose the husband first. In the usual interaction, the wife is more verbal. Thus, this intervention partially serves to interrupt a usual interactional sequence.

The husband replies, "She should be a good wife and manage her home like other women. She shouldn't get sick. That interferes with my work."

The therapist intervenes quickly. "You have a variety of complaints and requests intermingled. Could you address what you want her to do? Try to be specific."

*Comment.* The therapist quickly cut off the husband as he was beginning a long tirade of complaints. The longer he continued, the more angry his wife would become. Soon they would be back in a bitter, nonproductive battle. Also, the therapist is attempting to get the husband to state what he wants from his wife, rather than give orders.

The husband continues: "I want her to keep the home clean. From the first week of our marriage, the kitchen . . ."

The therapist intervenes: "Could you be specific? What in particular do you want done?"

*Comment.* Again the husband is interrupted. He is about to repeat a litany about how the house is never clean. His utterance isn't new information, as he's already summarized this particular viewpoint on numerous previous occasions. Allowing him to go on would be destructive.

The husband continues, "Well, the kitchen is a mess. Julie's [the daughter's] toys are everywhere and . . ." The wife interrupts: "You son of a bitch. You try staying home and raising a child. If you don't like my cleaning, you do it." Turning to the therapist, "He was spoiled by his mother and . . ."

The therapist turns to the wife: "That may be true. I also understand your irritation. You feel that you're trying to be a good wife and mother and that he doesn't appreciate it. Your feelings about this are important. But for now, we're trying to get a clear picture of what he wants. That doesn't mean that he will get it or that you're at fault. Nothing can be resolved until we determine what each of you wants. Then we'll be in a position to see how far apart you are and how much compromise is necessary. Can we go on?"

*Comment.* The wife apparently had an outburst upon hearing charges against her going unchallenged. Her outburst had to be interrupted and the therapist had to address her concerns for the sequence to proceed. It was important for the therapist to face the wife during this interchange. His last question to her forces her to tacitly agree to be quiet.

The therapist turns back to the husband. The husband continues: "Well, the meals are never ready and . . ." The therapist intervenes: "That's another issue. Which is more important? Meals or a clean house? Let's stay on one issue at a time. We'll get to meals later on or you can change the subject. It's up to you."

*Comment.* A common pitfall is the intermingling of numerous interdependent requests. If too many topics are raised at once, solution is impossible. The therapist points this out, then returns control to the husband by asking him which topic he prefers to discuss.

The husband continues: "The house is important. It's a pigsty. It embarrasses me to have people from work drop by . . ." The wife intervenes: "He's always been too concerned with others' opinions. It related back to his relationship with . . ."

The therapist interrupts: "You might be right, but that's irrelevant right now. Each of your wishes from the other is related to your idiosyncratic pasts. The point is, how do we work a current compromise?"

*Comment.* The therapist purposely redirects the conversation flow back to the present. At this point, the exploration of past issues would be a diversion (defense) against trying to solve contemporary problems. At a later point in the therapy, an exploration of how their past experiences bias their perceptions of similar events may be important. At this point, shifting blame appears more important to the spouses than mutual understanding. For this reason, the therapist maintains a current focus.

The therapist faces the husband again. After a pause, the husband continues: "I want the house clean. That's an absolute. I won't tolerate . . ." The therapist interrupts the husband. "A clean house is important to you for a variety of reasons. OK. You have a young child. That complicates matters. You know, toys, and all that. There will always be things amiss. If your wife faces an impossible task, she may just say the hell with it. What we need is an explicit set of guidelines which she either meets or doesn't. That way she knows when she's done a good job."

The wife interrupts: "Wait a minute. He can't tell me how to clean house. I don't tell him what to do at work."

The therapist replies: "That's true. All we're trying to do right now is to find out exactly what he wants. The way it is now, no matter what you do, you always fall short of his expectations. If we make the expectations explicit, maybe this won't have to happen. Let's see."

*Comment.* The therapist's interruption of the husband was to prevent an escalating battle. All the therapist is attempting to do at this point is to obtain a set of clear expectations of the other's behavior without a battle escalating. With a set of expectations clearly stated, an attempt at compromise is possible. Compromise will interrupt the behavioral sequences that maintain the status quo. A clear set of expectations will also interrupt the pattern of the husband's always disapproving of his wife's conduct.

The therapist looks again to the husband.

MR. P: Well, the house looks terrible when I come home. Magazines are all over the floor . . .

MRS. P (interrupting): Those are your magazines . . .

THERAPIST (interrupting): For now, we want to find out what he wants. Mr. P, please continue.

MR. P: The house is a mess. Magazines are everywhere. It hasn't been vacuumed. The beds aren't made. Toys are everywhere.

MRS. P (interrupting): That's not true . . .

THERAPIST: We're not after truth. We're only concerned right now with his desired situation. (Turning to Mr. P) Is vacuuming once a week OK?

MR. P: Sure.

THERAPIST: Magazines up and beds made. How often? By when?

MR. P: Before I return home. I want to come home to a clean house. Nobody in her family . . .

THERAPIST (interrupting firmly): OK. So far, vacuum once a week. Pick up magazines and make beds before you return. That's fairly clear. The child's toys are more difficult. What if she picks them all up before you come home and Julie brings them back out? How do we resolve that?

MRS. P: That happens all the time. He never . . .

THERAPIST (interrupting Mrs. P and continuing to face Mr. P): Well, how do we handle that? We need a clear set of expectations that your wife either meets or doesn't meet. Otherwise, the two of you can continue fighting, feeling justifiably that you've done your part.

MR. P: OK. I guess the toys are impossible.

THERAPIST: Are you sure? It's important that your position is clear.

MR. P: Yes, that's OK. I kind of enjoy Julie wandering about with the toys.

THERAPIST: Let me paraphrase. You would like your wife to vacuum once a week, pick up magazines, and make beds before you return home. You want these things from her (turns to the wife while making these statements).

*Comment.* At this point, the therapist is modeling how to express wishes in a direct manner. Later, he will coach both spouses in this technique.

MR. P: I forgot about the dishes. There's always a stack in the kitchen a couple of days old. I worry about disease . . .

THERAPIST: You would like your wife to wash these dishes more regularly. Perhaps daily before you return. Anything else?

MR. P: That's enough, but she will never . . .

THERAPIST (turning away from husband and facing Mrs. P): These are things your husband wants from you. Are these possible?

MRS. P: Of course, but I'm not going to do these things if he continues to criticize me.

THERAPIST: I agree. We're trying to find a way to solve that. Now he's mentioned several things—vacuuming, picking up magazines, making beds, washing dishes. Four separate things. Are there things that you want from him? Maybe some things of equal relative importance to you?

MR. P: Wait a minute, these are things a wife is supposed to do. I'm not bartering . . .

THERAPIST: Your rules are different from hers. Our task is to eventually agree on a joint set of rules. That takes the clear expression of both your viewpoints (turns to face the wife).

MRS. P: Well, we never do anything together. Before we were married, we used to have picnics, trips in the woods to see the leaves change . . .

MR. P: If you would run the household properly, I would have time to go to work and then we could do these things. But, goddammit, you are so disorganized and . . .

THERAPIST: She let you express your opinion. It's only fair that you give her a chance.

*Comment.* The therapist emphasizes fairness for a purpose. The husband is clearly a man who feels that life should be lived by a set of moral rules. The therapist temporarily disarms the husband by applying these rules to the husband's behavior. The therapist turns back to the wife. His looking away from the husband signifies that the therapist feels the matter between them is clear-cut and requires no more discussion.

THERAPIST: You were mentioning leisure time together.

MRS. P: I really miss those things. The brilliant golds and reds of the autumn forest. The beauty and tranquillity of being in the woods. I had those things before I met him.

THERAPIST: This is something you want from your husband. For him to take you on weekend trips.

*Comment.* The therapist is attempting to convert a global statement of disappointment into a specific request by the wife from the husband. Global statements of disappointment implicitly attribute blame without identifying a solution. Thus, they help to maintain the current interaction.

MRS. P: Yes.

THERAPIST: You would be willing to do the four things he mentioned in return for trips in the country? How often? What's a reasonable trade-off from your viewpoint?

MR. P: Wait a minute. I'm not going to take a weekend off from work just to get her to do things that . . .

THERAPIST (quickly interrupting): We're just trying to find out how she views the situation. We're exploring solutions. Brainstorming, if you will.

MR. P: One of my colleagues, a divorce lawyer, was talking about behavior therapy. Is that what this is?

THERAPIST: In a way . . . we're trying to work out a way for each of you to honor and appreciate the other's private universe. That's what our bartering is about.

MRS. P: A reasonable trade-off would be no nagging, his coming home from work on time, his staying home when I'm sick, his going to work on time, going for walks in the woods, weekends in the country . . .

THERAPIST: He's mentioned four things mainly to do with housework. We're looking for things from him that would involve a similar degree of inconvenience. The trade-off needs to be reasonably equitable from each perspective or it won't work. Make him an offer. We have to start somewhere.

MRS. P: You know, I'd keep the house clean if he would help.

THERAPIST (noting that husband is looking angry and about to speak, and quickly intervening): Like how?

MRS. P: Well, if he would pick up his own magazines and papers from work and entertain Julie while I'm preparing dinner.

THERAPIST (looking at husband): That seems like a reasonable deal. What do you think?

*Comment.* The therapist is attempting to force a compromise.

MR. P: The minute I return from work, the kid is under my feet. I don't even get a chance to mix a drink.

MRS. P: What about me? I'm stuck at home all day.

THERAPIST: Would 15 minutes to unwind make a difference?

MR. P: Yeah, a lot.

THERAPIST: Agreeable to you, then? House vacuumed, beds made up. You pick up your own magazines and you take care of your daughter before dinner, allowing 15 minutes to unwind first. In return, you're also home from work on time. Oh, what time is "on time"? (A conversation ensues. Eventually, with help, 6:00 p.m. is agreed upon as a mutually acceptable compromise time. The therapist repeats the bargain, makes sure that all agree and understand. He recommends that both uphold their side of the agreement, regardless, implicitly hinting that induced guilt in the partner might be a satisfactory punishment.) Well, we've solved that one. What are some of the other minor battles that take up so much time?

*Comment*

In the preceding section, the therapist's intervention is modeled after behavioral interventions known as reciprocity counseling (Azrin *et al.*, 1973) and contingency contracting (Jacobson and Margolin, 1979). In this sequence, the therapist helps the couple to choose an area to work on and actually suggests solutions. The choice of content area is relatively unimportant. The main point is to choose an initial topic where a solution is possible. The goal of the therapist is to disrupt the interactional struggle and to restore hope that compromise is possible. In subsequent sessions, this technique is utilized to disrupt other interactional struggles. These struggles include Mr. P's desire that Mrs. P take her medication regularly, Mrs. P's desired weekend trips in the country, Mr. P's desire to have friends from work drop by, and Mrs. P's desire to have her husband help with other household chores. In these sessions, the therapist gradually titrates his withdrawal from the interaction, intervening only when escalation is otherwise imminent. He is attempting to teach them a way of resolving these nonproductive struggles on their own. This teaching is accomplished by coaching their interaction, having them rehearse alternative strategies, and emphasizing general rules of negotiation.

Dynamically oriented therapists may be uncomfortable with the degree of activity and control exerted by the therapist. In the presence of severe discord, the therapist has no option unless he concludes that this case is untreatable. Other therapists might suggest that true intimacy will be impossible for this couple. This is a reasonable hypothesis, but prematurely made. In severe discord, the therapist needs to disrupt the recurring behavioral sequences before he can make any realistic appraisal of the participants involved. A way of conceptualizing the therapist's activity in this sequence is to use the model of Ezriel (1952), which was introduced in a previous chapter. According to this model, impulse becomes the avoided relationship and defense the required relationship. In other words, the disturbed interactional pattern of the couple is the required relationship. Rather than interpret the defense as one might do in individual psychotherapy, the therapist disarms or disallows the defense, using a behavioral intervention. This form of intervention is necessary because of the action–reaction patterns prevalent in disturbed relationships between intimates.

## Modifying Specific Interactional Problems

Negotiation training is used to eliminate some of the recurring areas of disagreement. Once the spouse have begun to compromise, the interactional climate eases to the point where other interventions are also possible. At this point, the therapist wishes to focus on the style of negotiation and communication as well as the actual commodities being exchanged. In most marital disputes, it appears that the style of communicating feelings and wishes, more than the actual content of the change desired in the mate, is the problem area. The interventions used by the therapist resemble those of behavior therapists who stress modification of dysfluent marital communication (e.g., Thomas, 1977; Gottman et al., 1976). In this case, the therapist attempts to modify specific interactional problems for this couple.

In the first sequence, the interactional pattern of Mr. P's continually diverting his wife away from subjects she wishes to discuss and its consequences are outlined for the couple. In particular, Mrs. P learns that she is not helpless when this occurs and that alternative behaviors are available to her. In this particular sequence, Mrs. P is discussing the relationship of her daughter with her husband. This discussion obviously mirrors the relationship of Mrs. P with her father. The therapist purposely avoids pointing this out. He is more concerned with process than content.

## Specific Communication Problems

MRS. P: I worry about Julie. She seems so lonely. You know she hardly
    ever sees her father. Is this good for her development? You're
    a psychiatrist.
THERAPIST: What do you want from your husband?

*Comment.* The therapist redirects the question to the husband. The therapist's opinion is irrelevant. The couple needs to learn how to negotiate differences.

MRS. P: I want you to spend more time with Julie. I'm worried . . .
MR. P: She's only lonely because you indulge her. Children need to learn
    about life.
MRS. P: You're only concerned about your work. You don't care about
    us. We're stuck at home and so lonely (looks on the verge of
    tears).
MR. P: (looking uncomfortable at first and then beginning to get angry):
    "I really don't care how you . . .
THERAPIST: OK. Let's stop and examine what's going on. This is a fre-
    quent pattern. Both of you are upset and neither has what
    you want. What happened here? Mr. P?
MR. P: She should . . .
THERAPIST: Mrs. P?
MRS. P: He's still impossible. It's just . . .
THERAPIST: OK. I'll replay it for you. You asked your husband for some-
    thing. He didn't answer your question. You became helpless
    and he became unyielding. The whole sequence is unnec-
    essary. Mr. P, you could have answered her or asked her to
    clarify what she wanted. Mrs. P, when he diverted the sub-
    ject, you could have brought him back to your question. Let's
    try it again. Mrs. P, you start.

MRS. P (turning toward therapist): But you know what I mean. Why is
    he so dense?
THERAPIST: I'm not positive that I know what you mean. Besides, its
    important that your husband understand. Can you explain
    it to him?

*Comment.* This is simply an attempt to shift the conversation flow
back between the spouses. The therapist judges that he was worked
enough individually with Mrs. P and that perhaps now he can get her
to express her wishes to her husband.

Mrs. P. looks at her husband with a skeptical facial expression and
then with an irritated voice says, "It never works with you. What's the
use?"
Before the husband can reply, the therapist intervenes: "Look at
what just happened. You expressed your disappointment without saying what you wanted. You didn't give him a chance. How about trying
again. This time focus on your feelings and what you want from him."
Mrs. P, looking at the therapist, says, "All I want is . . ."
The therapist nonverbally gestures toward the husband and turns
to face the husband, breaking eye contact with Mrs. P.
Mrs. P persists, "But he never . . ."
The therapist, continuing to look at the husband, counters, "The
way you're starting off, he won't. Give him a fair chance. If he blows
it, it's his fault. But at least you've given him a fair chance."

*Comment.* The therapist at this point is concerned that by the time
he has coached Mrs. P into expressing herself differently, Mr. P will be
so angry that her new behavior won't be rewarded.

Mrs. P continues: "I want to feel that you care." She then hangs
her head and cries softly.
Mr. P at first looks hurt, then angry. He starts to speak.
The therapist intervenes: "You expressed what you wanted. But
then you turned away before seeing whether it was possible. What you
missed was the pained expression on your husband's face as you cried.
Mrs. P looks up. At this point, Mr. P looks first uncomfortable, than
angry, "Look, dammit. Of course I care or I wouldn't have married her.
What's this got to do with the house . . ."
The therapist stops him: "Hold it a minute. How did you feel when
she cried and then turned away from you?"
Mr. P responds, "She always does that. Cries and then withdraws.
I get so damned frustrated. All women ought to learn how . . ."

Again the therapist intervenes: "Hold it. You said 'frustrated.' Maybe cut off and lonely as well."

Mr. P answers, "Yeah. Why the hell God didn't have the sense to teach women . . ."

The therapist repeats: "Isolated and lonely. The same as your wife felt. That loneliness could only be helped by the other. Yet the two of you drive each other off when you need each other the most. That's sad, truly sad."

*Comment.* The therapist is attempting an emotional bridging, pointing out their similar feelings. He emphasizes the sadness, de-emphasizing the shame and anger. The sadness may help to foster further reaching out. This intervention is both an attempt to shift the intervention pattern and an attempt to get the spouses to perceive one another differently.

THERAPIST (continuing): Let's summarize what we've learned. Mrs. P, your husband does the same thing, but we'll concentrate on you, as what you did is more clear-cut in this interaction. You originally attacked your husband instead of saying what you wanted. In this way, you reduced the chances of getting what you wanted. Later, when you did ask more directly, you looked away so soon that you didn't realize that you may be able to get what you want from him. He was upset by your pain. I assume that he cares. Mr. P, you got angry instead of expressing your feelings. Anger was only part of what you felt. If I hadn't so rudely interrupted, you two would have been in a fight again. The lesson is simple. Give each other a chance. Be sure of what the other is saying before jumping to conclusions.

MR. P: I want to talk about her taking her asthma medications. I have a big court case to prepare for and . . .

THERAPIST (to Mrs. P): Are you willing to discuss this now?

MRS. P: OK!

*Comment.* The therapist redirects the communication between the participants. It appears that Mr. P is nervous about the intimacy and this prompts his abrupt change of subject. The therapist doesn't comment on this, as he doesn't feel Mr. P is ready to be engaged on that level.

MR. P: Well, I have this big case; Western Electric is being sued by some
    industrial customers. It's my first big case for the firm and . . .
THERAPIST: It's important to you and your career.


*Comment.* The therapist intervenes to underscore the central point.
Mr. P has a tendency to go off on long monologues during which it is
difficult to follow him. Mrs. P's attention usually beings to wander.
When Mr. P notices this, his monologue appears to stretch on indefi-
nitely. Thus, the therapist acts promptly to prevent this.


MR. P: You're damn' right. And if my wife gets sick, I can't go to work.
    I can't trust her to not get sick. She always . . .
THERAPIST: You're doing the same thing as your wife. You want some-
    thing from her, but your way of asking makes it unlikely
    that you'll get it. (Turning to the wife) Do you see what he's
    doing? It's the same thing you do. You're probably feeling
    the same way he did a few minutes ago.


*Comment.* The therapist is again emphasizing the similarity of their
feeling states and using the interaction to educate them as to their influence on one another.


THERAPIST: Mr. P, how about trying that again. Remember the mistake
    your wife made and try to avoid that. Just say what you want
    and how you feel without making her angry.
MR. P: Well if that's possible.
THERAPIST (laughing): Come on, now.


*Comment.* The therapist senses a relaxing in Mr. P's guard and purposely jokes with him a bit. The humor is that they both know better
than to take seriously what he is saying.


MR. P (slightly disgruntled): OK. This job is important. I need to devote
    my full energy to it. If you get sick, everything will foul up for
    me. I want you to take your asthma medication, run the house
    without bugging me, complaining, and take care of yourself.
MRS. P: I can't promise not to get sick. It's beyond my control. My mother
        . . .
THERAPIST: Of course not. He's not asking that. What did you hear him
    say?

Mrs. P: He said that his work is more important than me or the child and . . .

Therapist (looking at Mr. P): Did you say that? Hold your temper a minute and repeat what you just said.

Mr. P: I said that the job and the next few weeks are extremely important to me. I want your help. If you get sick like you . . .

Therapist (to Mr. P): Hold it. The job's important. You want your mate to help you. That's enough.

Mr. P: I need your help. It's the least my wife . . .

Therapist: Don't blow it. Try again.

Mr. P: I need your help. I want you to try to stay well so I have time to do this job. If I do it right, then we can relax.

Mrs. P: And take a trip to the Smokies. Camp out like we used to.

Mr. P: Sure. But first you need to run the house. You should . . .

Therapist: Don't blow it, now. You've almost got her cooperation. If you revert to orders, we'll be back at square one.

Mr. P: I need you to try to help. I want you to get rest and to take your medications. I don't want you to get sick again. I worry about you and this job is important.

Mrs. P (in a negative voice tone and looking out the window): All right, I'll do it.

Mr. P: And I don't want any . . .

Therapist: Hold it a minute. Do you believe her?

Mr. P: No. She always . . .

Therapist: Why go back to that? Why don't you find out what she's thinking?

Mr. P: OK, what's going on?

Mrs. P: What do you mean?

Mr. P (frowns and looks out the window).

Therapist (to Mrs. P): When you agreed to go along with your husband's request, you seemed irritated. We're both confused. Do you mean that you won't go along with him or do you mean that you will, but you're disappointed and a little irritated?

Mrs. P: It's just the same old thing. He always gets his way. It's always . . .

Therapist: That may be true, but could you answer my question before getting into that?

Mrs. P: What was the question again?

Therapist: You remember. What did you mean a minute ago when you said . . .

Mrs. P: Why should I always give in?

THERAPIST: You don't have to. You could have said no.

MRS. P: No.

THERAPIST: That's too final. It's a dead end. Leave some room for discussion. How come? Is it negotiable?

MRS. P: (in a tone of resignation, looking out of the window): Of course.

THERAPIST: On what terms, then?

MRS. P: Oh, I give up!

THERAPIST: That's a cop-out.

MRS. P: Goddammit. That bastard always has his way.

THERAPIST: Only if you let him. What do you want right now? How are you feeling?

MRS. P: It's his work again. Its always his work.

THERAPIST: It's important to him. What's important to you?

MRS. P: A family. A normal home.

THERAPIST: Could you be more specific?

MRS. P: We haven't camped out in over a year since he took that damn' job.

THERAPIST: That means a lot to you?

MRS. P: Yes.

THERAPIST: Surely there's a way that both of you can get what you want.

SILENCE

THERAPIST: Mr. P, if your wife made a real effort to help for the next . . . how long will the case last—only three more weeks . . . well, if your wife really tried to help because this means so much to you even though she couldn't care less, would you be willing to take a long weekend for a camping trip? And try to enjoy yourself on it even?

*Comments.* The therapist is quite active here. As a resolution is approached, the system breaks down. Thus, the therapist works hard for this transaction to reach a satisfactory outcome. A demonstration in action that alternative behaviors pay off is now more important than interpretation of the underlying dynamics. He even suggests the logical compromise. He also stresses that each is giving in to please the other. The perception of positive intent may be as important as the actual behavior exchanged.

After the couple reaches a compromise, the therapist then outlines how Mrs. P's elusive answer almost disrupted the sequence. He also outlines how the husband colluded by not forcing his wife to stay on the subject. This clarification of interaction remained on the manifest level, i.e., the behavior and the elicited response.

*Summary*

In the previous sequences, the interventions employed by the therapist resemble those used by therapists emphasizing the role of communication skills in marriages. The difference is that the therapist facilitates interaction around current issues, pinpoints the maladaptive pattern, and actively restructures this interaction. As well as prompting new behavior, he pinpoints and labels difficulties on the assumption that this will facilitate generalization. The prompting of new behavior is based on the assumption that demonstration in action will be more effective than instruction. Clearly, the sequence outlined will be repeated with minor variations on numerous occasions until the interaction sequence is aborted.

## Cognitive Restructuring

The therapeutic thrust to this point has mainly been to prevent escalation in conflict (prevent "runaways") and to promote a shift in the interactional pattern. This was accomplished by helping the couple to negotiate compromises and to adopt a more useful communication style. Earlier in the therapy, the couple was locked into a rigid interactional pattern and a fixed way of perceiving one another. At this point, attempts at cognitive relabeling of their interaction or of their perceptions of each other would have been ineffective. The therapist's relabeling or clarification of event sequences would have been contradicted by their current experiences. Once the severe discord is tempered a bit and the interactional sequences are a bit in disequilibrium, the therapist begins a conscious effort at relabeling each spouse's perception of the other. If the interactional sequence is shifted, discrepant information is being perceived—i.e., events are occurring that don't fit their rigid perceptions of one another. At this point, the therapist's attempts at relabeling have a chance of having an impact.

Two facets of cognitive restructuring need emphasis. First, the timing of this intervention strategy is dependent on the therapist's perception of the couple's possible receptivity to a cognitive reappraisal of events. In some couples, the therapist may begin such an attempt earlier in the therapeutic context. If couples are severely limited in their interactional sequences, an interruption of the fixated behavioral sequences is usually necessary before cognitive restructuring is possible, The therapist throughout is making tentative efforts at cognitive restructuring. His first attempts will probably elicit disbelief, vociferous denial, or total inattention to his comments. Later, he will note that the spouses pause reflectively before denying his comment. At this point, the therapist has a foot in the door. The artistry of the therapist is his gauging of the tempo at which he can proceed, while still maintaining his credibility to the couple. In other words, I am not uniformly recommending that reciprocity training and communication training procede cognitive re-constructuring. In more cases, the therapist will attempt all three ap-proaches and the couple's differential receptivity to one or the other will determine the timing and emphasis on his intervention.

The concept of relabeling in marital therapy was introduced by Haley (1963). Haley recommended that the therapist simply disagree with the spouses' cognitions in order to throw the system into disequi-librium. This seeming casual disregard for the truth of the therapist's comments has been upsetting for some more traditional therapists. Also, the therapist's initial flat contradiction of a spouse's statement may not be the most efficient use of the therapist's power.

What I am suggesting is that the therapist wants to lead the spouses into seeing each other differently. A gradual effort to accomplish this may be more effective than a flat contradiction. The truthfulness of the therapist's comments is a difficult issue. His comments have to be plau-sible to even be considered. In severe discord, couples tend to concep-tualize one another and their interaction in relatively narrow and fixated ways. These conceptualizations are usually unrealistic. For example, few husbands are totally insensitive and few wives are totally dependent or helpless. When the therapist focuses on opposite perceptions, he is emphasizing what is not being seen, to challenge the fixated perceptions. The therapist's comments thus facilitate the generation of disequilibrium within the behavioral-cognitive system. This disequilibrium is necessary for the couple to evolve more satisfactory ways of relating.

In this case, the therapist made a conscious effort to gently begin disagreeing with the spouses' fixated misperceptions of one another. These interventions are spread over numerous sessions. Therefore, an exact listing of case material would be an inefficient way to explicate this intervention. Instead, the sequence of interventions will be de-scribed as they occurred in therapy.

Mrs. P was quite dogmatic in her assertion that her husband was insensitive, cold, and emotionally unavailable. In certain ways, this did characterize Mr. P's manner of relating in the marriage. Of course, Mrs. P was unaware of how she contributed to her husband's seeming in-sensitivity. From the therapist's perspective, Mr. P was a somewhat emotionally removed man who became totally inaccessible when his wife began a series of interpersonal maneuvers that defined her as help-less, inducing guilt in Mr. P for not helping more. In these instances,

Mr. P would become increasingly angry, rigid, and unyielding. The therapist had already pointed out to the couple how their interactional style perpetuated their discord and had been successful in shifting the couple partially to different ways of interacting. However, they persisted in their fixated descriptions of one another. Over a series of sessions, the therapist began to challenge the description of Mr. P as insensitive.

During a discussion of their daughter's need for more attention from her father, Mr. P had insisted that "life is tough and kids need to learn how to take it." Mrs. P had turned to the therapist, saying, "See how insensitive he is?" At this point, the therapist simply said, "Well, he's certainly gruff today." In other words, the therapist agreed with Mrs. P but added an element of uncertainty. After the statement Mr. P had made, no greater redirection of emphasis would have been credible. At this point, Mrs. P was too angry and defensive to examine how she had contributed to her husband's current interactional position. Thus, "gruff today" was the maximal allowable intervention. At another point, when Mrs. P commented on Mr. P's insensitivity, the therapist agreed that Mr. P occasionally had trouble dealing with his feelings. Thus, in a series of moves, the therapist agreed with the spouse while gradually shifting the focus of agreement.

Throughout this sequence, the therapist searches for material to support his contention. For example, once after Mrs. P had characterized her husband as insensitive to his daughter's feelings, the therapist asked Mr. P directly how he felt about his daughter's adjustment. Mr. P stammered a bit and began a confused dialogue in which his concern for his daughter was embedded. Of course, Mrs. P heard only the part that supported her view of her husband. Therefore, the therapist repeated in a paraphrased manner the husband's expression of concern for his daughter, making certain that Mrs. P heard it correctly. In a slightly offhand manner, to avoid direct confrontation with Mrs. P, the therapist mused, "I guess there might be a sensitive guy under that bastard facade." A series of similar intervention used to challenge the fixated perception of the husband: "He has difficulty expressing his feelings, maybe it wasn't safe in his family to express feelings; maybe he can learn from you how to express his feelings"; etc.

As well as gently and consistently sprinkling comments that disagree slightly with Mrs. P's description of her husband, the therapist searches for current interaction that is contradictory to the personality description. For example, Mrs. P described how her husband didn't go to his best friend's funeral because he had work to do. The therapist, of course, knows that such situations are usually more complicated. Also, he noted that the husband looked sad for a moment when his wife discussed the best friend's death. At this point, the therapist turned to the husband and asked, "How old was he? How did he die? How long had you known him?" etc. In other words, the therapist approached the husband in a factual way first and gently approached the husband's feelings about his friend. Over the next few minutes, the husband was able to verbalize how he had skipped the funeral because he was afraid of seeing the grief in his friend's wife's eyes. Gradually, the husband was able to describe how much he missed his friend and the only way he knew how to cope with the pain was to return to work. During this interchange, the wife looked at first skeptical and then puzzled, as if she didn't know how to process the information. Then the husband reverted back to his usual self and said, "Well, he's dead and I have the Western Electric case to work on." His wife looked relieved and commented again how insensitive her husband was. The therapist repeated his observation as to what happened and how Mr. P uses a gruff facade to cover over disturbing feelings. He asked Mr. P if he had desired an opportunity to discuss his feelings shortly after hearing of his friend's death. Mr. P replied that he had but that his wife had seemed uninterested. Mrs. P looked genuinely confused and then became angry, saying that her husband had not made any overtures in this regard. Mr. P stated that he had, and an escalation appeared imminent. The therapist intervened, saying that Mr. P was so unused to seeking emotional comfort that his signals may easily have been misread. The therapist nodded sadly, saying, "That's too bad." His intent was to signify that the couple could obtain much more from one another than they currently do.

Throughout these sequences, the therapist is aware that Mrs. P is really concerned with Mr. P's expression of love for her. This issue is temporarily avoided for strategic reasons.

Mr. P always characterizes his wife as dependent and helpless, never realizing the part he plays in forcing her to adopt this interpersonal stance. For example, the therapist notes that Mrs. P usually reverts to a helpless interpersonal stance when attempts to relate to Mr. P in a more adult manner fail. Thus, the therapist strives to break the confirmatory interpersonal sequence while at the same time disagreeing with Mr. P's characterization of his wife. His disagreement is at first gentle and peripheral and then progressively more direct and confrontational.

For example, during one sequence of disagreement about Mr. P's not helping with household chores, Mr. P describes his wife as helpless. The therapist agrees by saying that she is temporarily overwhelmed by the magnitude of the tasks she is taking on all at once. Later, the therapist emphasizes how Mrs. P is stuck at home with a new child in a city where she has few friends. He emphasizes the stress of her ill health and the child's frequent illnesses. The therapist notes in passing that most people might feel overwhelmed by this and turn to a spouse for support. In this sequence, the therapist agrees with the husband's observation, yet emphasizes the temporary nature of things. As the husband operates by a system of logic, emphasizing rules and correct codes of behavior, the therapist turns this against him, noting that most women would have been overwhelmed by the same events. If most women would have been similarly affected, then by inference, perhaps his wife isn't as unusually weak as he tends to think. In later sequences, when the husband characterizes his wife as weak, the therapist emphasizes her struggle and need for support.

As the therapist is sprinkling the husband with novel ways of perceiving his wife, the therapist also looks for disconfirmatory information. For example, the wife had been complaining that the husband never told the next-door neighbors to turn down the record player. This demonstrated how little he cared about their child. Further questioning revealed that Mr. P was too embarrassed to confront the neighbor about this, and his wife had finally confronted the neighbor. She had done this in a surprisingly competent way, which even her husband had temporarily admired. The therapist listened, smiled, and then looked at Mr. P with a twinkle in his eye: "You mean this helpless, incompetent, dependent, weak wife of yours did that? A superwoman underneath, perhaps." The therapist purposely exaggerated the ambivalence with a tinge of humor. With a little probing, other instances of the wife's real competence were readily elicited.

## A Return to the Past

As emphasized in the previous chapter, this model tends to focus on solving contemporary problems. In many ways, a couple's persistent tendency to bring up the past can be conceptualized as a defense against confronting contemporary real problems. For strategic reasons, the therapist focuses on current problems, emphasizing that he can't change the past but that he can help them to make the future different. Too often, discussions of past marital events are attempts to prove moral positions rather than solve problems. Another problem with discussions of the past is that the therapist wasn't there and the two spouses' versions of the past usually differ. Therefore, the therapist is often put into a helpless position. Thus, past marital problems are usually avoided if possible. Like all rules of therapy, this one was broken as well.

The therapy of Mr. and Mrs. P had reached a state where each was able to relate better to the other and even express affection on occasion.

The new equilibrium could perhaps best be described as an uneasy truce, with each spouse on guard for a return of the old patterns and associated pain. At about this time, Mrs. P made the statement "Things may be working out now. In fact, maybe we can even make things work out in the long run. But I'll never be able to completely forgive my husband for totally abandoning me and Julie when we moved to Chicago." This, of course, is a common occurrence in couple therapy. Just as things look as if they are about to work out, one spouse diverts onto another subject or expresses some ultimate reservation about the marriage. Many therapists would conceptualize this as a fear of intimacy. An easily plausible assumption is that in the absence of severe turmoil, each spouse's hope and wishes for the relationship are rekindled. In this state, they seek unreal reassurances that it is again safe to trust in the relationship.

At any event, Mrs. P returned to the theme of her abandonment several years ago and its lasting impact on her ability to trust her husband. The therapist chose to explore this past issue for several reasons: It was a recurring theme, those events seemed to symbolize something to Mrs. P, the climate was such that it might be explored now without catastrophe, and the therapist felt that he knew the couple well enough to conceptualize their probable actions toward one another. Therefore, the therapist said, "OK, I give up. Let's go back to two years ago one last time and resolve this once and for all. I'm getting tired of this."

*Comment.* The therapist exaggerates his defeat while looking at Mrs. P. As the therapist has had no difficulty keeping control so far, Mrs. P knows quite well that she hasn't overpowered the therapist. However, she enjoys his token giving in to her fantasy. Mr. P is puzzled by the interaction but identifies with the therapist's sense of exasperation, although not appreciating the subtle meaning.

The therapist asks, "What is it that actually happened?"

Mrs. P replies, "Well, we just moved to Chicago. Julie was sick. I had asthma. He was never home and he didn't care about us. He just walked out of the house as if he had no responsibility."

The therapist pursues it: "OK. Let's get the facts straight. This happened every day. Did he come home at night? What exactly happened for what frequency and over what period of time? Be as specific as possible."

Mr. P looks irritated and begins to interrupt. The therapist cuts him off with "No, you're the villain. Villains don't get to talk." The therapist purposely exaggerates the meaning of the sequence in this manner for the husband's benefit. The therapist's statement of this reassures the husband that his interests are being protected.

In a lengthy series of questions, diversions, and requests for clarification, a coherent picture begins to evolve that resembles reality without exaggeration. When the couple initially moved to Chicago, Mrs. P had suffered from frequent, extreme asthmatic attacks and Julie had recurrent ear infections. Mr. P had stayed home from the office to assist on some occasions after the move to Chicago. After that, Mr. P had become more resistant to helping and Mrs. P even more demanding that he help.

One event of particular emotional significance occurred approximately 3 months after that move. Mr. P had stayed home late for several weeks and people in his office were beginning to question his performance. On this particular morning, Mrs. P had insisted that he stay and he had refused. Later that day, he had telephoned to find out how things were going. The neighbor answered the phone to say that his wife had been hospitalized. As soon as the conference at his office was over, Mr. P returned home to see his wife. She never forgave him for that.

On a close-grained analysis of the events, it became obvious that on previous occasions Mrs. P had been more preoccupied with Mr. P's expression of concern than with his actual staying home. Mr. P had interpreted her helplessness as a need for him to stay home, which he did with resentment and reluctance. As Mrs. P had not obtained what she wanted, she increased her demands. As Mr. P began to feel that her demands were unreasonable and in excess of her actual physical incapacitation, he began to become totally unyielding to her demands. The sequence then evolved into a self-perpetuating cycle. The more unresponsive her husband appeared to be, the more demanding the wife became. The more demanding his wife became, the more insensitive and unyielding Mr. P became. Mrs. P began to see her husband as withdrawn and unavailable; Mr. P began to see Mrs. P as clinging and unavailable. Both had opposite-sex parental images facilitating this perception.

The therapist helped each of them to look at the sequence of events now that time had toned down some of the emotional significance. He also engaged each in the perspective that his or her version of reality was true but that each version left out the part that each had played. The therapist pointed out how the polarizations of their characters had been a consequence of their interaction. Then he helped them to figure out ways to prevent such cyles from recurring. One obvious preventive measure is to verbalize that one is angry and confused and to engage the other in trying to decipher what is going on. The manner in which each of the spouses reacts against demands was emphasized. The resulting power struggle catapulted each into a polarized position that neither liked, yet neither knew how to escape.

## Discrimination Training

The earlier interventions were structured to alter the behavioral interactions of the couple so that it assumed a new form. This alteration of usual behavioral patterns led to a situation in which the spouses were observing behaviors in the mate that were difficult to assimilate to old representational patterns. The modification of communication patterns led to a situation where new information from the spouse was received and processed. Again, this information is often different from old representational patterns. The therapist augments this process by cognitive relabeling, emphasizing aspects of the spouses' personalities that are difficult to assimilate to old patterns. At this point in the therapy, the therapist is prepared to force a discrimination between inner representational images and the current reality of the spouse's personality. The whole thrust of therapy has been toward this goal. The timing of particular forms of intervention are, of course, determined by the therapist's judgment of the couple's receptivity.

The goal of the therapy is to help the spouses experience each other in a way more greatly resembling the totality of their beings rather than in the somewhat encapsulated forms mandated by inner representational models from previous experiences. The structuring of the therapy to this point has had this goal in mind. The actual behavior of the spouses has to change before a discrimination between inner and external reality is possible. Once the behavior has shifted, a discrimination is possible. In many ways, the discrimination sought is similar to what occurs in individual psychotherapy during the interpretation of the transference. In individual psychotherapy, the therapist is an unequal participant in the interaction and thus can usually deduce the irrational characterization of his personality. Because the interpersonal interaction of the therapist and the patient is structured and time-limited, the therapist remains somewhere between a blank screen and a full-participant observer. The spouse, of course, is a full participant and, most often, not even a true observer. This difference from marital and psychotherapy mandates the different procedures employed earlier in therapy. Once the therapist has been truly effective in restructuring the behavioral system, he is prepared to make interventions resembling transference interpretations. His goal is not so much to interpret the transference as to force a discrimination between transference and actual reality.

In many couples, a bilateral disproof of the transference may be necessary. In other couples, a strong unilateral disproof may suffice. Clearly, if one spouse changes dramatically, the interactional system and the other spouse must accommodate, strive to maintain the status quo, or seek escape from the interaction. If the bond between the spouses appears stable, it may suffice to disrupt the transference reaction in one spouse. The spouse chosen will depend on accessibility and motivation for change, as well as the role played by the spouse in the marital interaction.

In the case of Mr. and Mrs. P, Mrs. P appeared clearly to be the dominant interpersonal force in the marriage. Her husband was willing to compromise on most issues as long as it did not necessitate great emotional energy and diversion from his own career goals. He had little motivation for internal change. His wife, however, was quite dissatisfied, and her dissatisfaction clearly pervaded the marital interaction. Thus, the therapist made a tactical decision to modify the system by helping Mrs. P to form critical internal discriminations.

The process by which this occurred included emphasizing unnoticed aspects of her husband's personality, accentuating the discrepancies between her inner representational model and her husband's behavior, astutely monitoring their interaction for critical instances of this, and searching for moments of emotional poignancy that highlighted the discrepancy. In passing, it is of note that Mrs. P tended to comprehend Mr. P at the level of his defenses and assimilate this information into her transferential reference system. Mr. P, unwittingly or collusively, complied with her strategy on most occasions.

At this point in the therapy, Mr. P was returning home from work at a regular time and Mrs. P was coping well with running the house, making few demands on her husband's time. The emotional atmosphere was considerably less charged. At about this time, Mr. P mentioned that his wife was somewhat irregular in her taking of antibiotics. In a confused monologue, Mr. P expressed his concern about this. He mentioned his concern about his wife's health as well as his fear that she might become ill again and the probable impact of this on his work and their relationship. To the therapist, it was clear that Mr. P was concerned about his wife's health and their newfound marital tranquillity as well as his own work schedule. As might be expected, Mrs. P heard only the part of his statement that fit her inner representational model for him.

MRS. P (angrily): I was right all along. He's only concerned about his work.

THERAPIST: Wait a minute. I didn't hear it quite that way. I heard him express concern for you first and concern about his work second. As a matter of fact, I was surprised. (Turning to face Mr. P) You didn't come across as your usual bastard self. You caught me off guard. It looks like you caught your wife off guard too. She's still seeing you the old way. (Mrs. P is silent but looks puzzled during this interchange.)

*Comment.* The therapist is beginning to drive a wedge between inner and external reality for Mrs. P. At this point, the wedge is limited to perceptions in the present and immediate past. The therapist purposely agrees with Mr. P yet says that maybe things are different now. The therapist talks to Mr. P, to keep his anger from escalating. Mr. P's elicited anger would preclude further discrimination training.

THERAPIST: Mr. P, could you repeat what you just said? As close as possible.

MR. P (looking irritated): Well, I said I was concerned about her health and . . .

THERAPIST: To your wife.

MR. P: Dammit. You've been sick too much and . . .

THERAPIST: Like you said it before.

MR. P: Dammit all, Joan. You've had a rough year. I don't want you to get sick again. I wonder about your possibly having permanent lung damage. You need to take better care of yourself. (He looks uncomfortable). A direct expression of caring is a somewhat unusual experience for Mr. P.) And next week, the case of Genentec versus . . .

THERAPIST: Stop. She knows all of that. The first part she doesn't know. (Turning to Mrs. P) What did you just hear?

MRS. P: He's concerned about his work and my being ill would be an inconvenience.

THERAPIST: That's what you heard or what you think he meant, perhaps. But that's not what he said. Mr. P, could you repeat what you said?

MR. P: This is silly (continues and paraphrases what he has just said).

THERAPIST (to Mrs. P): Could you repeat what he said? Just the words. Not your interpretation.

MRS. P (looking irritated): He said he cares for me, but he doesn't mean it because . . .

THERAPIST: What he said, only . . .

MRS. P: He said that he is concerned about my health.

THERAPIST: I believe him. He cares about you. Flat and simple.

MRS. P: And his work.
THERAPIST: His work too, of course.

Mrs. P looks a little confused at this point and attempts to provoke her husband's hostility. The therapist intervenes, labeling her maneuver and enlisting the husband not to comply. In a series of such maneuvers, Mrs. P's fixated perception of her husband begins to shift. As it shifts, her husband offers direct expressions of caring a little more frequently. Each time that this spontaneously occurs, the therapist ascertains if Mrs. P has heard her husband correctly. Eventually, Mrs. P gets irritated with the therapist's repetitive labeling of events and says, "Oh, all right, he does care, I guess. But he's lousy at expressing it." At this point, the therapist engages the couple in reviewing their interaction to see how the wife could encourage and reward her husband's attempts to express affection.

In a subsequent session, Mrs. P was quite upset because her father had a severe heart condition and refused to seek medical care. Her mother had just called in tears, expressing her fear that the father would die at work because he was too stubborn to admit that he was ill. Mrs. P began crying as she related this event. As his wife was crying, Mr. P looked uncomfortable and then angry. Finally, Mr. P interrupted his wife's crying: "The old bastard ought to know better. If he's going to die, he's going to die. If he dies, you'll fall apart and I won't get any work done."

This brief interjection by the husband appeared likely to destroy all of the previous work of the therapist. The therapist suspected that Mr. P's reaction was a result of Mr. P's discomfort with strong emotions. Thus, the therapist quickly intervened about Mr. P's relationship with his father-in-law and what he liked about the stubborn, difficult old man. Mr. P clearly identified strongly with the father-in-law. As he spoke, he eventually became tearful and voiced his concern for the man. Mrs. P looked away at this time, complaining about her husband's insensitivity. The therapist insisted that she look at her husband, assuming that her husband's facial expression would be a more powerful disproof of her transference distortion than would a verbal intervention.

The next several sessions were uneventful by comparison. These sessions were used to review what had been learned. The therapist was thinking about an early termination when he received a call from Mrs. P requesting an emergency session, as her husband was the same again. The therapist assumed that Mrs. P had provoked her husband into being angry again and scheduled a session.

During this session, Mrs. P was extremely angry, complaining that her husband was cold, insensitive, and selfish. She followed this with a litany of associated complaints. The therapist was unable to identify precipitating events in their relationship. During this session, Mr. P appeared genuinely concerned, tried to be supportive, and actually reached out to touch his wife on several occasions. She rebuffed or ignored all of his efforts. The therapist could discern nothing in the couple's present interaction to explain the reemergence of the old representational model. Therefore, he assumed that a past figure must be the problem. Shooting in the dark, he inquired as to the health of Mrs. P's father. Mrs. P related that her father was scheduled for open-heart surgery (mitral valve replacement) and that the surgeons in a different city felt that his chances for survival were limited. At this point, Mrs. P started crying, saying, "He'll die and I'll never make contact with him. He never really cared about me." The therapist replied, "That's not necessarily true of your husband. Would you look at him now?" Reluctantly, Mrs. P turned to look at her husband, appeared confused, and then embraced him tearfully.

The last two sessions were used to consolidate both cognitive and behavioral learning that had occurred. Of course, the author contacted the surgeons for a realistic appraisal of Mrs. P's father's condition and relayed this to the couple.

Systematic follow-up is lacking on this couple. However, several months later, the author was referred another member of Mrs. P's family for psychotherapy. During this therapeutic contact, information suggested that the marriage of Mr. and Mrs. P had stabilized at a new and better equilibrium.

## Comment

I will briefly review the therapist's action in this case and how it relates to the author's conceptual model. This couple presented for therapy demonstrating considerable anger and disappointment. Their interaction was mainly characterized by mutual recriminations and inability to cooperate. Certain cognitive perceptual abnormalities were posited to coexist with these behavioral disturbances. The husband was described by his wife as rigid and emotionally unavailable. He characterized her as helpless and dependent. Both of these descriptions were partially true but were relatively undifferentiated images of the other's personality. Information that did not fit these perceptual models was consistently overlooked. The therapist assumed that these personality

predispositions were exaggerated as the result of years of marital interaction. He did not agree with the couple that these personality traits
were unmodifiable. Mr. P had a capacity for greater emotional expressiveness and Mrs. P had demonstrated her competence in other areas
of her life.

The therapist's first interventions were to modify the interactional
system. These interventions were made on the assumption that the
current interaction was confirmatory to each spouse's inner representational world. Thus, the therapist moved to modify these interactional
patterns. Two general processes seemed to characterize the initial interaction: escalating battles and repetitive arguments without resolution
or compromise. The therapist was quite active in preventing escalations
since they seemed nonproductive, to have minimal informational value,
and not to challenge the spouse's usual ways of seeing one another.
The early interaction was also characterized by each spouse expressing
anger at the other for not complying with some wish. The therapist
worked to convert these mutual recriminations into requests for change.
Then he assisted quite actively in assisting the couple in working out
compromises. These interventions were effective in changing the interactional climate.

The therapist assumed that each spouse elicited behavior from the
other that was confirmatory to inner representational models. His next
interventions were specifically structured to interrupt these behavioral
sequences. Mrs. P saw her husband as rigid and ungiving. Her way of
asking things from her husband tended to evoke this in him. Her requests were usually comingled with anger and attempts to evoke guilt
in her husband. This strategy reliably elicited her husband's rigidity and
noncompliance. At other times, she would make requests in a whining
little-girl voice. This reliably evoked anger in her husband, confirming
her image of him. This pattern was specifically modified and her husband became more pliable as a result. Mr. P tended to issue orders rather
than make requests of his wife. His wife usually responded by passive
noncompliance, confirming his view of her as helpless and useless. Mr.
P also tended to be nonspecific about what he wanted. He was never
satisfied as a result and blamed this on his wife's inefficiency. Each
partner contributed to the other's misperception, and these patterns
likewise had to be modified. Whenever Mrs. P made a request of her
husband, he tended to divert the subject. This reinforced her view that
she could not obtain things from her husband. She "colluded" in this
by not forcing her husband to answer questions directly. Likewise, Mr.
P allowed his wife to get away with passive noncompliance without

directly confronting her about this. Interruption of these patterns facilitated disconfirmatory experiences.

The author purposely used cognitive relabeling of events to point out aspects of the spouse that did not fit with the inner representational model. He specifically pinpointed and emphasized events that were unambiguously discrepant. In these interventions he focused on the complexity of motivations and the positive intent of the spouse. The final stage of the therapy consisted of helping Mrs. P discriminate between her inner representational image and the personality of her husband.

I think that it is accurate to conclude that the therapist flexibly employed concepts and techniques from behavioral, general systems, and psychoanalytic approaches and that these techniques were employed in a unified and systematic manner. I think that it is also accurate to emphasize that the empirically oriented therapist does not have to ignore hypothetical events within the organism.

## REFERENCES

Azrin, N. H., Naster, B. J., and Jones, R. Reciprocity counseling: a rapid learning-based procedure for marital counseling. *Behavior Research and Therapy*, 1973, *11*, 365–382.

Ezriel, H. Notes on psychoanalytic group therapy: II. Interpretation and research. *Psychiatry*, 1952, *15*, 119–129.

Gottman, J., Notarius, C., and Markman, H. Behavior exchange theory and marital decision making. *Journal of Personality and Social Psychology*, 1976, *34*, 14–23.

Haley, J. Marriage therapy. *Archives of General Psychiatry*, 1963, *8*, 213–234.

Jacobson, N. J., Margolin, G. *Marital therapy*. New York: Brunner/Mazel, 1979.

Thomas, E. J. *Marital communication and decision making*. New York: Free Press, 1977.

# Index

Abreaction, 131–133
Alcoholism and marital status, 31–32
Ambivalence, 249–250
Assimilative projection, 177
Assortive mating, 39–40, 180–181
Aversive conditioning, 104
Aversive stimuli, 109, 179

Behavior therapy
  description 103–107
  elicited memories 131–134, 207–208
  relationship to psychoanalytic therapy
    72–73
Behavioral marital therapy
  cognition, 119–120
  critique, 6–7, 99, 116–120, 128–129
  procedures and assumptions, 5–7,
    96–99, 107–116, 167–168
  relationship to general system theory,
    78, 90–91, 97–98
Behavioral trap, 105
Behaviorism, 99–102, 154
Borderline personality disorder, 176

Chair placement, 244
Channel inconsistency, 86, 116
  See also Communication; Deficits;
    Incongruence
Childhood experiences and adult
    psychopathology, 173–175
Children
  and divorce, 40–42
  and marital discord, 43–45

Circular causality, 81, 92, 153
Classical conditioning, 101–102, 103
Closed system, 80, 134–135
Coercive cycles and marriage, 109, 184,
    219
Cognition
  definition, 163
  interpersonal perception, 135–139,
    165–169, 171–178
  See also Schema; Transference
Cognitive behaviorism, 8, 89, 93, 106–107
  See also Social learning theory
Cognitive complexity, 164–165, 175–177,
    187–188
Cognitive marital therapy techniques
  behavioral rehearsal example, 273–282,
    241–242
  cognitive relabeling, 89, 201–202,
    233–235, 245, 282–286
  discrimination training, 204–208,
    238–241, 289–293
  disconfirmatory experiences, 239–240
  goal, 213–214
  labeling, 241–242
  modeling, 268
  provisional hypotheses, 221–223
  shaping, 229
  See also Marital therapy techniques
Cognitive social psychology, 10–13, 93,
    141–143, 148, 152
Communication deficits
  content shifting, 114, 115, 228

Communication deficits (*cont.*)
  cross complaining, 86
  failure to validate, 226
  incomplete messages, 227
  incongruence, 116, 227–228
  overgeneralization, 114, 226–227
  presumptive attribution, 86, 116,
    229–230
  pronouns (first person plural), 230
  rules, 228
  summarizing self, 230–231
  vague references, 111, 227
Communication training, 90–91, 113–116,
    185–187, 226–231, 271–282
Complementary needs, 180–181
Complementary reactions. *See* Response
    determined stimulus effect; Self-
    fulfilling prophesy
Concordance of mental illness in
    marriage, 39–40
Conjugal relationship therapy, 114
Constructive alternativism, 139
Constructs, *See* Personal constructs
Contingency contracting. *See* Negotiation
    training
Contracting. *See* Negotiation training
Core symbols, 119–120
Cybernetics, 82–83

Defensiveness, 217–219
Desensitization, 103–104
Deterioration of well spouse, 64, 181
Disconfirmatory experiences, 161, 185,
    187–188, 206–208
  *See also* Cognitive marital therapy;
    Disconfirmatory experiences; Inner
    representational world and
    behavior change
Discrimination learning, 175
Discrimination training, 142, 204–208,
    238–241, 289–293
  *See also* Cognitive marital therapy;
    Discrimination training
Discriminative stimulus, 102
Divorce
  children, and 40–42
  sex differences, 45–46
  elderly, 30
  statistics, 49–50
Double bind hypothesis, 84

Early childhood experiences and adult
    psychopathology, 173–175
Eclectic marital therapy, 3–4, 66–67
Elicited behavior from others. *See*
    Response determined stimulus
    effect; Self-fulfilling prophesy
Enmeshment, 119
Extinction, 105
Eye Contact, 244

Family rules, 87–88
  *See also* General system therapy
Family therapy, 65, 83–84, 149, 242
Fixed role therapy, 139
Flooding, 103

General system therapy
  critique, 91–93, 128
  definition and history, 76–82
  relationship to behavioral marital
    therapy, 78, 90–91, 97–98
  relationship to cognitive social
    psychology, 89
Good faith agreement, 112

Happiness and marital status, 30–31
Homeostasis, 83
  *See also* General system theory; Family
    rules
Hope, restoration of, 220–221

"I" Statements, 114, 246–247
  *See also* Communication training
Idealization, 178
Incidence
  definition, 22
Individual psychopathology and marriage,
    5, 37–40, 58–59
  *See also* Psychoanalytic marital therapy
Inner representational world
  description, 137–141
  and behavior change, 130–135, 187–188,
    18
  and social behavior, 135–136, 182–183
  *See also* Objects relations theory;
    Schema; Disconfirmatory
    experiences
Instrumental conditioning. *See* Operant
    conditioning
Interaction hypothesis, 35, 37–40, 181
Internal speech, 156
Interpersonal perception. *See* Schema

Introject, 68, 156
   *See also* Objects relations theory; Inner
      representational world, description
Isomorphism, 81

Longevity and marital status, 34–36
Love, 243

Malevolent transformation, 143
Marital discord
   and individual psychopathology, 37
   and personality, 3, 165
Marital happiness, predictors, 3, 37–40,
      165
Marital therapy
   indications, 209–210
   non-specific factors, 242–250
   relationship to individual therapy, 13,
      161, 197–199, 213–215, 239–240,
      242, 245, 271, 289
   stages, 214–242
Marital therapy technique
   co-therapy, 213
   individual sessions, 212–213
   length, 210–211
Marriage contract, 67, 84
Marriage neurosis, 167
   *See also* Transference
Mate selection, 72, 180–181
Medical visits and marital status, 27–28
Metaphors, 245–246
Mind reading. *See* Communication
      deficits; Presumptive attribution
Morphogenesis, 81
Morphostasis, 81

Negative reinforcement, 97, 102, 184
Negotiation training, 97, 110, 111–113,
      117, 231–233, 264–271
Nonverbal communication. *See*
      Communication deficits;
      Incongruence; Channel
      inconsistency

Objects-relations marital therapy, 69–70
Objects-relations therapy, 67–70, 168
   *See also* Projective identification
Open system, 80, 134
Operant Conditioning, 101–102, 104–106
Outcome studies. *See* Psychotherapy
      outcome studies

Outpatient psychiatric treatment and
      marital status, 26–27

Palo Alto school, 76–77
Parent–child separation, 40–45
   *See also* Early childhood experiences
Parent loss. *See* Parent–child separation
Payoff matrix, 108
Person–environment interaction, 153–154
   *See also* Inner representational world;
      Response-determined stimulus
      effect; Circular causality
Personal constructs, 138–139
   *See also* Schema
Personality, definition, 150–153
Personification, 141, 156
Phobias, 103–104, 133
Polemical disputes
   individual psychotherapy, 7–9, 130–131
   marital therapy, 5, 127, 130–131
Positive reinforcement, 102, 105, 111–113
Power, 247
Prevalence, definition, 22
Projective identification, 12, 68–70,
      167–168
   *See also* Objects-relations therapy
Protection hypothesis, 46–47
Psychiatric hospitalization and marital
      status, 24–26
Psychoanalytic marital therapy
   collaborative, 65
   conjoint, 5, 65–67
   consecutive, 64
   critique, 5, 127–128
   individual, 4–5, 59–60
Psychoanalytic psychotherapy
   brief therapy, 158
   critique, 63, 70–73
   relationship to behavior therapy, 72–73
   relationship to cognitive social
      psychology, 63–64, 141–142,
      168–169
   technique and assumptions, 4–5, 61–62,
      66, 135, 141, 152, 156, 158
Psychopathology and marital status,
      29–30, 36–37
Psychotherapy outcome studies, 89,
      116–117, 157–158, 211
Punishment, 97, 109
   *See also* Coercive cycles

Quid pro quo, 84–85, 97, 112

Rapprochement
    psychoanalysis and behavior therapy,
        7–9, 131–135
    research and practice, 251–253
Reciprocal determinism. *See* Circular
        causality
Reciprocity, 97, 108–109, 115, 119
Reciprocal interpersonal responses. *See*
        Response determined stimulus
        effect and self-fulfilling prophesy
Reciprocity training, 110–113
    *See also* Negotiation training
Respondent conditioning. *See* Classical
        conditioning
Response chain, 102, 183
Response-determined stimulus effect, 10,
        11, 12–13, 16, 92, 136, 142–144, 154,
        179–182, 202–203, 204–205
    *See also* Self-fulfilling prophesy
Role construct repertory test, 138–139,
        164–165, 176–177
Runaways, 83
    *See also* Coercive cycles

Schema, 11–12, 72, 138–143, 145, 164, 169,
        171–175
Selection hypothesis, 35, 46, 49
Self-control, 156
Self-fulfilling prophesy, 10–12, 140–141,
        142–145, 178, 188
    *See also* Response determined stimulus
        effect
Self-perpetuating behavior. *See also* Self-
        fulfilling prophesy and Response
        determined stimulus effect
Sexual behavior, 112, 133, 202–203

Sex differences, reaction to divorce 45–46
Sex therapy, 104, 106, 132
Side-tracking. *See* Communication deficits;
        content shifting
Single parent families, 50
    *See also* Divorce; children
Social exchange theory, 6, 107–108
Social influence and psychotherapy,
        158–160
Social learning theory, 8, 13, 15, 107,
        137–138, 141, 153, 155
Stages of marital therapy
    early, 214–223
    middle, 223–235
    end, 238–242
Stimulus control, 106
Suicide
    and marital distress, 33–34
    and marital status, 33
Symptom substitution, 134
Systematic desensitization. *See*
        Desensitization

Template, *See* Schema
Terminal hypothesis, 111
Therapeutic alliance, 214–216
Therapist training and marriage, 50
Theory
    purpose, 129–130, 71
    and marital therapy, 1–3, 127, 148
Token economy and marriage, 112
Transference, 4, 17, 60, 62–63, 66–67, 127,
        134, 138, 140–141, 143, 145,
        160–161, 168, 173, 175, 204, 211
Transient marital discord, 161–162

Widows, 47–48